AF806479

Multimodal Management of Upper and Lower Extremity Lymphedema

Mark V. Schaverien • Joseph H. Dayan
Editors

Multimodal Management of Upper and Lower Extremity Lymphedema

Springer

Editors
Mark V. Schaverien
Department of Plastic Surgery
The University of Texas MD Anderson
Cancer Center
Houston, TX, USA

Joseph H. Dayan
Division of Plastic and Reconstructive Surgery
Memorial Sloan Kettering Cancer Center
New York, NY, USA

ISBN 978-3-030-93038-7 ISBN 978-3-030-93039-4 (eBook)
https://doi.org/10.1007/978-3-030-93039-4

This Springer imprint is published by the registered company Springer Nature Switzerland AG
The registered company address is: Gewerbestrasse 11, 6330 Cham, Switzerland

Preface

Although our understanding of the pathogenesis of lymphedema and its treatment have traditionally languished behind that of rarer diseases, currently there is rapidly growing interest in lymphedema paralleled by an increase in the number of experts treating and investigating it, placing us at the dawn of tremendous advances for a condition that has been relatively neglected in medicine. Advances in non-surgical and surgical treatments have ameliorated the functional and psychosocial disability of lymphedema. The treatment of lymphedema has traditionally resided with the lymphedema therapist alone; however, rapid advances in the last 5–10 years in imaging, surgical instruments, and surgical techniques have led to the development of modern surgical and supermicrosurgical procedures that work in concert with optimized conservative treatment to improve the magnitude and consistency of outcomes from lymphedema surgery.

Recently, there has been growing interest in lymphedema due to an increase in the number of centers with specialist teams assembled to treat the condition, supported by an increasing evidence-base demonstrating the effectiveness of surgical techniques that continues to provide higher-level supportive evidence through better conducted and controlled studies. In around a quarter of patients with limb swelling, a diagnosis other than lymphedema accounts for their condition, leading to improper or delayed treatment. Thus, there is an urgent healthcare need for wider availability of, and greater access to, specialist centers with expertise in evaluation of the patient presenting with limb swelling, and that offer the full complement of non-surgical and surgical treatments for the condition.

There is a strong evidence base supporting the effectiveness of lymphedema surgical procedures in reducing symptoms, limb volume excess, extracellular fluid, and episodes of cellulitis, and in improving limb function and the patient's quality of life. No single procedure is equally effective in all patients, and it is imperative that the surgical team provides the full spectrum of the modern surgical treatments available, complemented by skilled conservative therapy, including lymphovenous bypass (LVB), vascularized lymph node transplantation (VLNT), and suction-assisted lipectomy (SAL) debulking surgery with continuous compression therapy (CCT), to maximize outcomes. Indocyanine green (ICG) lymphography has become an important and practical tool for aiding in decision-making between the available surgical options. Many patients with breast cancer–related lymphedema (BCRL) have comorbid axillary contracture limiting range of motion, and lysis of axillary scar adhesions and orthotopic proximal VLNT to the axilla is an important component of their lymphedema surgical treatment. In patients with early obstructive lymphedema confined to the upper arm, axillary adhesiolysis and orthotopic transplantation of groin lymph nodes as a composite with the deep inferior epigastric artery perforator (DIEP) flap for postmastectomy breast reconstruction, or microsurgical omental lymphatic flap transfer, can provide significant benefit. In appropriately selected patients with significant fibroadipose soft tissue excess that affects function, who are continuously complaint with compression garments and have minimal pitting edema, SAL can achieve tremendous improvements in quality of life and limb function with minimal morbidity.

In the developed world, lymphedema predominantly affects survivors of breast, gynecologic, or urologic cancers, for whom it may be their greatest survivorship burden. Caring for lymphedema imposes a significant time burden on patients and their carers, and leads to cumulative and cascading economic consequences from the costs of lymphedema management and compression garments, the treatment of infections, and the loss of work productivity. Modern-day management of lymphedema recognizes the superior effectiveness of the multimodal multidisciplinary team approach in improving patient outcomes. This includes risk-reduction strategies and prophylactic surgeries (immediate lymphatic reconstruction) to reduce the risk of developing lymphedema, optimization of conservative therapy in established lymphedema to reduce progression, and combined surgical approaches including physiological and debulking procedures, where appropriate, to maximize outcomes. These should be delivered within lymphedema centers offering the highest standard of best practice multi-team comprehensive care.

In this book – *Multimodal Management of Upper and Lower Extremity Lymphedema* – world experts in the field of lymphedema concisely and comprehensively detail all of these non-surgical and surgical approaches. The chapters uniquely provide a step-by-step practical multidisciplinary approach and framework for performing each aspect of the multimodal management of the lymphedema patient, as well as comprehensive instruction for those treating such patients, accompanied by key video contributions from the authors. It also provides a framework for collecting outcomes measures for these patients to improve the consistency of outcomes data and allow for comparisons between the different treatments and across institutions internationally. In addition to the array of treatment options for this currently incurable disease, new therapies that target inflammation and fibrosis to prevent and treat lymphedema, either primarily or in conjunction with surgical modalities, are reviewed – the outcomes of translational research studies are eagerly awaited to more effectively treat patients and reduce their morbidity.

Houston, TX, USA — Mark V. Schaverien
New York, NY, USA — Joseph H. Dayan

Acknowledgments

We owe the authors of chapters in this book an enormous debt of gratitude for their contributions to this landmark book on the multimodal management of upper and lower extremity lymphedema that details the current state of lymphedema science, patient evaluation, and treatment. We especially want to acknowledge the lymphedema therapists, nurses, physicians, and surgeons, who have dedicated their careers to tirelessly treating patients suffering with lymphedema to improve their quality of life.

We want to thank our project coordinators, Nishanthini Vetrivel and Sasirekka Nijanthan, at Springer Nature, our project manager, ArulRonika Pathinathan, and our editor, Asja Rehse, at Springer, who have provided invaluable support for this project from conception to completion – without them, this book would not have been possible. We also wish to thank the graphics team at Springer for their wonderful illustrations to accompany the chapters to communicate key anatomical concepts.

Houston, TX, USA　　Mark V. Schaverien
New York, NY, USA　　Joseph H. Dayan

Contents

Contributors

Jane M. Armer University of Missouri, Sinclair School of Nursing, Ellis Fischel Cancer Center, Columbia, MO, USA

Håkan Brorson Lymphedema Center, Plastic and Reconstructive Surgery, Skåne University Hospital, Malmö, Sweden

Department of Clinical Sciences, Malmö, Lund University, Lund, Sweden

Corrado Cesare Campisi Plastic, Reconstructive and Aesthetic Surgery, Private Consultant, Genoa, Italy

University of Catania, Genoa & Catania, Italy

Corradino Campisi General Surgery, Vascular Surgery and Emergency Surgery, Clinical Lymphology, Lymphatic Surgery and Microsurgery, School of Medical Sciences and Pharmaceutics, Department of Surgical Sciences and Integrated Diagnostics – DISC, University of Genoa, Genoa, Italy

David W. Chang Department of Surgery, Section of Plastic and Reconstructive Surgery, University of Chicago, Chicago, IL, USA

Dawn N. Chen MD Anderson Cancer Center – West Houston, Rehabilitation Services, Houston, TX, USA

Hung-Chi Chen Department of Plastic Surgery, China Medical University Hospital, Taichung, Taiwan

Ming-Huei Cheng Department of Plastic and Reconstructive Surgery, Mayo Clinic, Jacksonville, FL, USA

Section of Plastic Surgery, The University of Michigan, Ann Arbor, Michigan, USA

Carrie K. Chu Department of Plastic Surgery, The University of Texas MD Anderson Cancer Center, Houston, TX, USA

Joseph H. Dayan Division of Plastic and Reconstructive Surgery, Memorial Sloan Kettering Cancer Center, New York, NY, USA

Pietro Giovanni di Summa Department of Plastic, Reconstructive and Hand Surgery, Centre Hospitalier Universitaire Vaudois (CHUV), Lausanne, Switzerland

Rosie Friedman Boston Lymphatic Center, Division of Plastic and Reconstructive Surgery, Beth Israel Deaconess Medical Center, Harvard Medical School, Boston, MA, USA

Rebecca M. Garza Department of Surgery, Section of Plastic and Reconstructive Surgery, University of Chicago, Chicago, IL, USA

Melisa D. Granoff Boston Lymphatic Center, Division of Plastic and Reconstructive Surgery, Beth Israel Deaconess Medical Center, Harvard Medical School, Boston, MA, USA

Jay W. Granzow Division of Plastic Surgery, Department of Surgery, Harbor-UCLA Medical Center, Torrance, CA, USA

Arin K. Greene Boston Lymphatic Center, Department of Plastic and Oral Surgery, Boston Children's Hospital, Harvard Medical School, Boston, MA, USA

Ryoko Hamaguchi Harvard Medical School, Boston, MA, USA

Akitatsu Hayashi Lymphedema Center, Kameda General Hospital, Kamogawa, Chiba, Japan

Olivia Ho Department of Plastic and Reconstructive Surgery, Chang Gung Memorial Hospital, College of Medicine, Chang Gung University, Taoyuan, Taiwan

Kavan S. Johal Department of Plastic Surgery, China Medical University Hospital, Taichung, Taiwan

Department of Plastic Surgery, St Thomas' Hospital, London, UK

Elizabeth Kiwanuka Department of Surgery, Division of Plastic and Reconstructive Surgery at Memorial Sloan Kettering Cancer Center, New York, NY, USA

Jaume Masia Plastic and Reconstructive Surgery, Hospital de la Santa Creu i Sant Pau and Clinica Planas, Barcelona, Spain

Babak Mehrara Department of Surgery, Division of Plastic and Reconstructive Surgery at Memorial Sloan Kettering Cancer Center, New York, NY, USA

Marc A. Miller MD Anderson Cancer Center, Rehabilitation Services, Houston, TX, USA

Lidia Molinari General Surgery, Private Consultant, Genoa, Italy

Ketan M. Patel Center for Advanced Lymphedema Treatment & Surgery, Division of Plastic and Reconstructive Surgery, Department of Surgery, Keck School of Medicine, University of Southern California, Los Angeles, CA, USA

Cristhian Pomata Plastic and Reconstructive Surgery, Clinica Planas, Barcelona, Spain

Gemma Pons Plastic and Reconstructive Surgery, Hospital de la Santa Creu i Sant Pau and Clinica Planas, Barcelona, Spain

Anjali C. Raghuram Division of Plastic Surgery, City of Hope National Medical Center, Duarte, CA, USA

Stanley G. Rockson Stanford Center for Lymphatic and Venous Disorders, Division of Cardiovascular Medicine, Stanford University School of Medicine, Stanford, CA, USA

Jose Ramon Rodriguez Department of Plastic and Reconstructive Surgery, Center Hospital of National Center for Global Health and Medicine, Tokyo, Japan

Department of Plastic and Reconstructive Surgery, Clinica Las Condes, Santiago, Chile

Mark V. Schaverien Department of Plastic Surgery, The University of Texas MD Anderson Cancer Center, Houston, TX, USA

Akira Shinaoka Department of Human Morphology, Okayama University, Graduate School of Medicine, Dentistry and Pharmaceutical Sciences, Okayama, Japan

Department of Plastic and Reconstructive Surgery, Okayama University, Graduate School of Medicine, Dentistry and Pharmaceutical Sciences, Okayama, Japan

Robert C. Sibley Stanford Center for Lymphatic and Venous Disorders, Division of Cardiovascular Medicine, Stanford University School of Medicine, Stanford, CA, USA

Dhruv Singhal Boston Lymphatic Center, Division of Plastic and Reconstructive Surgery, Beth Israel Deaconess Medical Center, Harvard Medical School, Boston, MA, USA

Roman Skoracki Department of Plastic Surgery, Arthur G. James Cancer Hospital and Richard J. Solove Research Institute and Comprehensive Cancer Center, The Ohio State University Wexner Medical Center, Columbus, OH, USA

Nicole L. Stout West Virginia University Cancer Institute, School of Medicine, Department of Hematology Oncology, Morgantown, WV, USA

Hiroo Suami Australian Lymphoedema Education, Research and Treatment (ALERT), Faculty of Medicine, Health and Human Sciences, Macquarie University, Sydney, NSW, Australia

Duane Wang Division of Plastic and Reconstructive Surgery, Department of Surgery, University of Washington School of Medicine, Seattle, WA, USA

Alex K. Wong Division of Plastic Surgery, City of Hope National Medical Center, Duarte, CA, USA

Takumi Yamamoto Department of Plastic and Reconstructive Surgery, Center Hospital of National Center for Global Health and Medicine, Tokyo, Japan

Introduction

1

Mark V. Schaverien and Joseph H. Dayan

Overview

Lymphedema is a common, chronic, and debilitating condition resulting from disruption of the lymphatic system by a myriad of causes, including inherited or sporadic genetic mutations or surgical injury. The disease is a major burden to healthcare systems because it is chronic and incurable. It is typically a progressive condition, the complications of which can be life-threatening. Caring for lymphedema imposes a significant time burden on patients and their carers and is a significant economic burden on them due to the direct costs of lymphedema therapist-delivered conservative care, compression garments and bandages, and pneumatic compression devices, as well as the indirect costs for the treatment of cellulitis including hospitalization, lost time at work, productivity in the home, and leisure time, as well as the cost of managing associated comorbidities. These costs impact savings and may result in delayed retirement, reduced employment, and decreased ability to access needed lymphedema care [1, 2]. Lymphedema also imposes a lifelong substantial negative impact on quality of life, with some cancer survivors describing the burden of living with lymphedema as greater than the cancer itself [3].

Lymphedema affects up to 250 million people worldwide – around 1 in 30 [4–6]. This is predominantly secondary to the parasitic infection filariasis that causes lymphedema by direct lymphatic obstruction. In the West, approximately 99% of individuals with lymphedema have secondary disease, most commonly following lymphadenectomy and/or radiation therapy for the treatment predominantly of breast, gynecologic, or urologic cancers [7]; primary lymphedema is rare, resulting from genetic or developmental abnormalities in the lymphatic system, in some cases from genetic mutations in the signaling pathway for vascular endothelial growth factor-C (VEGFC). Current oncologic treatment algorithms require lymphadenectomy in the axillary, inguinal, or pelvic lymph nodal basins in patients with regional metastatic involvement, often leading to significant lymphatic disruption and subsequent failed function. In the United States, up to ten million people are affected by lymphedema, with around 200,000 new cases diagnosed each year.

Advances in our understanding of the anatomophysiology of the lymphatic system, as well as in the pathogenesis underlying lymphedema, have led to the development of effective surgical techniques to ameliorate the symptoms and disability of patients with lymphedema and reduce the risk of future episodes of cellulitis. Physiological procedures, most commonly lymphovenous bypass (LVB) or vascularized lymph node transplantation (VLNT), can improve lymphatic fluid drainage within the affected area. Once established, the chronic lymphedema phenotype is characterized by hypertrophy of fibroadipose soft tissues, which can only be removed directed by suction-assisted lipectomy (SAL) or excisional procedures to restore limb function and improve appearance. Immediate lymphatic reconstruction (ILR) at the time of lymphadenectomy has the potential to reduce the risk of lymphedema developing.

Anatomophysiology of the Lymphatic System

As detailed in Chap. 2, the lymphatic system is a component of the circulatory system, the main purpose of which is maintaining fluid homeostasis and transporting protein-rich interstitial fluid, enabling migration and transport of immune cells, regulation of inflammatory responses, and allowing

M. V. Schaverien (✉)
Department of Plastic Surgery, The University of Texas MD Anderson Cancer Center, Houston, TX, USA
e-mail: mvschaverien@mdanderson.org

J. H. Dayan (✉)
Division of Plastic and Reconstructive Surgery, Memorial Sloan Kettering Cancer Center, New York, NY, USA
e-mail: dayanj@mskcc.org

M. V. Schaverien, J. H. Dayan (eds.), *Multimodal Management of Upper and Lower Extremity Lymphedema*,
https://doi.org/10.1007/978-3-030-93039-4_1

dietary absorption of fat. Networks of lymphatic vessels begin as lymphatic capillaries and transport interstitial fluid unidirectionally via a valved peristaltic system ultimately back to the venous circulation. The venous system is responsible for absorption of more than 90% of the extracellular fluid produced as a consequence of cellular metabolism and capillary perfusion – the remaining 10% is transported by the lymphatic system. The lymphatic system has a large reserve for fluid transport and mild disturbances in function usually do not result in fluid accumulation. When the system is damaged or overloaded, however, then interstitial fluid accumulation can occur, manifesting as pitting edema. As described in Chap. 3, this fluid can have major adverse effects on local cellular behavior, resulting in local and systemic activation of inflammatory cascades, and localized adipose cell differentiation.

Pathophysiology of Lymphedema

Lymphedema results from dysfunction of the lymphatic system, characterized by lymphatic vessel ectasia leading to valve dysfunction, and then reflux, of lymphatic fluid into the interstitial space. This lymphatic fluid stasis leads to a localized chronic inflammatory process, resulting in remodeling and fibrosis of the extracellular matrix, adipose tissue differentiation with hypertrophy, and progressive proliferation of smooth muscle cells surrounding the lymphatics with collagen deposition and sclerosis, and then eventual obliteration, of the lymphatic vessel lumen [8, 9].

The inflammatory cell accumulation around the lymphatic vessels results in inducible nitric oxide synthase (iNOS)-mediated decreased lymphatic vessel contractility and consequent lymphatic fluid transport, and cytokine expression via the T helper 2 cell-biased response impairs collateral lymphatic vessel formation by hindering lymphatic endothelial cell proliferation, as well as tubule formation, migration, and function. Chronic inflammation and fibrosis affecting the skin and subcutaneous soft tissue including the muscle fascia are therefore the histological characteristics of lymphedema. The multiple episodes of cellulitis that typically occur result in a cycle of progressive impairment of functioning lymphatic channels via inflammation, fibrosis, and obliteration.

Lymphedema Classification

Lymphedema can be categorized as either primary or secondary. Primary lymphedema is caused by abnormal development of, or pathological changes intrinsic to, the lymphatic system, and has a prevalence of approximately 1 in 100,000 [10]. The lymphatic morphology can be characterized as hypoplasic/aplasic (≈90%) or hyperplasic (≈10%) [11]. These developmental abnormalities may relate to genetic mutations that either directly or indirectly regulate lymphatic differentiation and function involving the VEGFC–VEGFR3 ligand–receptor signaling complex and its downstream signaling pathways [12–14]. Around 15% of patients with primary lymphedema have hereditary and/or syndromic lymphedema, such as Milroy disease, Noonan syndrome, or Turner syndrome, and the clinical presentation may indicate the most likely causative gene. Primary lymphedema can be classified by the age of presentation (i.e., congenital lymphedema, lymphedema praecox, or lymphedema tarda if after age 35) although this classification does not correlate with the identified genetic mutations [15, 16]. Individuals most often develop swelling after infancy, with only around 20% of patients developing lymphedema in adulthood. Females are affected twice as often as males and the lower extremities are involved in over 90% patients, bilaterally in around 50% of cases [17]. Approximately 60% of patients have progression of their disease, and patients with unilateral lower extremity lymphedema have an up to 25% risk of developing the condition in their contralateral extremity [11]. In the pediatric population, 70% of conditions mistaken for lymphedema are other types of lymphatic and/or vascular anomalies or other etiologies of limb swelling [18, 19]. Patients with primary lymphedema are best managed by a multidisciplinary team focused on the condition.

Secondary lymphedema is the most common cause of lymphedema and results from either direct or indirect injury to the lymphatic system by surgery, radiation, trauma, or infection. The most common form of secondary lymphedema worldwide is filariasis, a parasitic infection (*Wuchereria bancrofti*) that occupies the lymphatic vasculature, obstructing the flow of lymph fluid. In the West, lymphedema is predominantly secondary to lymphadenectomy for the treatment of cancer, in particular breast cancer. Radiation therapy is frequently used as an adjunct to lymphadenectomy in the treatment of a variety of cancers, increasing the risk of lymphedema by as much as tenfold through radiation-induced fibrosis mechanisms and decrease in the density of small vessel lymphatics [20, 21]. Around 30% of women who undergo axillary lymphadenectomy and receive radiation therapy develop breast cancer-related lymphedema (BCRL), with the risk doubled when the axilla is included in the radiation field compared with radiation to the breast and supraclavicular nodes only [22, 23]. Other risk factors for BCRL include mastectomy and taxane-based chemotherapy, with obesity the most significant modifiable risk factor [24, 25]. Obese patients have a threefold greater risk of developing lymphedema than patients with a BMI <25 [26]; a randomized-controlled trial found that patients who underwent weight loss had significant reductions in arm volumes and upper arm lymphedema when compared to control patients [27]. Super morbidly obese patients (BMI >59) may develop spontaneous lower extremity lymphedema, and those at higher obesity classes (BMI >65) are at risk of developing spontaneous upper extremity lymphedema. Obesity can also rarely result in a large, localized area of overgrowth termed massive localized lymphedema [28]. Around three-quarters of patients that develop BCRL do so within 3 years [29–31]. Late-onset secondary lymphedema is rare, and typically occurs following significant secondary insult such as infection or trauma. Around 15% of patients overall who undergo treatment for other solid tumors such as melanoma, sarcoma, and gynecological malignancies also develop lymphedema [32]. Rarely, sentinel lymph node biopsy (SLNB) alone can result in lymphedema, and excisional surgeries that injure the lymphatics, especially when combined with radiation therapy, or trauma, can result in lymphedema distally. Infection often precedes the development of lymphedema and may cause progressive damage to the lymphatic system, with a history of cellulitis a significant factor associated with increased limb volume [33]. Once lymphedema develops, there is variability in the rate at which pathologic changes occur; in some cases, lymphedema has a slow progression with a gradual increase in limb volume, while in others there is rapid disease progression leading to gross limb swelling.

Approximately one-fourth of patients presenting with a swollen extremity are misdiagnosed as having lymphedema, most commonly confused with lipedema, obesity, venous disease, or vascular anomalies [34] (Chap. 5). Physiological lymphatic imaging modalities [i.e., indocyanine green (ICG) lymphography, magnetic resonance lymphangiography, radionuclide lymphoscintigraphy] are sensitive and specific for the diagnosis of lymphedema and exclusion of other causes of limb swelling. Systemic conditions (e.g., cardiac, renal, hepatic, rheumatological) typically cause bilateral lower limb edema. Lipedema is bilateral, occurs almost exclusively in females, most commonly affects the lower extremities, occurs in the absence of lymphatic surgery, and spares the dorsum of the foot when the lower extremity is involved [34].

The majority of studies of genetic risk factors for the development of lymphedema have been performed in patients with primary lymphedema, where over 20 gene mutations have been linked to its development. Recent studies have also suggested that secondary lymphedema may be influenced by genetic predisposition due to the observation that some patients with BCRL exhibit abnormalities in lymphatic transport even in their unaffected extremity [35, 36].

Morbidity of Lymphedema

Lymphedema is characterized by constant symptoms including swelling, heaviness, discomfort, and paresthesia that may be exacerbated by certain activities, and which serve as a continual reminder for survivors of their cancer diagnosis. The increased limb size leads to both appearance concerns and functional impairment which negatively impact a patient's psychosocial well-being, body image, and sexuality, and severely disrupts their activities of daily living from loss of function in the affected extremity – the more severe the disease, the greater the negative impact, in particular if the dominant arm is affected. Lower extremity lymphedema can be severely debilitating due to dependency of the limb and the impact on gait and ambulation. The increased limb size may lead to issues with clothes fitment, especially shoes in leg lymphedema, and lead to secondary effects on the musculoskeletal system due to decreased ability to use the limb for routine activities and increased stress on the joints due to the extra weight of the extremity from muscle and bone hypertrophy secondary to the extra subcutaneous tissue and skin.

Patients with secondary lymphedema have an approximately 70 times increased risk of infection in the affected versus the unaffected limb due to impaired immunosurveillance and a proteinaceous environment favorable for bacterial growth. Superficial cellulitis can develop rapidly into a systemic infection and sepsis. In one study, around one-third of patients reported an episode of cellulitis within the past 12 months, and one-fourth required hospitalization for intravenous antibiotics [6]. Chronic lymphedema can predispose to lymphangiosarcoma in the affected extremity with a poor prognosis due to pulmonary metastasis and local recurrence, although the risk is very low [37]. In the most severe cases, high-output congestive cardiac failure may develop due to shunting of blood flow to a massive lymphedematous lower extremity.

Treatment of Lymphedema

Conservative Therapy

The progression of lymphedema and disability is dependent on patient compliance with their conservative therapy. Established techniques of complex (complete) decongestive therapy (CDT) have proven effective when combined with daily compressive garment use (Chap. 6). Individuals should maintain a normal body weight, lead an active lifestyle, protect the extremity from trauma/infections, and use compression garments and a pneumatic compression device (if indicated). Exercise promotes proximal flow of lymphatic fluid by muscle contraction against the resistance of a compression garment. Obese individuals have more complications from lymphedema compared to those of normal weight due to reversible adverse effects on lymphatic function, and dietary/nutrition support may be required for patients to attain and maintain a normal body weight.

Surgical Treatment of Lymphedema

Advances in surgical microscopes and the development of supermicrosurgical instruments and techniques have resulted in the widespread adoption of LVB, with surgical techniques on the supermicrosurgical scale utilizing distal lymphatic vessels and venules overcoming previous failed efforts due to high venous pressure gradients intrinsic to the larger veins (Chaps. 8 and 9). There are a plethora of options currently available for VLNT, a significant advance that allows for augmentation of the compromised lymphatic function within an affected extremity by transferring lymph nodes that can be spared without causing donor site lymphedema, perfused by microsurgical reestablishment of their intrinsic blood supply (Chaps. 13, 14, 15, 16, and 17); these include transplants from within the peritoneal cavity that avoid any risk of donor extremity lymphedema and that may lend themselves to minimally invasive harvest techniques including laparoscopic or robotic techniques (Chaps. 18 and 19). The advent of reverse lymphatic mapping, developed from SLNB techniques, has revolutionized VLNT from within regional lymphatic basins by reducing the risk of iatrogenic donor extremity lymphedema [38] (Chap. 11).

The adipose soft tissue hypertrophy that accumulates in the subcutaneous compartment of a lymphedematous limb can only be removed directly by SAL or excisional procedures. Because the underlying physiological abnormality is only minimally improved by reducing the burden on the compromised lymphatic system, lifelong compression is typically required to prevent lymph fluid stasis and disease recurrence. It is effective and consistent, with a near total reduction of the limb volume excess in the upper extremity typically achieved by 1 year postoperatively that is maintained long term without recurrence; the reduction in limb volume in the lower extremity is slightly less although is still maintained without recurrence through follow-up (Chap. 20). Combined approaches – performing SAL either following or in preparation for physiological surgeries (LVB and/or VLNT) – have demonstrated improved outcomes by extending the indications for physiological surgery to those with significant soft tissue excess (Chap. 21).

Staged direct excisional surgeries are reserved for severe advanced lymphedema characterized by severe soft tissue fibrosis (Chap. 22). Perforator- and lymphatic-sparing excisional techniques excise the subcutaneous tissue and deep fascia; however, this surgical approach is characterized by long surgical incisions with consequent high operative morbidity. The Charles procedure, whereby resection of all skin, subcutaneous tissue, and fascia is performed and the muscle is covered with split-thickness skin grafts, is characterized by significant morbidity including recurrent graft breakdown, lymphorrhoea, severe cosmetic deformity, and a high rate of amputation, and is generally reserved as a last resort.

There is current investigation into ILR, including the LYmphatic Microsurgical Preventive Healing Approach (LYMPHA), at the time of axillary lymphadenectomy to reduce the risk of development of lymphedema (Chap. 23). Axillary reverse lymphatic mapping (ARM) allows identification and preservation of the afferent lymphatic vessels to the SLN(s) draining the upper extremity. The available data suggests that this procedure may reduce the risk of lymphedema by around two-thirds [39].

Lymphedema surgeries are effective at improving the patient's quality of life and reducing the incidence of cellulitis (Chap. 24). Although the heterogeneous populations presenting for lymphedema surgery limit evaluation of comparative techniques, these are consistent within studies, and patients presenting for lymphedema surgery have exhausted conservative therapy and therefore outcomes can be attributed to the effects of the surgical intervention. These specialist treatments should ideally be delivered within lymphedema centers offering the highest standard of comprehensive best-practice multidisciplinary care (Chap. 28).

New and Emerging Therapeutics

Chronic lymphedema is characterized by inflammatory and fibrotic tissue changes that impair lymphangiogenesis and lymphatic function, and pro-lymphangiogenic, anti-inflammatory, and anti-fibrotic targets are emerging as treatments for the prevention and treatment of lymphedema (Chaps. 26 and 27). Effective pharmacological therapeutics, either used primarily or in conjunction with other treatments, are anticipated to revolutionize lymphedema treatment, improve outcomes, and reduce the morbidity of this chronic disease.

Future Directions

Results from future comparative outcomes studies are awaited to better define patient selection, and to progress and refine surgical treatment algorithms, in particular for newer and combination therapies, as well as from clinical studies of novel surgical treatments. Developments in imaging techniques and surgical equipment will parallel and underpin these. Advances in our understanding of the molecular basis of lymphedema are anticipated to result in biomarker profiling to better define treatments and prognosis, and lead to much needed viable translational pharmaceutical therapeutics to improve outcomes. With the increasing recognition of the role of the lymphatic system in multiple disease processes, spotlighting the lymphatic system through basic science research will have a more far-reaching impact than for the lymphedema population alone.

References

1. Stout NL, Pfalzer LA, Springer B, et al. Breast cancer-related lymphedema: comparing direct costs of a prospective surveillance model and a traditional model of care. Phys Ther. 2012;92:152–63.
2. Lopez M, Roberson ML, Strassle PD, et al. Epidemiology of lymphedema-related admissions in the United States: 2012-2017. Surg Oncol. 2020;35:249–53.
3. Fu MR, Ridner SH, Hu SH, Stewart BR, Cormier JN, Armer JM. Psychosocial impact of lymphedema: a systematic review of literature from 2004–2011. Psychooncology. 2013;22:1466–84.
4. Rockson SG. Estimating the population burden of lymphedema. Ann N Y Acad Sci. 2008;1131:147–54.
5. Mendoza N, Li A, Gill A, Tyring S. Filariasis: diagnosis and treatment. Dermatol Ther. 2009;22:475–90.
6. Moffatt CJ. Lymphoedema: an underestimated health problem. QJM. 2003;96:731–8.
7. Nguyen TT, Hoskin TL, Habermann EB, et al. Breast cancer-related lymphedema risk is related to multidisciplinary treatment and not surgery alone: results from a large cohort study. Ann Surg Oncol. 2017;24:2972–80.
8. Mihara M, Hara H, Hayashi Y, Narushima M, Yamamoto T, Todokoro T, et al. Pathological steps of cancer-related lymphedema: histological changes in the collecting lymphatic vessels after lymphadenectomy. PLoS One. 2012;7:e41126.
9. Zampell JC, Aschen S, Weitman ES, Yan A, Elhadad S, De Brot M, et al. Regulation of adipogenesis by lymphatic fluid stasis: part I. Adipogenesis, fibrosis, and inflammation. Plast Reconstr Surg. 2012;29:825–34.
10. Smeltzer DM, Stickler GB, Schirger A. Primary lymphedemas in children and adolescents: a follow-up study and review. Pediatrics. 1985;76:206–18.
11. Wolfe J, Kinmonth JB. The prognosis of primary lymphedema of the lower limbs. Arch Surg. 1981;116:1157–60.
12. Mendola A, Schlogel MJ, Ghalamkarpour A, Irrthum A, Nguyen HL, Fastre E, et al. Mutations in the VEGFR3 signaling pathway explain 36% of familial lymphedema. Mol Syndromol. 2013;4:257–66.
13. Connell FC, Ostergaard P, Carver C, Brice G, Williams N, Mansour S, Mortimer PS, Jeffery S. Analysis of the coding regions of VEGFR3 and VEGFRC in Milroy disease and other primary lymphoedemas. Hum Genet. 2009;124:625–31.
14. Gordon K, Spiden SL, Connell FC, Brice G, Cottrell S, Short J, et al. FLT4/VEGFR3 and Milroy disease: novel mutations, a review of published variants and database update. Hum Mutat. 2013;34:23–31.
15. Allen EV. Lymphedema of the extremities. Classification, etiology and differential diagnoses. A study of 300 cases. Arch Intern Med. 1934;56:606–24.
16. Connell FC, Gordon K, Brice G, Keeley V, Jeffery S, Mortimer PS, et al. The classification and diagnostic algorithm for primary lymphatic dysplasia: an update from 2010 to include molecular findings. Clin Genet. 2013;84:303–14.
17. Schook CC, Mulliken JB, Fishman SJ, Grant F, Zurakowski D, Greene AK. Primary lymphedema: clinical features and management in 138 pediatric patients. Plast Reconstr Surg. 2011;127:2419–31.
18. Schook CC, Mulliken JB, Fishman SJ, Alomari AI, Grant FD, Greene AK. Differential diagnosis of lower extremity enlargement in pediatric patients referred with a diagnosis of lymphedema. Plast Reconstr Surg. 2011;127:1571–81.
19. Maclellan RA, Couto RA, Sullivan JE, Grant FD, Slavin SA, Greene AK. Management of primary and secondary lymphedema: analysis of 225 referrals to a center. Ann Plast Surg. 2015 Aug;75(2):197–200.
20. Avraham T, Yan A, Zampell JC, Daluvoy SV, Haimovitz-Friedman A, Cordeiro AP, et al. Radiation therapy causes loss of dermal lymphatic vessels and interferes with lymphatic function by TGF-beta1- mediated tissue fibrosis. Am J Physiol Cell Physiol. 2010;299:C589–605.
21. Jackowski S, Janusch M, Fiedler E, Marsch WC, Ulbrich EJ, Gaisbauer G, et al. Radiogenic lymphangiogenesis in the skin. Am J Pathol. 2007;171:338–48.
22. Gärtner R, Mejdahl MK, Andersen KG, Ewertz M, Kroman N. Development in self-reported arm lymphedema in Danish women treated for early stage breast cancer in 2005 and 2006 – a nationwide follow- up study. Breast. 2014;23:445.
23. Hayes SB. Does axillary boost increase lymphedema compared with supraclavicular radiation alone after breast conservation? Int J Radiat Oncol Biol Phys. 2008;72:1449–55.
24. Dayangac M, Makay O, Yeniay L, Aynaci M, Kapkac M, Yilmaz R. Precipitating factors for lymphedema following surgical treatment of breast cancer: implications for patients undergoing axillary lymph node dissection. Breast J. 2009;15:210–1.
25. Yen TW, Fan X, Sparapani R, Laud PW, Walker AP, Nattinger AB. A contemporary, population-based study of lymphedema risk factors in older women with breast cancer. Ann Surg Oncol. 2009;16:979–88.
26. Helyer LK, Varnic M, Le LW, Leong W, McCready D. Obesity is a risk factor for developing postoperative lymphedema in breast cancer patients. Breast J. 2010;16:48–54.
27. Shaw C, Mortimer P, Judd PA. A randomized controlled trial of weight reduction as a treatment for breast cancer-related lymphedema. Cancer. 2007;110:1868–74.
28. Greene AK, Grant FD, Slavin SA. Lower-extremity lymphedema and elevated body-mass index. N Engl J Med. 2012;366: 2136–7.
29. Johansson K, Branje E. Arm lymphoedema in a cohort of breast cancer survivors 10 years after diagnosis. Acta Oncol. 2010;49:166–73.
30. Petrek JA, Senie RT, Peters M, Rosen PP. Lymphedema in a cohort of breast carcinoma survivors 20 years after diagnosis. Cancer. 2001;92:1368–77.
31. McLaughlin SA, Wright MJ, Morris KT, et al. Prevalence of lymphedema in women with breast cancer 5 years after sentinel lymph node biopsy or axillary dissection: patient perceptions and precautionary behaviors. J Clin Oncol. 2008;26:5220–8.
32. Cormier JN, Askew RL, Mungovan KS, et al. Lymphedema beyond breast cancer: a systematic review and meta-analysis of cancer-related secondary lymphedema. Cancer. 2010;116:5138–49.

33. Vignes S, Arrault M, Dupuy A. Factors associated with increased breast cancer-related lymphedema volume. Acta Oncol. 2007;46:1138–42.
34. Rudkin GH, Miller TA. Lipedema: a clinical entity distinct from lymphedema. Plast Reconstr Surg. 1994;94:841–7.
35. Newman B, Lose F, Kedda MA, Francois M, Ferguson K, Janda M, et al. Possible genetic predisposition to lymphedema after breast cancer. Lymphat Res Biol. 2012;10:2–13.
36. Miaskowski C, Dodd M, Paul SM, West C, Hamolsky D, Abrams G, et al. Lymphatic and angiogenic candidate genes predict the development of secondary lymphedema following breast cancer surgery. PLoS One. 2013;8:e60164.
37. Sharma A, Schwartz RA. Stewart-Treves syndrome: pathogenesis and management. J Am Acad Dermatol. 2012;67:1342–8.
38. Dayan JH, Dayan E, Smith ML. Reverse lymphatic mapping: a new technique for maximizing safety in vascularized lymph node transfer. Plast Reconstr Surg. 2015;135:277–85.
39. Johnson AR, Kimball S, Epstein S, et al. Lymphedema incidence after axillary lymph node dissection: quantifying the impact of radiation and the lymphatic microsurgical preventive healing approach. Ann Plast Surg. 2019;82:S234–41.

Anatomy of the Lymphatic System and Structural Changes in Lymphedema of the Extremities

2

Akira Shinaoka and Hiroo Suami

Current Understanding of Lymphatic Anatomy

Hippocrates described 'white blood' in the body in the year 5 BCE, and this is considered to be the oldest account of the lymphatics. The first discovery of the lymphatics in academia is credited to Gaspare Aselli and his canine study in 1622 was published posthumously in 1627 [1]. The word 'lymphatics' was coined by Thomas Bartholin in 1653 in his book *Vasa Lymphatica*, in which he stated that the lymphatics were a vascular system independent to the blood system [2]. Anton Nuck (1691) developed a new technique to visualize the lymphatics in cadavers using mercury, and his technique enabled anatomists to investigate the lymphatics for the next three centuries [3]. Anatomical study of the lymphatic system reached its pinnacle around the early twentieth century with several notable publications: Sappey (1874), Delamere et al. (1903), Bartels (1909) and Rouviere (1932) [4–7]. These seminal works provided us with fundamental knowledge about normal lymphatic anatomy. However, their anatomical descriptions did not include any morphological changes that occur in pathological conditions such as lymphedema.

Kubik conducted a review of lymphatic anatomical studies and collated them in a chapter in Foldi's book for physicians and lymphedema therapists [8]. One of his achievements was a body chart of skin lymphatic territories. His chart has become a popular educational resource to guide lymphedema therapists in applying manual lymphatic drainage (MLD) for lymphedema patients. The author (HS) coined the term 'lymphosome' to describe a skin lymphatic territory divided by their corresponding node group and created a lymphosome chart (Fig. 2.1) [9, 10]. Lymphosomes provide an overview of normal lymphatic anatomy and are also a useful way of comparing and contrasting the lymphatics between species in animal research.

The lymphatics are described as a two-layer system, consisting of superficial and deep systems separated by the deep fascia. Each system is independent from the other except at a few sites, but they unite in the deep axillary or intrapelvic regions. The superficial lymphatic system transfers lymph fluid from the skin and subcutaneous tissue, and the deep lymphatic system carries lymph fluid from the musculoskeletal tissue. The tissue changes that occur in lymphedema represent an accumulation of fluid and adipose tissue and fibrosis, but these changes are identified predominantly in the superficial soft tissue above the deep fascia. Thus, the superficial lymphatic system has a special significance for understanding the pathology of lymphedema. As a result, this chapter focuses primarily on the anatomy of the superficial lymphatics in both the normal condition and lymphedema.

Imaging Options for the Diagnosis of Lymphedema

Lymphedema is a chronic swelling of soft tissue caused by lymph stasis. The pathophysiology of lymphedema is not yet fully understood. Damage to the lymphatic system following lymph node dissection, radiotherapy or filariasis provokes lymphatic dysfunction and retention of lymph fluid in the affected limbs. Lymph stasis triggers structural damage in the lymphatic vessels, giving rise to progressive change such

A. Shinaoka
Department of Human Morphology, Okayama University, Graduate School of Medicine, Dentistry and Pharmaceutical Sciences, Okayama, Japan

Department of Plastic and Reconstructive Surgery, Okayama University, Graduate School of Medicine, Dentistry and Pharmaceutical Sciences, Okayama, Japan

H. Suami (✉)
Australian Lymphoedema Education, Research and Treatment (ALERT), Faculty of Medicine, Health and Human Sciences, Macquarie University, Sydney, NSW, Australia
e-mail: hiroo.suami@mq.edu.au

M. V. Schaverien, J. H. Dayan (eds.), *Multimodal Management of Upper and Lower Extremity Lymphedema*,
https://doi.org/10.1007/978-3-030-93039-4_2

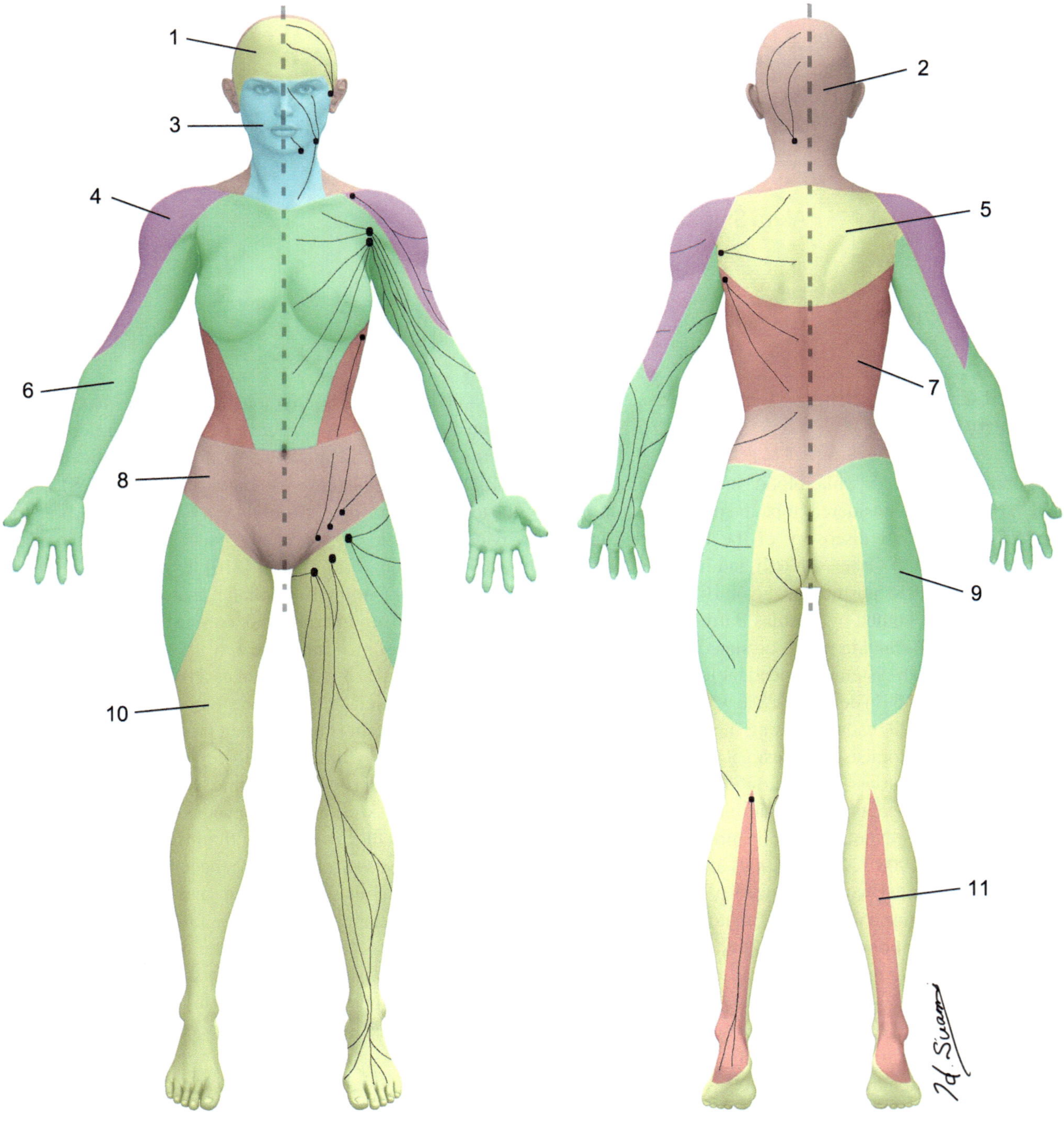

Fig. 2.1 Lymphosomes of the body. The lymphatic territories are demarcated according to their corresponding lymphatic basins: 1. temporal, 2. occipital, 3. submental, 4. subclavicular, 5. subscapular, 6. lateral axillary, 7. pectoral, 8. superior inguinal, 9. lateral inguinal, 10. inferior inguinal, 11. popliteal. (Reproduced with permission of Hiroo Suami)

as fibrosis of vessel walls, a narrowing lumen and a reduction in smooth muscle cells which are a feature of lymphedema [11].

There are several imaging techniques that can identify anatomical change in the lymphatic system and aid the development of diagnostic criteria for lymphedema. The first of these, and the current gold standard for diagnostic imaging for lymphedema, is lymphoscintigraphy. It is a form of nuclear medicine imaging developed in the 1950s and demonstrates lymph nodes as hot spots [12]. The reduction or absence of nuclear tracer in the lymph nodes is a criterion of lymphedema. Although lymphoscintigraphy has been used in lymphedema diagnosis for several decades, the poor-resolution, two-dimensional images produced are not ideal for evaluating the condition of the lymphatic vessels. In advanced lymphedema, the nuclear tracer commonly moves only a short distance from the injection site, and no imaging information can be obtained in the proximal body regions.

Lymphangiography is an imaging technique developed by Kinmonth in 1952 [13]. It is no longer used for lymphedema diagnosis because one of its side effects was to make lymphedema worse. However, the high-resolution images produced by this technique provided the most detailed information about the lymphatic vessels in lymphedema.

Indocyanine green (ICG) fluorescence lymphography has been widely adopted as a new way to conduct lymphatic imaging. The camera system uses near-infrared technology and it was first applied to the lymphatics in 2005 [14]. ICG dye injected into dermal or subcutaneous tissue is spontaneously absorbed into the lymphatic capillaries and fluoresces when excited by near-infrared light. The camera and filter system selectively picks up the near-infrared rays and identifies lymphatic structures within a depth of 2 centimetres from the surface of the skin. The use of photoacoustic imaging with ICG dye has the advantage of demonstrating the lymphatics as a three-dimensional image [15].

Lymphatic imaging technology continues to develop, with each development providing further detailed images of the lymphatics. Although significant advances have been made in lymphatic imaging techniques, the relationship between the tracer injection site and the lymphatic pathway has not been much discussed. When different techniques use different injection sites, it is difficult to compare the images obtained. To address this issue, we undertook anatomical studies of the lymphatic system in cadaver legs using both CT lymphography and ICG lymphography [16]. We found that standard injection sites at the web spaces between the toes did not help visualize some lymph nodes of the leg. Additional injection sites in the medial, lateral and posterior aspect of the foot were required for evaluating the whole lymphatic pathways. We would like to stress the importance of developing a precise knowledge of normal lymphatic anatomy because this knowledge enables us to distinguish the structural changes that occur in lymphedema.

Normal Lymphatic Anatomy in the Lower Extremity

To understand the normal anatomy of the lymphatics in the lower extremity, a knowledge of embryological development of the cutaneous veins and lymphatic vessels is crucial. The superficial lymphatic vessels run alongside the superficial veins, and the superficial lymph nodes are located near the junction of the great saphenous vein (GSV) and the common femoral vein. Recent articles have revealed that the peripheral lymphatic vessels develop before lymph nodes [17, 18]. In the foetus, lymph node anlages emerge at the junction of the GSV and the common femoral vein and fuse to the lymphatic vessels. Thus, lymph nodes in the lower extremity are concentrated in the inguinal region, and the superficial lymphatic vessels along the GSV connect to these nodes.

The superficial lymphatic vessels are distributed circumferentially around the foot. Our anatomical studies using fresh cadaver specimens indicate that the superficial lymphatic vessels in the lower leg are classified into four subgroups according to their anatomical relationship with the cutaneous veins (Fig. 2.2) [16, 19, 20]. These four distinct subgroups are the posteromedial, anteromedial, anterolateral and posterolateral groups. In our study, three of the four – the anteromedial, anterolateral, and posteromedial – connected to the inguinal nodes. Both posteromedial and anteromedial groups of vessels connected to the same superficial lymph nodes in the medial inguinal region, but the anterolateral group connected to different inguinal lymph nodes located in the lateral inguinal region (Fig. 2.3). The posteromedial group of vessels ran along the

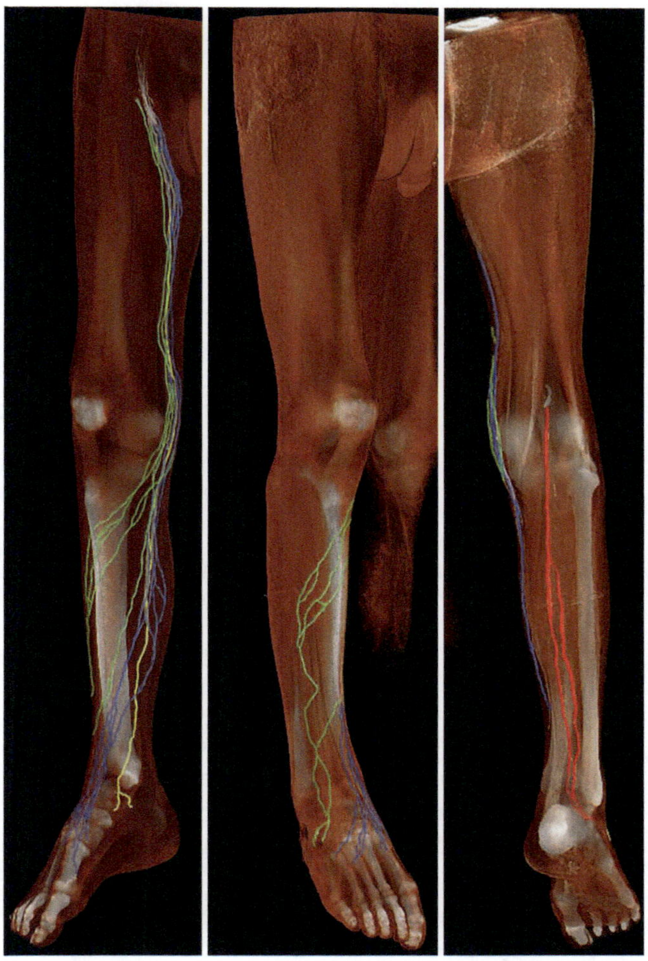

Fig. 2.2 CT-lymphangiography images of four lymphatic groups in a cadaveric lower extremity. Lymphatic vessels were divided into four groups according to their anatomical features: posteromedial (yellow), anteromedial (blue), anterolateral (green) and posterolateral (red)

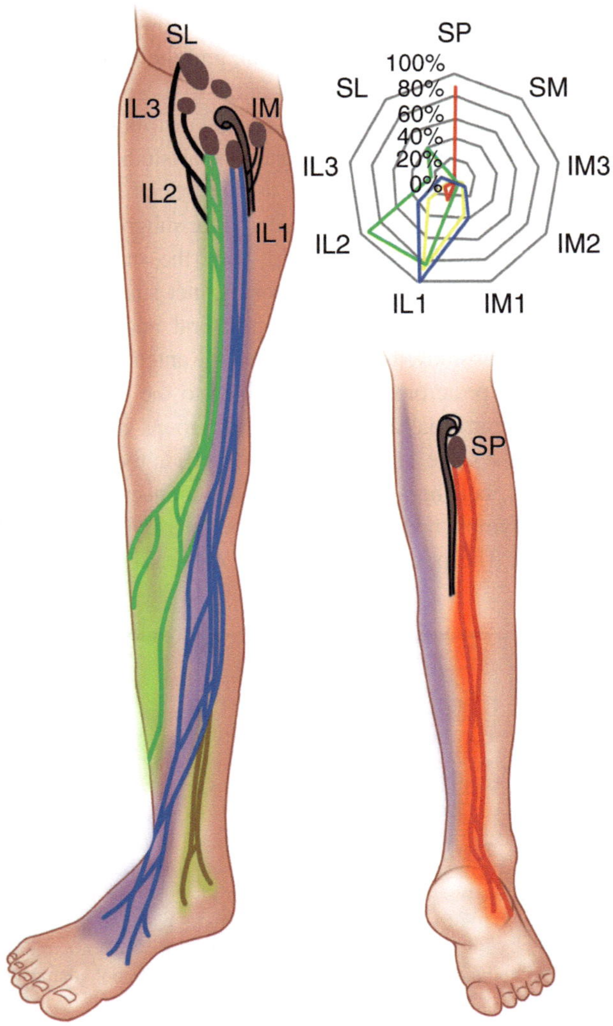

Fig. 2.3 A schematic diagram of detailed lymphosomes in the lower extremity and the correlation between a lymphosome and the location of the first-tier lymph node. Lymphatic groups are color-coded using the same scheme as in Fig. 2.2. Three regional lymph nodes received most of the lymphatic fluid in the lower limbs: inferior lateral (IL) 1 and 2 and superficial popliteal (SP). IM = inferior medial, SL = superior lateral, SM = superior medial

main trunk of the GSV, while the vessels in the anteromedial and anterolateral groups ran along branches of the GSV. The posterolateral group of vessels alone ran along the lesser saphenous vein (LSV) and connected to the popliteal lymph nodes. The posterolateral and posteromedial groups of vessels were composed of only a few lymphatic vessels. Their diameter was larger and they ran deeper than the vessels in the other two groups. The lymphatic vessels in the anteromedial group originated in the dorsum of the foot and were greater in number than the other groups in the lower leg. The lymphatic vessels in the anterolateral group originated in the lateral foot. They ran along a lateral branch of the GSV in the lower leg and then along a lateral accessory branch of the GSV in the thigh.

To provide a comprehensive imaging examination, it is important that all four subgroups can be identified. The ICG dye must be injected into four specific sites: below the medial and lateral malleolus, at the first toe web and at the midpoint between the head of the fifth metatarsal bone and below the lateral malleolus.

Anatomical Changes in Lower Extremity Lymphedema

The pathology of cancer-related lymphedema is explained as the obstruction of superficial lymphatic vessels at different levels in the lower extremity that causes collateral pathways to form to maintain lymph flow. Lymph fluid in the affected vessels spills backwards into the dermal lymphatics at the obstructed site in a phenomenon known as 'dermal backflow' (Fig. 2.4). Dermal backflow is a specific criterion in diagnosing lymphedema and enables a connection to be made between the obstructed vessel and a nearby patent vessel. However, dermal backflow is not the only mechanism to maintain lymph flow. An alternative type of collateral pathway creation is lymphangiogenesis, whereby a new lymphatic vessel develops from the stump of an obstructed vessel and extends towards the remaining lymph nodes [21].

Imaging studies of the lymphatics have reported anatomical changes in lymphedema. Kinmonth performed lymphangiography in primary leg lymphedema patients and classified the cases into two categories, 'proliferative' and 'aplastic', according to the number of lymphatic vessels identified [22]. Maegawa et al. classified the severity of leg lymphedema through lymphoscintigraphy [23]. Their findings indicated that deterioration of the lymphatic vessels commenced in the inguinal region and extended distally as lymphedema progressed. All lymphatic vessels eventually disappeared, and the tracer did not move beyond the injection site in the most advanced stage.

Conservative management known as comprehensive decongestive therapy (CDT) or complex lymphedema therapy (CLT) has been the mainstay of lymphedema treatment. The axillo-inguinal pathway has routinely been used in the MLD sequence for leg lymphedema to move extra-cellular fluid from the affected leg to the axillary region. However, lymphatic imaging in leg lymphedema rarely demonstrated this pathway, but often only demonstrated the pathway to the contralateral inguinal region. This suggests that there is a discrepancy between the general principle of conservative management and imaging findings. Further imaging investigations into the altered anatomy in lymphedema will shed light on the pathophysiology of lymphedema and help develop an evidence-based management plan.

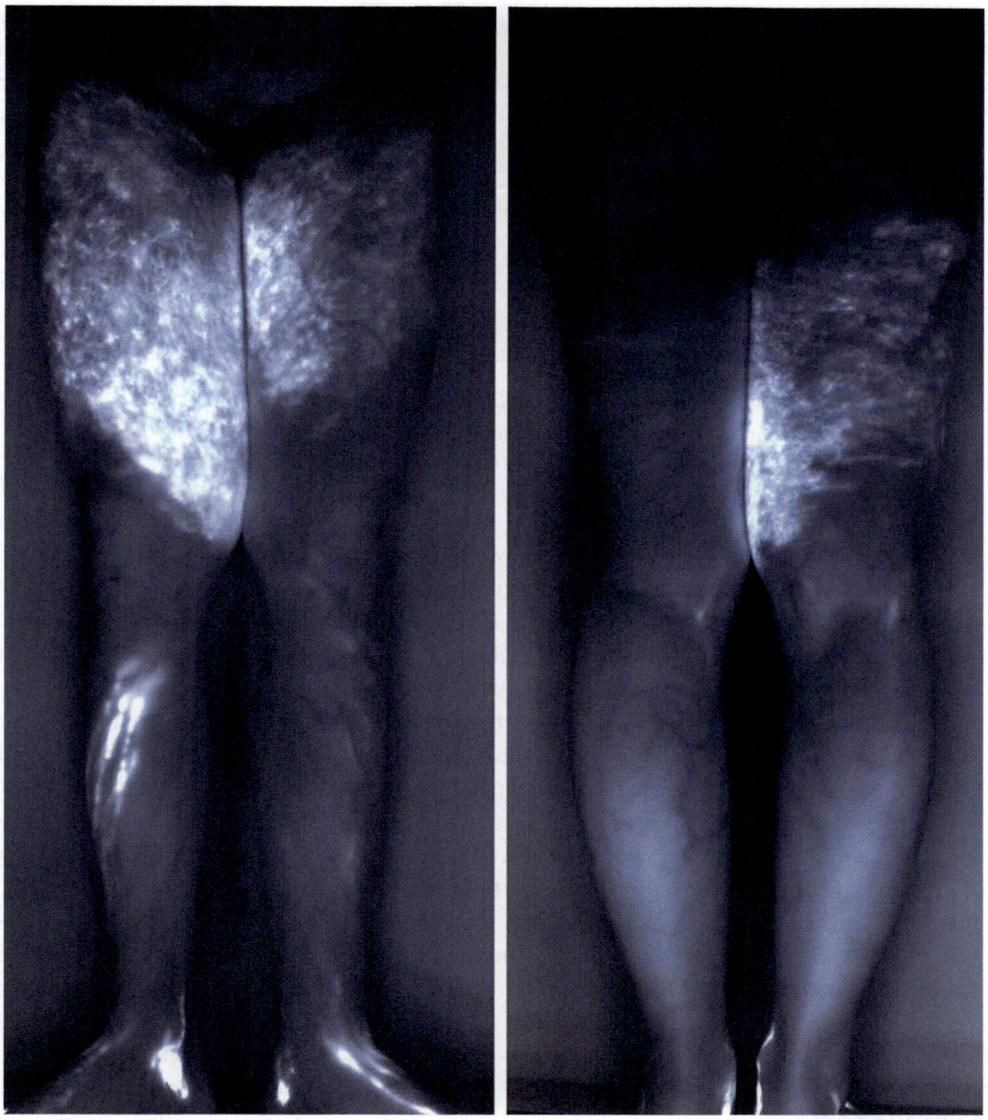

Fig. 2.4 ICG fluorescent lymphography images of a patient with bilateral lower limb lymphedema. Dermal backflow covered the anterior thigh in both legs, and the anterolateral lymphatic group was only identified in the lower leg

Normal Lymphatic Anatomy in the Upper Extremity

The lymphatics in the upper extremity originate in the lymphatic capillaries in the dermis of the fingertips and palm. Those vessels in the fingertips converge at the level of the distal interphalangeal joint to form one or two lymphatic vessels on each side. All lymphatic vessels from the fingers run in the dorsum of the hand. Those in the palm converge to form several lymphatic vessels at the anterior wrist. These superficial lymphatic vessels are arranged circumferentially around the wrist. The lymphatic vessels originating at the anterior wrist run straight towards the axilla. The lymphatic vessels originating at the dorsal hand run along the posterior forearm and divide into two courses distally from the olecranon (Fig. 2.5). They gradually change their course to the medial upper arm en route to the axilla.

The superficial lymphatic pathway connecting to the axillary lymph nodes is the dominant pathway, but an alternative pathway to the clavicular nodes exists as an anatomical variation. The lymphatic vessels running along the cephalic vein pass through an interval lymph node named the deltopectoral lymph node at the deltopectoral groove. The vessels run below the head of the pectoralis major and connect to the supraclavicular nodes. This lymphatic pathway was described by Sappey and Mascagni [4, 24]. Anatomical studies were conducted by Kubik and LeDuc [25, 26]. As this lymphatic pathway bypasses the axillary nodes, knowledge about it is important in skin cancer management to help identify cancer metastatic sites.

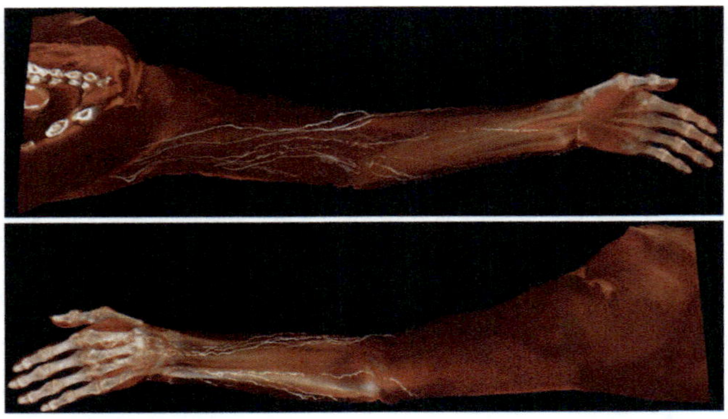

Fig. 2.5 CT-lymphangiography images of the superficial lymphatic vessels in a cadaveric upper extremity. The lymphatic vessels originating in the dorsal hand run along the posterior forearm and divide into two courses distally from the olecranon

The deep lymphatic system is located below the deep fascia. The deep vessels run along the major arteries, including the ulnar, radial and humeral arteries. The superficial and deep vessels are generally independent of each other without any direct connection between them, but they are very close to each other at the anterior elbow. The superficial lymphatic vessels located along the basilic vein sometimes run together with the vein and merge with the deep lymphatic vessels.

In order to identify all lymphatic vessels running towards the axilla, the tracer injection needs to be given at multiple sites circumferentially around the hand. If the tracer is injected into the finger webs alone, only the lymphatic vessels in the posterior forearm are revealed, missing those in the anterior forearm.

Anatomical Changes in Upper Extremity Lymphedema

Lymphedema in the lower extremity is representative of various causes, including congenital maldevelopment and primary idiopathic, traumatic or cancer-related disorders. However, upper extremity lymphedema is predominantly caused by breast cancer treatment. Axillary surgery is the major factor in lymphedema development, and radiation given in addition to surgery increases lymphedema risk [27]. The pathology of upper extremity lymphedema has conventionally been explained as the blockage of arm lymphatic drainage provoked by surgical intervention that subsequently causes swelling of the arm. The current principle of conservative management is based on this theory, and MLD for arm lymphedema is performed to shift excess lymph fluid from the affected arm to other intact nodal regions by massaging it downwards to the ipsilateral inguinal region and horizontally to the contralateral axilla. However, our recent ICG lymphography study in breast cancer-related lymphedema (BCRL) revealed that more than two-thirds of arm lymphedema still drained to the ipsilateral axilla, the site of the breast surgery [28]. These results suggest that axillary node dissection does not always block the lymphatic drainage pathway to the axilla. Therefore, it is reasonable to reconsider that is the limitation of lymph flow to the axilla, rather than total blockage, that causes arm lymphedema.

In normal anatomy, there are two bypassing lymphatic pathways – one to the supraclavicular nodes via the deltopectoral groove and the other to the deep lymphatic system at the anterior elbow – that play a key role in maintaining lymph flow in BCRL and help prevent lymphedema progression [21]. Lymph fluid in lymphedema is often diverted through these pathways when the superficial lymphatic pathway to the axilla is damaged or obstructed. Lymphedema is caused by damage to the superficial lymphatic vessels followed by identification of dermal backflow at the site. As a definite imaging criterion for lymphedema diagnosis, dermal backflow is often considered to be a negative sign. However, dermal backflow enables lymph fluid in the affected lymphatic vessels to be transported to the unaffected region, so it should be considered to be a positive reaction by the body to maintain lymph fluid drainage. The patterns of lymphatic drainage in BCRL found in our study are summarized in Fig. 2.6 [29].

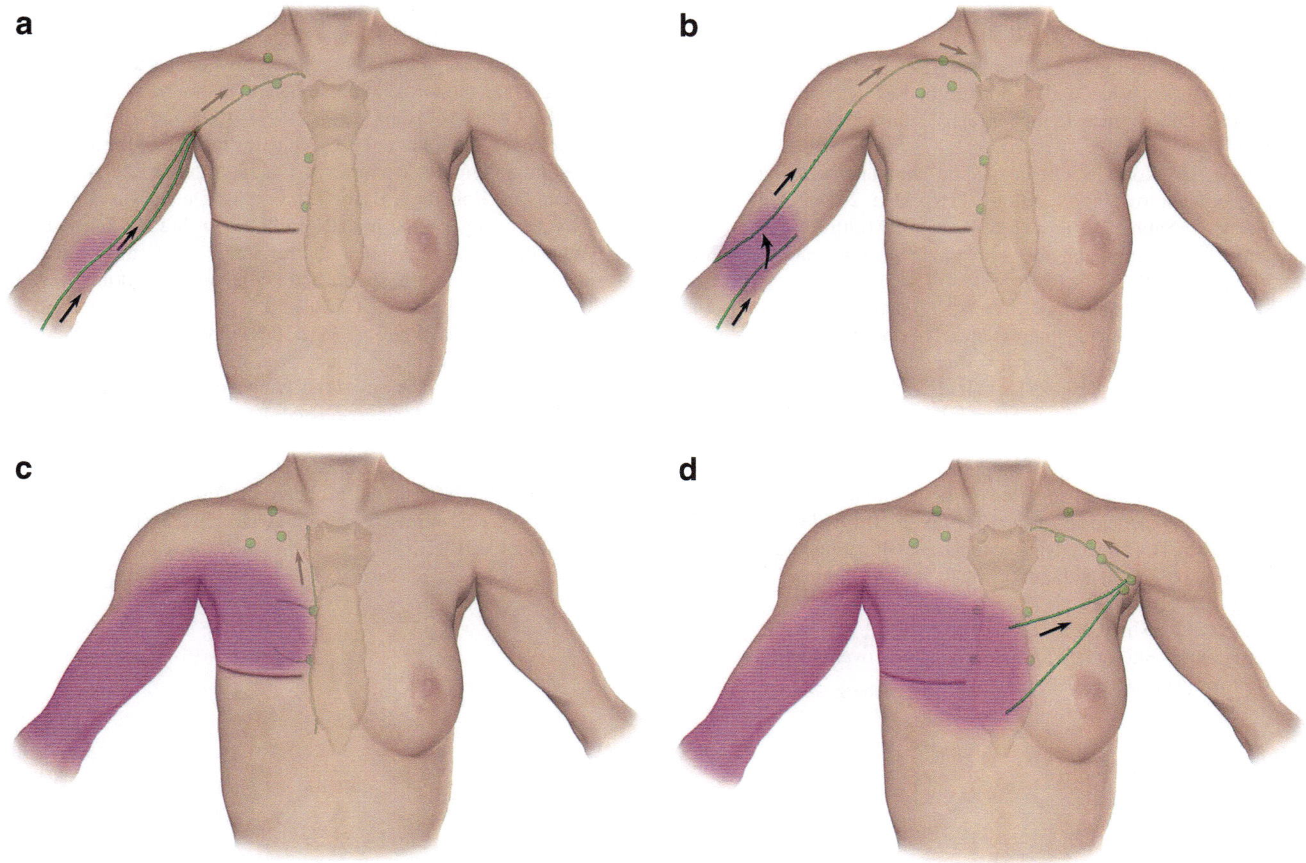

Fig. 2.6 Schematic diagrams show the patterns of lymphatic drainage in upper extremity lymphedema. (**a**) The ipsilateral axillary region; (**b**) the clavicular region; (**c**) the parasternal region; (**d**) the contralateral axillary region. (Reproduced from Ref. 29 with permission)

Summary

This chapter describes both the normal anatomy of the superficial lymphatic system in the extremities and the altered anatomy in lymphedema. We have demonstrated that the human body has the flexibility to maintain lymph drainage via anatomical structural changes even when lymphedema has developed. While surgical procedures for lymphedema are being continually refined, conservative management strategies must also be updated to reflect recent imaging findings.

References

1. Aselli G. De Lactibus Sive Lacteis Venis. J.B. Bidellius: Milan; 1627.
2. Bartholin T. Vasa lymphatica nuper Hafniae in animalibus inventa et hepatis exsequiae. Petrus Hakius: Hafniae (Copenhagen); 1653.
3. Nuck A. Adenographia curiosa et uteri foeminei anatome nova. Jordan Luchtmans: Leyden; 1691.
4. Sappey MPC. Anatomie, Physiologie, Pathologie des Vaisseaux Lymphatiques consideres chez L'Homme et les Vertebres. Paris: Adrien Delahaye; 1874.
5. Delamere G, Poirier P, Cuneo B. The lymphatics. In: Charpy PP, editor. A treatise of human anatomy. Westminster: Archibald Constable and Co Ltd; 1903.
6. Bartels P. Das Lymphgefäßsystem. Handb. d. Anat. Verlag von gustav fischer: Jena; 1909.
7. Rouviére H. Anatomie des lymphatiques de l'homme. Paris: Masson; 1932.
8. Foldi M, Foldi E, Kubik S. Textbook of lymphology for physicians and lymphedema therapists. Urban & Fischer: Munchen; 2003.
9. Suami H. Lymphosome concept: anatomical study of the lymphatic system. J Surg Oncol. 2017;115(1):13–7.
10. Suami H, Scaglioni M. Anatomy of the lymphatic system and the lymphosome concept with reference to lymphoedema. Semin Plast Surg. 2018;32:5–11.
11. Koshima I, Kawada S, Moriguchi T, Kajiwara Y. Ultrastructural observations of lymphatic vessels in lymphedema in human extremities. Plast Reconstr Surg. 1996;97:397–405.
12. Sherman AI, Ter-Pogossian M. Lymph-node concentration of radioactive colloidal gold following interstitial injection. Cancer. 1953;6:1238–40.
13. Kinmonth JB. Lymphangiography in man; a method of outlining lymphatic trunks at operation. Clin Sci. 1952;11:13–20.
14. Unno N, Inuzuka K, Suzuki M, et al. Preliminary experience with a novel fluorescence lymphography using indocyanine green in patients with secondary lymphedema. J Vasc Surg. 2007;45:1016–21.
15. Suzuki Y, Kajita H, Konishi N, et al. Subcutaneous lymphatic vessels in the lower extremities: comparison between photoacoustic

lymphangiography and near-infrared fluorescence lymphangiography. Radiology. 2020;295:469–74.
16. Shinaoka A, Koshimune S, Yamada K, et al. Correlations between tracer injection sites and lymphatic pathways in the leg: a near-infrared fluorescence Lymphography study. Plast Reconstr Surg. 2019;144:634–42.
17. Petrova TV, Koh GY. Organ-specific lymphatic vasculature: from development to pathophysiology. J Exp Med. 2018;215:35–49.
18. Bovay E, Sabine A, Prat-Luri B, et al. Multiple roles of lymphatic vessels in peripheral lymph node development. J Exp Med. 2018;215:2760–77.
19. Shinaoka AA, Koshimune S, Yamada K, et al. A fresh cadaver study on indocyanine green fluorescence lymphography: a new whole body imaging technique for investigating the superficial lymphatics. Plast Reconstr Surg. 2018;141:1161–4.
20. Shinaoka A, Koshimune S, Suami H, et al. Lower-limb lymphatic drainage pathways and lymph nodes: a CT lymphangiography cadaver study. Radiology. 2020;294(1):223–9.
21. Suami H. Anatomical theories of the pathophysiology of cancer-related lymphoedema. Cancers (Basel). 2020;12:1338.
22. Kinmonth JB. Primary lymphedema: classification and other studies based on oleo-lymphography and clinical features. J Cardiovasc Surg. 1969;10(suppl):65–77.
23. Maegawa J, Mikami T, Yamamoto Y, et al. Types of lymphoscintigraphy and indications for lymphaticovenous anastomosis. Microsurgery. 2010;30:437–42.
24. Mascagni P. Vasorum Lymphaticorum Corporis Humani Historia et Ichonographia. P. Carli: Sienne;1787.
25. Kubik S. The role of the lateral upper arm bundle and the lymphatic watersheds in the formation of collateral pathways in lymphedema. Acta Biol Acad Sci Hung. 1980;31:191–200.
26. Leduc A, Caplan I, Leduc O. Lymphatic drainage of the upper limb. Substitution lymphatic pathways. Eur J Lymphol. 1993;4:11–8.
27. Naoum GE, Roberts S, Brunelle CL, et al. Quantifying the impact of axillary surgery and nodal irradiation on breast cancer-related lymphedema and local tumor control: long-term results from a prospective screening trial [published online ahead of print, 2020 Jul 30]. J Clin Oncol. 2020:JCO2000459.
28. Suami H, Heydon-White A, Mackie H, Czerniec S, Koelmeyer L, Boyages J. A new indocyanine green fluorescence lymphography protocol for identification of the lymphatic drainage pathway for patients with breast cancer-related lymphoedema. BMC Cancer. 2019;19(1):985.
29. Suami H, Koelmeyer L, Mackie H, Boyages J. Patterns of lymphatic drainage after axillary node dissection impact arm lymphoedema severity: a review of animal and clinical imaging studies. Surg Oncol. 2018;27:743–50.

Pathophysiology and Molecular Research in Lymphedema

3

Elizabeth Kiwanuka and Babak Mehrara

Introduction

Lymphedema is a progressive disease characterized by abnormal lymphatic drainage that leads to the accumulation of interstitial fluid and fibrofatty tissue deposition [1]. The lymphatic system is a network of vessels connecting the lymphoid organs of the body and plays a key role in immune surveillance, clearance of inflammatory cells, dietary fat absorption, cholesterol metabolism, and fluid hemostasis [2]. The lymphatic network runs parallel to the venous circulation and begins as blind-ended lymphatic capillaries. In the tissues, the proteins and immune cells that are too large to enter the venous system are absorbed by the lymphatic capillaries which in turn empty into larger collecting lymphatic vessels [3]. The collecting lymphatics have luminal valves and are lined by smooth muscle cells, facilitating the unidirectional flow of the lymphatic fluid via connections of the thoracic duct to the internal jugular vein [4].

Lymphedema can occur either as a primary condition or secondary to injury or insults to the lymphatic system. Primary lymphedema presents during infancy, childhood, or adolescence and is caused by genetic mutations that directly or indirectly regulate lymphatic differentiation and function [5]. Less frequently, primary lymphedema can appear after age 35 and is known as lymphedema tarda [2, 6]. Secondary lymphedema is the most common type of lymphedema and develops in response to direct or indirect injury to the lymphatic system resulting from infectious diseases (filariasis), trauma or cancer surgery, or obesity [2, 7, 8]. Both primary and secondary lymphedemas share similar pathologic features, including chronic swelling, inflammation, adipose deposition, and fibrosis; however, there is great variability in the rate of disease progression, severity of lymphedema, and response to treatment.

Etiology and Staging of Lymphedema

Primary lymphedema is often classified based on the patient's age at presentation. Congenital lymphedema presents within the first 2 years of life, lymphedema praecox presents at puberty, and lymphedema tarda is diagnosed after age 35 years. The phenotype of primary lymphedema varies with age of onset, anatomical location, inheritance patterns, and underlying genetic cause [9].

Congenital lymphedemas account for 10–25% of all cases of primary lymphedema and occur most commonly in the lower extremity of females. The most common form of congenital primary lymphedema is Milroy's disease and accounts for approximately 2% of all lymphedemas [9]. Patients with this disease present with bilateral lower extremity lymphedema that is, in some cases, accompanied by hydroceles. Milroy's disease is a familial, sex-linked disease that is caused by a mutation of FLT4, thereby inactivating the gene that encodes for the receptor for VEGF-C (vascular endothelial growth factor receptor-3 (VEGFR-3) [9]. VEGFR-3 signaling is necessary for lymphatic endothelial cell development, proliferation, differentiation, and migration, and as a result, patients with Milroy's disease have hypoplastic lymphatic vessels. Another common genetic cause of lymphedema is lymphedema-distichiasis syndrome and is caused by an autosomal dominant mutation in the FOXC2 gene. These patients often present with lower extremity lymphedema and an extra row of eyelashes [10].

The most common form of sporadic primary lymphedema is lymphedema praecox, also known as Meige's disease. Most patients diagnosed with lymphedema praecox are female (ratio of 4:1 with males), and symptoms most commonly present at the time of puberty, highlighting the role of female sex hormones in developing lymphedema [11, 12].

E. Kiwanuka · B. Mehrara (✉)
Department of Surgery, Division of Plastic and Reconstructive Surgery at Memorial Sloan Kettering Cancer Center, New York, NY, USA
e-mail: mehrarab@mskcc.org

M. V. Schaverien, J. H. Dayan (eds.), *Multimodal Management of Upper and Lower Extremity Lymphedema*,
https://doi.org/10.1007/978-3-030-93039-4_3

Although pathologic changes in the lymphatic system in patients with lymphedema praecox are highly variable, most patients have decreased lymphatic capillaries and hypoplastic collecting vessels.

Secondary lymphedema develops as a result of direct or indirect injury to the lymphatic system. The most common cause of secondary lymphedema worldwide is lymphatic filariasis, caused by infection with roundworms. Mosquitos commonly transmit roundworms, and their larvae cause injury to the lymphatic system by occluding the vessels. In addition, the inflammatory response leads to the progression of the disease with devastating limb swelling as a result. The treatment for filariasis is primarily antiparasitic medications, but patients with severe filariasis-induced lymphedema often require surgery [13].

In Western countries, most patients develop secondary lymphedema after an iatrogenic injury to the lymphatic system in the course of their cancer treatment. Breast cancer, due to its high prevalence, is the most common cause of secondary lymphedema. Estimates of the rates of lymphedema in breast cancer survivors following axillary lymph node dissection vary widely—ranging from 15% to 50%—due to heterogenous methods used for diagnosis and follow-up time [14–16]. However, it is important to note that even minor disruption of the lymphatic system such as sentinel lymph node biopsy can cause lymphedema in 5–7% of patients [17–19]. Lymphedema is also not limited to breast cancer survivors and occurs commonly following treatment for gynecological/urologic tumors, melanoma, sarcoma, and pelvic tumors [8, 20, 21]. On average, breast cancer-related lymphedema usually develops approximately 8 months following surgery, and nearly 80% of patients who will develop the disease do so within the first 3 years following lymphadenectomy [22]. In contrast, lower extremity lymphedema tends to develop more rapidly, usually presenting within 3–4 months of surgery [23].

The progression of lymphedema is highly variable. Initially, affected patients may notice the edema as swelling or heaviness of the affected limb, and this can later advance to pitting edema. With the progression of the disease, the skin becomes dry and firm, and the pitting decreases secondary to cutaneous fibrosis and adipose deposition. The skin becomes thicker and progresses to hyperkeratosis, acanthosis, lichenification, and verrucae (Fig. 3.1). In severe cases, patients develop skin fissures, lymphorrhea, and recurrent infections [24].

There are various classification systems used to describe the severity of lymphedema. The most commonly used is the International Society of Lymphology (ISL) staging system, and it takes into account the pliability of the tissue and the volume of the affected limb. ISL Stage 0 is a subclinical stage without swelling of the affected limb despite impaired lymph transport. Although most patients are asymptomatic, some patients may report subjective complaints of heaviness in the limb or mild aching and tightness. ISL Stage I is mild lymphedema with the accumulation of interstitial fluid that subsides with compression. The skin is typically soft with no dermal fibrosis, and pitting edema is present. This is often called the reversible stage since the edema resolves within 24 h with compression. ISL Stage II is moderate lymphedema characterized by the development of derma fibrosis. In Stage II, the edema does not subside with elevation or compression. ISL Stage III is severe lymphedema with permanent limb swelling and trophic skin changes such as fat deposits, acanthosis, and verrucae [25].

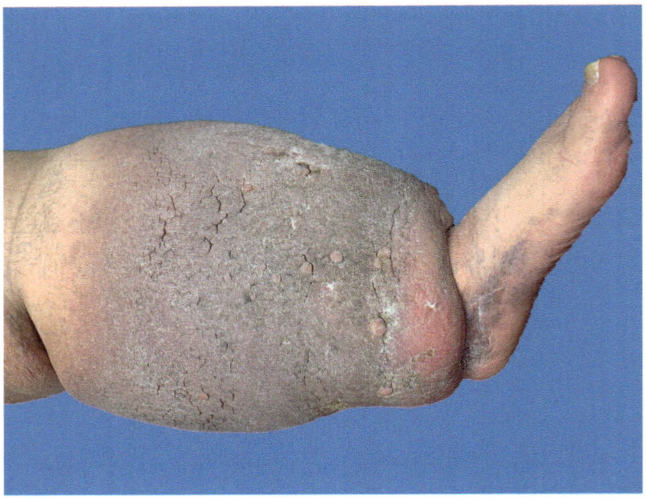

Fig. 3.1 Skin changes in a patient with International Society of Lymphology (ISL) Stage III lymphedema of the lower extremity. Note the hyperkeratosis, acanthosis, lichenification, and verrucae

Although there is some debate regarding the efficacy or timing of conservative treatments in preventing the development of lymphedema, early diagnosis and aggressive physical therapy/compression are helpful in most patients and should be instituted as soon as possible [26, 27].

Pathophysiology of Lymphedema

Historically, it was thought that lymphedema was caused by injury to the lymphatic system and the subsequent failure of the lymphatics to regenerate or form collateral pathways that bypass the zone of injury. This hypothesis was supported by in vivo studies that showed that growth factors, such as vascular endothelial growth factor (VEGF), promoted lymphatic regeneration with the resolution of lymphedema [28]. However, recent studies have shown that lymphedema is a progressive disease of the entire lymphatic vascular tree rather than an isolated injury at the site of lymph node dissection. The pathophysiology of secondary lymphedema is complex and affects different tissue compartments manifesting as chronic inflammation, fibrosis, inhibition of collateral lymphatic vessel formation, and adipose tissue deposition [29, 30].

Chronic Inflammation and Fibrosis

Fibrosis is characterized by the excessive deposition of extracellular matrix, eventually leading to tissue and organ dysfunction. In chronic lymphedema, the lymphatic vessels become progressively fibrosed with proliferation of smooth muscle cells, valvular dysfunction, and collagen deposition eventually obliterating the vessel lumen [30–33]. The dermal capillary lymphatic vessels also become leaky and encased in fibrous tissue with resultant dilatation of the lumen and formation of "lymphatic lakes." These changes are responsible for interstitial fluid backflow in the skin and abnormal changes on indocyanine green lymphography [30, 34]. There is also substantial fibrosis of the skin and adipose tissue as evidenced by increased deposition of type I and type III collagen in the papillary and reticular dermis and subcutaneous fat (Fig. 3.2) [35, 36].

Recent studies have highlighted the important role of inflammatory cells in the pathogenesis of fibrosis [36–39]. Clinical and experimental lymphedema models have identified CD4+ cells as the dominating inflammatory cell type in chronic lymphedematous tissues [40]. CD4+ cells can be categorized as T-helper cells, natural killer cells, and T-regulatory cells; T-helper cells can be further subclassified into many other subtypes including T-helper type 1 (Th1), Th17, and Th2 cells. Th1 and Th17 cells protect against bacterial pathogens by producing cytokines such as interferon-gamma, while Th2 responses play an essential role in the responses to parasite infections. In vitro and in vivo studies show that Th2 cells play a central role in regulating the fibrotic response that drives lymphatic dysfunction [39]. Th2-deficient transgenic mice do not develop lymphedema and fibrosis. Furthermore, inhibition of Th2 differentiation but not Th1 or Th17 differentiation effectively prevents the development of lymphedema [39, 41].

TGF-β1 is a well-known profibrotic agent, and increased levels of TGF-β1 have been detected in lymphedematous tissue of both mice and patients [42–44]. TGF-β1 stimulates the production of collagen proteins, increases fibroblast proliferation, and promotes the transition of fibroblasts to myofibroblasts. Inhibition of TGF-β1 leads to decreased Th2 cell migration and a subsequent decrease of profibrotic cytokines by Th2 cells suggesting that TGF-β1 can regulate inflammatory responses in lymphedema [44]. Recent studies suggest that capillary lymphatic vessel sclerosis might be induced via the TGF-β1 signaling cascade in lymphatic endothelial cells [44, 45]. In addition, TGF-β1 also promotes the accumulation of myofibroblasts and collagen fibers in the subcu-

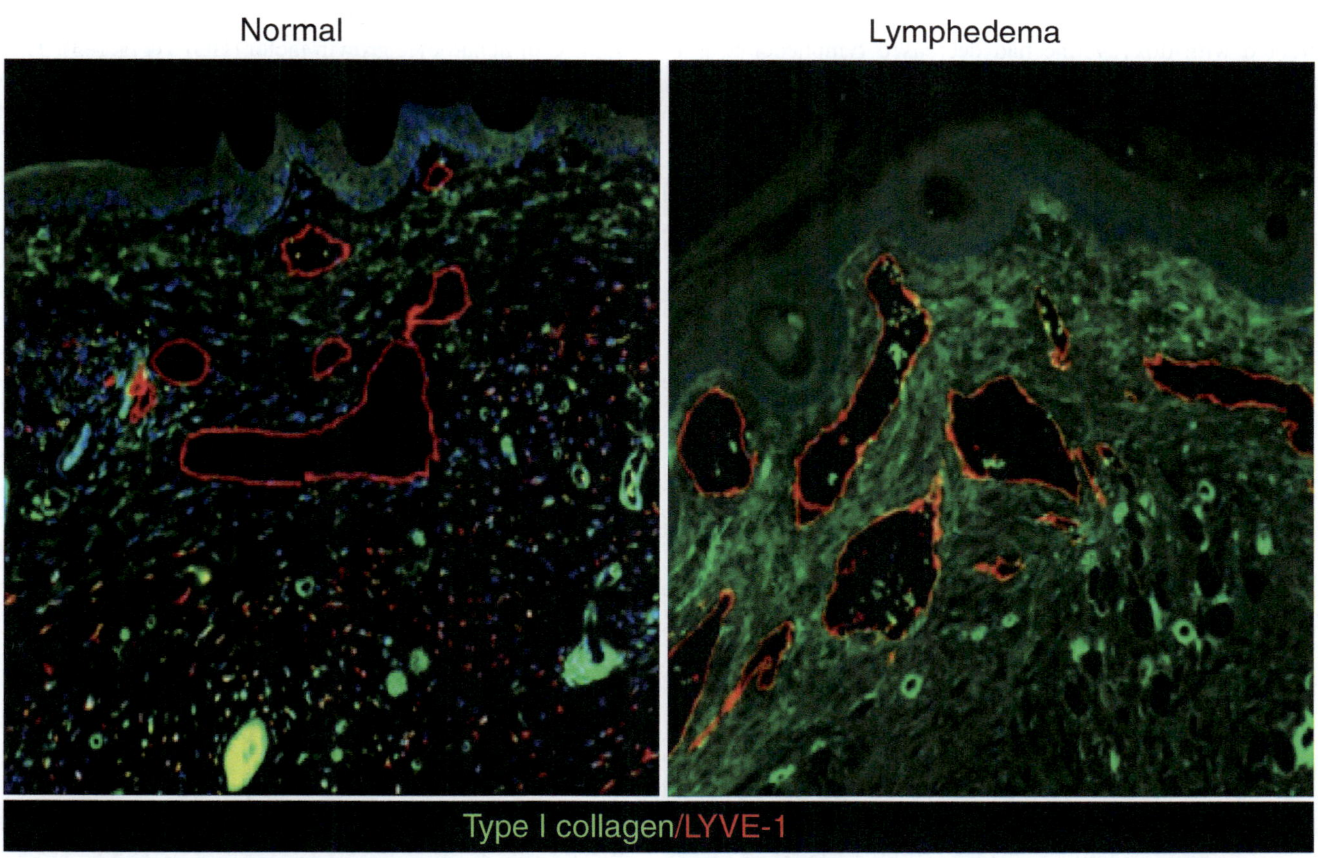

Fig. 3.2 Dilated lymphatic "lakes" trapped in scar tissue (type I collagen) in a mouse model of lymphedema. LYVE, lymphatic vessel endothelial receptor

taneous tissues, which is thought to impair the absorption of lymphatic fluid and drive lymphedema [46].

Investigators from Stanford University showed that inhibition of chronic inflammation with ketoprofen, a nonsteroidal anti-inflammatory drug (NSAID), decreased the severity of lymphedema in a mouse model of lymphedema [47]. These findings led to a clinical trial testing the efficacy of ketoprofen in 55 patients with primary or secondary lymphedema of the upper or lower extremity. Although treatment with ketoprofen failed to decrease excess limb volumes, biopsy specimens of the lymphedematous skin demonstrated decreased inflammation and improved skin histopathology. Subsequent studies from this group showed that the benefit of ketoprofen in lymphedema was derived from blockade of the leukotriene B4 pathway [48]. A phase II clinical trial with bestatin, a drug that preferentially blocks the leukotriene B4 pathway, was also recently completed, and the results from the study should be available soon.

Several recent studies have shown that doxycycline may be effective for the treatment of filariasis-induced lymphedema and that the efficacy of this treatment may be related to anti-Th2 effects of doxycycline [49, 50]. A randomized clinical trial of 162 patients showed that a 6-week treatment with doxycycline but not amoxicillin was associated with significant sustained reductions in the severity of lymphedema at 1- and 2-year follow-up. Nearly half of the patients treated with doxycycline had decreased lymphedema at 1 and 2 years; in contrast, only 3.2% and 5.6% of the control groups treated with either amoxicillin or placebo, respectively, showed any improvements at the 2-year time point [50]. A more recent study showed that improvements resulting from doxycycline treatment were related to decreased Th2 inflammatory responses in a mouse model of filariasis [49]. Taken together, these findings suggest that secondary lymphedema resulting from either surgical injury or filariasis may share a common pathophysiology.

Inhibition of Functional Lymphatic Vessel Regeneration by Chronic Inflammation

Cytokines expressed by T cells and inflammatory cells that infiltrate lymphedematous tissues—including IL4, IL13, interferon gamma (IFN-γ), and TGF-β—can directly inhibit lymphangiogenesis and prevent formation of lymphatic channels that bypass the zone of injury [39]. These cytokines act directly on lymphatic endothelial cells and decrease cellular proliferation, differentiation, migration, and tubule formation independent of lymphangiogenic cytokines such as VEGF-C [51, 52]. Inhibition of these inflammatory cytokines may therefore be a means of improving collateral lymphatic vessel formation without relying on delivery of pro-lymphangiogenic growth factors such as VEGF-C or hepatocyte growth factor (HGF) (Fig. 3.3). This

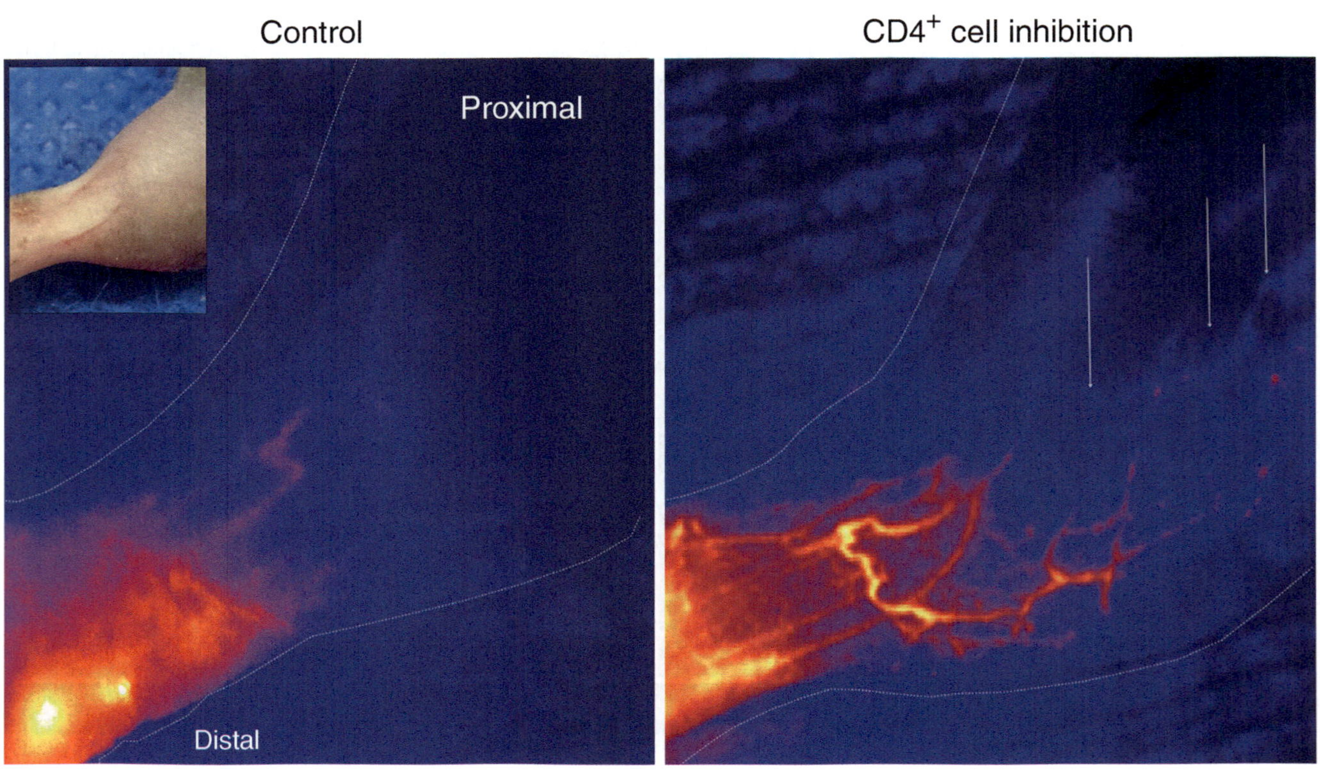

Fig. 3.3 Indocyanine green (ICG) lymphography in a mouse model of popliteal lymph node dissection. Control shows pooling of ICG in the injection site with few collateral lymphatics (left). Inhibition of CD4+ cells increases collateral vessel formation (arrows) (right)

is important since VEGF-C and HGF are important regulators of tumor growth and would require care when used in cancer survivors. In contrast, inhibiting inflammatory cytokines such as IL4, IL13, or TGF-B may be advantageous since this approach may also improve tumor immune responses and decrease the potential for tumor recurrence or metastasis [53].

Adipose Deposition in Lymphedema

Adipose deposition is a key and defining pathologic feature of lymphedema. Lymphatic fluid contains fatty acids that promote adipocyte differentiation and fat accumulation in vitro and in vivo [54, 55]. Interestingly, several studies have shown that lymphatic deficiencies can increase adipose deposition and tissue changes. For example, mice with heterozygous inactivating mutation of the Prospero homeobox protein 1 (Prox-1) gene have low level lymphatic dysfunction resulting in progressive subcutaneous tissue adipose deposition and obesity as adults [54]. These changes are responsible for the progressive deposition of adipose tissues in the affected extremities of patients with lymphedema.

Other studies have shown that the relationship between the lymphatic system and adipose tissues is bidirectional and that obesity can negatively regulate lymphatic function [56–58]. Indeed, clinical studies have shown that very obese patients can develop lymphedema even without lymphatic injury [6, 59]. The concept that lymphedema and obesity are related is also strongly supported by clinical studies demonstrating that obesity is a significant risk factor for lymphedema development after lymphadenectomy [60, 61].

Lymphatic vessels in obese mice have many characteristics that are reminiscent of lymphedema including increased leakiness, impaired collecting vessel pumping, and accumulation of perilymphatic inflammatory cells [56, 58, 62]. In addition, numerous studies have suggested that the inflammatory responses contribute to adipose deposition by directly regulating adipose tissue turnover and producing inflammatory cytokines (e.g., interleukin-6) that regulate adipose deposition [63]. Interestingly, obesity-induced lymphatic impairment in mice appears to be reversible with weight loss, aerobic exercise, or anti-inflammatory treatments suggesting that lifestyle changes or pharmacological treatments may be helpful (Fig. 3.4) [62, 64, 65]. This concept is supported by several level one, randomized clinical trials demonstrating that weight loss and resistance exercise are useful treatments for secondary lymphedema [66, 67]. Thus, exercise and weight loss regimens prior to, and following, surgical management of lymphedema are likely to improve outcomes. However, some studies on massively obese patients with lymphedema who undergo weight loss following gastric bypass surgery suggest lymphatic functional recovery in this patient population may be limited [68].

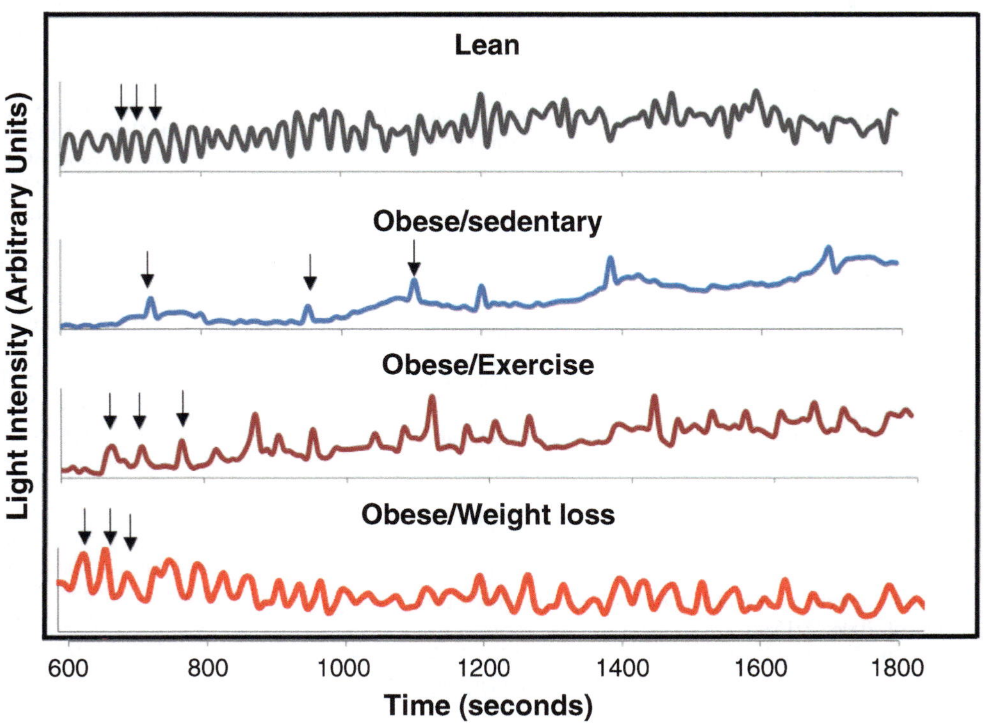

Fig. 3.4 Indocyanine green (ICG) lymphography and quantification of lymphatic pumping in lean mice as compared to obese/sedentary mice, obese/exercised mice, and obese mice following calorie reduction weight loss program. Arrowheads show changes in light intensity inside a lymphatic collector and correspond to lymphatic pumping. Note the significant decrease in pumping in obese/sedentary mice and improvements with exercise and weight loss

Conclusions

The lymphatic system plays a vital role in fluid homeostasis, and disruption can result in progressive interstitial fluid accumulation, fibrosis, chronic inflammation, and adipose deposition. The pathogenesis of secondary lymphedema is more complex than simple lymphatic injury, and the disease progression is driven by multiple cellular and molecular mechanisms. Much of the current knowledge in the pathophysiology of lymphedema is derived from animal models, and data shows that infiltration of lymphedematous tissues by CD4+ cells and differentiation along the Th2 lineage plays a key role in this process.

References

1. Hespe GE, Nitti MD, Mehrara BJ. Pathophysiology of lymphedema. In: Lymphedema. Springer International Publishing; 2015. p. 9–18.
2. Rockson SG. Lymphedema. Am J Med. 2001;110:288–95.
3. Suami H, Scaglioni MF. Anatomy of the lymphatic system and the lymphosome concept with reference to lymphedema. Semin Plast Surg. 2018;32:5–11.
4. Szuba A, Rockson SG. Lymphedema: anatomy, physiology and pathogenesis. Vasc Med. 1997;2:321–6.
5. Szuba A, Cooke JP, Yousuf S, Rockson SG. Decongestive lymphatic therapy for patients with cancer-related or primary lymphedema. Am J Med. 2000;109:296–300.
6. Greene AK, Maclellan RA. Obesity-induced upper extremity lymphedema. Plast Reconstr Surg Glob Open. 2013;1:e59.
7. Kim D-I. Cause and treatment of lymphedema. J Korean Med Assoc. 2004;47:966.
8. Cormier JN, Askew RL, Mungovan KS, Xing Y, Ross MI, Armer JM. Lymphedema beyond breast cancer. Cancer. 2010;116:5138–49.
9. Irrthum A, Karkkainen MJ, Devriendt K, Alitalo K, Vikkula M. Congenital hereditary lymphedema caused by a mutation that inactivates VEGFR3 tyrosine kinase. Am J Hum Genet. 2000;67:295–301.
10. Fang J, Dagenais SL, Erickson RP, Arlt MF, Glynn MW, Gorski JL, Seaver LH, Glover TW. Mutations in FOXC2 (MFH-1), a forkhead family transcription factor, are responsible for the hereditary lymphedema-distichiasis syndrome. Am J Hum Genet. 2000;67:1382–8.
11. Fontaine C, Morfoisse F, Tatin F, Zamora A, Zahreddine R, Henrion D, Arnal JF, Lenfant F, Garmy-Susini B. The impact of estrogen receptor in arterial and lymphatic vascular diseases. Int J Mol Sci. 2020;21(9):3244.
12. Choi I, Lee S, Hong YK. The new era of the lymphatic system: no longer secondary to the blood vascular system. Cold Spring Harb Perspect Med. 2012;2:a006445.
13. Babu S, Nutman TB. Immunopathogenesis of lymphatic filarial disease. Semin Immunopathol. 2012;34:847–61.
14. Sakorafas GH, Peros G, Cataliotti L, Vlastos G. Lymphedema following axillary lymph node dissection for breast cancer. Surg Oncol. 2006;15:153–65.
15. Starritt EC, Joseph D, McKinnon JG, Lo SK, de Wilt JHW, Thompson JF. Lymphedema after complete axillary node dissection for melanoma. Ann Surg. 2004;240:866–74.
16. Treves N. An evaluation of the etiological factors of lymphedema following radical mastectomy. An analysis of 1,007 cases. Cancer. 1957;10:444–59.
17. Ahmed RL, Schmitz KH, Prizment AE, Folsom AR. Risk factors for lymphedema in breast cancer survivors, the Iowa Women's Health Study. Breast Cancer Res Treat. 2011;130:981–91.
18. Armer J, Fu MR, Williams DA, Wipke-Tevis DD, Porock D, Wainstock JM, Zagar E, Jacobs L. Lymphedema following breast cancer treatment, including sentinel lymph node biopsy. Rehabilitation Oncol. 2003;21:21.
19. McLaughlin SA, Wright MJ, Morris KT, Giron GL, Sampson MR, Brockway JP, Hurley KE, Riedel ER, Van Zee KJ. Prevalence of lymphedema in women with breast cancer 5 years after sentinel lymph node biopsy or axillary dissection: objective measurements. J Clin Oncol. 2008;26:5213–9.
20. Todo Y, Yamamoto R, Minobe S, Suzuki Y, Takeshi U, Nakatani M, Aoyagi Y, Ohba Y, Okamoto K, Kato H. Risk factors for postoperative lower-extremity lymphedema in endometrial cancer survivors who had treatment including lymphadenectomy. Gynecol Oncol. 2010;119:60–4.
21. Gould N, Kamelle S, Tillmanns T, Scribner D, Gold M, Walker J, Mannel R. Predictors of complications after inguinal lymphadenectomy. Gynecol Oncol. 2001;82:329–32.
22. Petrek JA, Heelan MC. Incidence of breast carcinoma-related lymphedema. Cancer. 1998;83:2776–81.
23. Dessources K, Aviki E, Leitao MM Jr. Lower extremity lymphedema in patients with gynecologic malignancies. Int J Gynecol Cancer. 2020;30:252–60.
24. Burian EA, Karlsmark T, Franks PJ, Keeley V, Quéré I, Moffatt CJ. Cellulitis in chronic oedema of the lower leg: an international cross-sectional study. Br J Dermatol. 2021;185(1):110–8.
25. Kim G, Smith MP, Donohoe KJ, Johnson AR, Singhal D, Tsai LL. MRI staging of upper extremity secondary lymphedema: correlation with clinical measurements. Eur Radiol. 2020;30:4686–94.
26. Uzkeser H, Karatay S, Erdemci B, Koc M, Senel K. Efficacy of manual lymphatic drainage and intermittent pneumatic compression pump use in the treatment of lymphedema after mastectomy: a randomized controlled trial. Breast Cancer. 2013;22:300–7.
27. Brayton KM, Hirsch AT, O'Brien PJ, Cheville A, Karaca-Mandic P, Rockson SG. Lymphedema prevalence and treatment benefits in cancer: impact of a therapeutic intervention on health outcomes and costs. PLoS One. 2014;9:e114597.
28. Visuri MT, Honkonen KM, Hartiala P, Tervala TV, Halonen PJ, Junkkari H, Knuutinen N, Ylä-Herttuala S, Alitalo KK, Saarikko AM. VEGF-C and VEGF-C156S in the pro-lymphangiogenic growth factor therapy of lymphedema: a large animal study. Angiogenesis. 2015;18:313–26.
29. Li CY, Kataru RP, Mehrara BJ. Histopathologic features of lymphedema: a molecular review. Int J Mol Sci. 2020;21(7):2546.
30. Mihara M, Hara H, Hayashi Y, Narushima M, Yamamoto T, Todokoro T, Iida T, Sawamoto N, Araki J, Kikuchi K, Murai N, Okitsu T, Kisu I, Koshima I. Pathological steps of cancer-related lymphedema: histological changes in the collecting lymphatic vessels after lymphadenectomy. PLoS One. 2012;7:e41126.
31. Scallan JP, Zawieja SD, Castorena-Gonzalez JA, Davis MJ. Lymphatic pumping: mechanics, mechanisms and malfunction. J Physiol. 2016;594:5749–68.
32. Koshima I, Kawada S, Moriguchi T, Kajiwara Y. Ultrastructural observations of lymphatic vessels in lymphedema in human extremities. Plast Reconstr Surg. 1996;97:397–405.; discussion 406-397.
33. Ogata F, Fujiu K, Matsumoto S, Nakayama Y, Shibata M, Oike Y, Koshima I, Watabe T, Nagai R, Manabe I. Excess lymphangiogenesis cooperatively induced by macrophages and CD4+ T cells drives the pathogenesis of lymphedema. J Investig Dermatol. 2016;136:706–14.
34. Tashiro K, Feng J, Wu SH, Mashiko T, Kanayama K, Narushima M, Uda H, Miyamoto S, Koshima I, Yoshimura K. Pathological changes of adipose tissue in secondary lymphoedema. Br J Dermatol. 2017;177:158–67.

35. Rutkowski JM, Markhus CE, Gyenge CC, Alitalo K, Wiig H, Swartz MA. Dermal collagen and lipid deposition correlate with tissue swelling and hydraulic conductivity in murine primary lymphedema. Am J Pathol. 2010;176:1122–9.
36. Zampell JC, Yan A, Elhadad S, Avraham T, Weitman E, Mehrara BJ. CD4+ cells regulate fibrosis and lymphangiogenesis in response to lymphatic fluid stasis. PLoS One. 2012;7:e49940.
37. Ly CL, Nores GDG, Kataru RP, Mehrara BJ. T helper 2 differentiation is necessary for development of lymphedema. Transl Res. 2019;206:57–70.
38. Kataru RP, Wiser I, Baik JE, Park HJ, Rehal S, Shin JY, Mehrara BJ. Fibrosis and secondary lymphedema: chicken or egg? Transl Res. 2019;209:68–76.
39. Ly C, Kataru R, Mehrara B. Inflammatory manifestations of lymphedema. Int J Mol Sci. 2017;18:171.
40. García Nores GD, Ly CL, Cuzzone DA, Kataru RP, Hespe GE, Torrisi JS, Huang JJ, Gardenier JC, Savetsky IL, Nitti MD, Yu JZ, Rehal S, Mehrara BJ. CD4+ T cells are activated in regional lymph nodes and migrate to skin to initiate lymphedema. Nat Commun. 2018;9(1):1970.
41. Avraham T, Zampell JC, Yan A, Elhadad S, Weitman ES, Rockson SG, Bromberg J, Mehrara BJ. Th2 differentiation is necessary for soft tissue fibrosis and lymphatic dysfunction resulting from lymphedema. FASEB J. 2012;27:1114–26.
42. Russell NS, Floot B, van Werkhoven E, Schriemer M, de Jong-Korlaar R, Woerdeman LA, Stewart FA, Scharpfenecker M. Blood and lymphatic microvessel damage in irradiated human skin: the role of TGF-β, endoglin and macrophages. Radiother Oncol. 2015;116:455–61.
43. Ridner SH, Dietrich MS, Sonis ST, Murphy B. Biomarkers associated with lymphedema and fibrosis in patients with cancer of the head and neck. Lymphat Res Biol. 2018;16:516–24.
44. Avraham T, Daluvoy S, Zampell J, Yan A, Haviv YS, Rockson SG, Mehrara BJ. Blockade of transforming growth factor-β1 accelerates lymphatic regeneration during wound repair. Am J Pathol. 2010;177:3202–14.
45. Yoon SH, Kim KY, Wang Z, Park JH, Bae SM, Kim SY, Song HY, Jeon JY. EW-7197, a transforming growth factor-beta type I receptor kinase inhibitor, ameliorates acquired lymphedema in a mouse tail model. Lymphat Res Biol. 2020;18:433–8.
46. Sano M, Hirakawa S, Suzuki M, Sakabe JI, Ogawa M, Yamamoto S, Hiraide T, Sasaki T, Yamamoto N, Inuzuka K, Tanaka H, Saito T, Sugisawa R, Katahashi K, Yata T, Kayama T, Urano T, Tokura Y, Sato K, Setou M, Takeuchi H, Konno H, Unno N. Potential role of transforming growth factor-beta 1/Smad signaling in secondary lymphedema after cancer surgery. Cancer Sci. 2020;111:2620–34.
47. Nakamura K, Radhakrishnan K, Wong YM, Rockson SG. Anti-inflammatory pharmacotherapy with ketoprofen ameliorates experimental lymphatic vascular insufficiency in mice. PLoS One. 2009;4:e8380.
48. Tian W, Rockson SG, Jiang X, Kim J, Begaye A, Shuffle EM, Tu AB, Cribb M, Nepiyushchikh Z, Feroze AH, Zamanian RT, Dhillon GS, Voelkel NF, Peters-Golden M, Kitajewski J, Dixon JB, Nicolls MR. Leukotriene B4 antagonism ameliorates experimental lymphedema. Sci Transl Med. 2017;9(389):eaal3920.
49. Furlong-Silva J, Cross SD, Marriott AE, Pionnier N, Archer J, Steven A, Schulte-Merker S, Mack M, Hong YK, Taylor MJ, Turner JD. Tetracyclines improve experimental lymphatic filariasis pathology by disrupting interleukin-4 receptor-mediated lymphangiogenesis. J Clin Invest. 2021;131(5):e140853.
50. Mand S, Debrah AY, Klarmann U, Batsa L, Marfo-Debrekyei Y, Kwarteng A, Specht S, Belda-Domene A, Fimmers R, Taylor M, Adjei O, Hoerauf A. Doxycycline improves filarial lymphedema independent of active filarial infection: a randomized controlled trial. Clin Infect Dis. 2012;55:621–30.
51. Oka M, Iwata C, Suzuki HI, Kiyono K, Morishita Y, Watabe T, Komuro A, Kano MR, Miyazono K. Inhibition of endogenous TGF-{beta} signaling enhances lymphangiogenesis. Blood. 2008;111(9):4571–9.
52. Savetsky IL, Ghanta S, Gardenier JC, Torrisi JS, Garcia Nores GD, Hespe GE, Nitti MD, Kataru RP, Mehrara BJ. Th2 cytokines inhibit lymphangiogenesis. PLoS One. 2015;10:e0126908.
53. Shiao SL, Ganesan AP, Rugo HS, Coussens LM. Immune microenvironments in solid tumors: new targets for therapy. Genes Dev. 2011;25:2559–72.
54. Harvey NL, Srinivasan RS, Dillard ME, Johnson NC, Witte MH, Boyd K, Sleeman MW, Oliver G. Lymphatic vascular defects promoted by Prox1 haploinsufficiency cause adult-onset obesity. Nat Genet. 2005;37:1072–81.
55. Escobedo N, Proulx ST, Karaman S, Dillard ME, Johnson N, Detmar M, Oliver G. Restoration of lymphatic function rescues obesity in Prox1-haploinsufficient mice. JCI Insight. 2016;1(2):e85096.
56. Garcia Nores GD, Cuzzone DA, Albano NJ, Hespe GE, Kataru RP, Torrisi JS, Gardenier JC, Savetsky IL, Aschen SZ, Nitti MD, Mehrara BJ. Obesity but not high-fat diet impairs lymphatic function. Int J Obes. 2016;40:1582–90.
57. Kataru RP, Park HJ, Baik JE, Li C, Shin J, Mehrara BJ. Regulation of lymphatic function in obesity. Front Physiol. 2020;11:459.
58. Weitman ES, Aschen SZ, Farias-Eisner G, Albano N, Cuzzone DA, Ghanta S, Zampell JC, Thorek D, Mehrara BJ. Obesity impairs lymphatic fluid transport and dendritic cell migration to lymph nodes. PLoS One. 2013;8:e70703.
59. Mehrara BJ, Greene AK. Lymphedema and obesity: is there a link? Plast Reconstr Surg. 2014;134:154e–60e.
60. Helyer LK, Varnic M, Le LW, Leong W, McCready D. Obesity is a risk factor for developing postoperative lymphedema in breast cancer patients. Breast J. 2010;16:48–54.
61. Norman SA, Localio AR, Kallan MJ, Weber AL, Torpey HA, Potashnik SL, Miller LT, Fox KR, DeMichele A, Solin LJ. Risk factors for lymphedema after breast cancer treatment. Cancer Epidemiol Biomark Prev. 2010;19:2734–46.
62. Torrisi JS, Hespe GE, Cuzzone DA, Savetsky IL, Nitti MD, Gardenier JC, García Nores GD, Jowhar D, Kataru RP, Mehrara BJ. Inhibition of inflammation and iNOS improves lymphatic function in obesity. Sci Rep. 2016;6:19817.
63. Cuzzone DA, Weitman ES, Albano NJ, Ghanta S, Savetsky IL, Gardenier JC, Joseph WJ, Torrisi JS, Bromberg JF, Olszewski WL, Rockson SG, Mehrara BJ. IL-6 regulates adipose deposition and homeostasis in lymphedema. Am J Phys Heart Circ Phys. 2014;306:H1426–34.
64. Hespe GE, Kataru RP, Savetsky IL, Garcia Nores GD, Torrisi JS, Nitti MD, Gardenier JC, Zhou J, Yu JZ, Jones LW, Mehrara BJ. Exercise training improves obesity-related lymphatic dysfunction. J Physiol. 2016;594:4267–82.
65. Nitti MD, Hespe GE, Kataru RP, Garcia Nores GD, Savetsky IL, Torrisi JS, Gardenier JC, Dannenberg AJ, Mehrara BJ. Obesity-induced lymphatic dysfunction is reversible with weight loss. J Physiol. 2016;594:7073–87.
66. Shaw C, Mortimer P, Judd PA. A randomized controlled trial of weight reduction as a treatment for breast cancer-related lymphedema. Cancer. 2007;110:1868–74.
67. Kwan ML, Cohn JC, Armer JM, Stewart BR, Cormier JN. Exercise in patients with lymphedema: a systematic review of the contemporary literature. J Cancer Surviv. 2011;5:320–36.
68. Greene AK, Grant FD, Maclellan RA. Obesity-induced lymphedema nonreversible following massive weight loss. Plast Reconstr Surg Glob Open. 2015;3:e426.

4 Lymphedema Prospective Surveillance and Risk Reduction

Nicole L. Stout and Jane M. Armer

Introduction

Lymphedema most commonly occurs due to an insult to the lymphatic system. In the developed world, this is most likely to be a result of cancer treatments, including surgical removal of lymph nodes requisite for disease staging and prognostication, or radiotherapy to treat diseased lymph nodes [1, 2]. In developing countries of subtropical regions of the world, the most common insult to the lymphatic system is by virtue of a mosquito-borne vector, the *Wuchereria bancrofti*, which infiltrates the lymphatic vessels, grows, and blocks lymphatic fluid flow resulting in localized swelling [3]. For the purposes of this chapter, we will focus on the risk for and surveillance of the former, also termed secondary lymphedema.

When the integrity of the lymphatic system is disrupted, there is risk for congestion of lymph fluid in the interstitial tissue space leading to progressive tissue fibrosis and lymphedema. While this risk is ubiquitous among those experiencing common cancer treatments, not all of those at risk will develop lymphedema [1]. Current estimates of lymphedema incidence among various types of cancers range from 2% to 6% in early-stage breast cancer with sentinel lymph node biopsy only, to >60% in lower extremity melanoma, gastrointestinal, gynecological, and head-and-neck cancers where more extensive surgical and lymph node dissection commonly occurs [4–8]. This presents something of a conundrum for healthcare providers when trying to ascertain who is at greatest risk for developing lymphedema, and if that risk can be mitigated.

N. L. Stout (✉)
West Virginia University Cancer Institute, School of Medicine, Department of Hematology Oncology, Morgantown, WV, USA
e-mail: nicole.stout@hsc.wvu.edu

J. M. Armer (✉)
University of Missouri, Sinclair School of Nursing, Ellis Fischel Cancer Center, Columbia, MO, USA
e-mail: armerj@missouri.edu

The purpose of this chapter is (1) to outline the evidence for risk factors associated with the onset of lymphedema, (2) to provide insight to evidence-based risk-reduction strategies, and (3) to share a model for prospective surveillance that enables early detection and treatment of lymphedema.

Risk Factors Associated with Lymphedema

Today, we have over two decades' worth of published evidence outlining the association of some cancer treatments with the risk for developing lymphedema. Further, this body of research also highlights activities and behaviors at the individual level that may influence risk. Broadly, there are two categories of risk factors to consider when evaluating the risk for lymphedema: non-modifiable and modifiable risk factors.

Cancer treatments are highly effective, enabling >70% of individuals to achieve disease-free status 5 years after their diagnosis [9]. Since these treatments are considered required components of cancer care, they introduce non-modifiable risk factors for the development of lymphedema. Additional factors such as genetic predisposition and arm and hand dominance are also considered non-modifiable [10]. Cancer surgeries and treatments are planned events which comprehensively address local and systemic disease. An individual with cancer is likely to experience more than one type of cancer treatment that will negatively impact their lymphatic system, resulting in an accumulated burden of risk.

Modifiable risk factors are behaviors and activities that are, to a relatively high degree, under an individual's control and, therefore, can be manipulated or altered to change the level of risk. Modifiable risk factors include level of physical activity, body weight, and participation in activities that may

M. V. Schaverien, J. H. Dayan (eds.), *Multimodal Management of Upper and Lower Extremity Lymphedema*,
https://doi.org/10.1007/978-3-030-93039-4_4

Table 4.1 Modifiable and non-modifiable risk factors for lymphedema

Body region	Modifiable risk factors	Non-modifiable risk factors
Upper extremity and upper quadrant lymphedema	Body mass index >30 [11, 12] Cellulitis infection [12] Low-level limb volume progression >5% [12]	Extent of axillary lymph node dissection [11, 13] Volume of radiation therapy [11, 14] Taxane-based chemotherapy [11]
Lower extremity, genital, and lower quadrant lymphedema	Body mass index >35 [6] Younger age at cancer treatment [15] Postoperative lymphocyst [16] Low levels of physical activity prior to cancer diagnosis [17] Preexisting peripheral vascular disease [8]	Number of lymph nodes surgically removed [7, 8, 16] Surgical approach [18, 19] Postoperative radiotherapy [18] Disease stage [20] Number of lymph node dissection surgeries [20]
Head and neck lymphedema	High body mass index [21] Postsurgical and progressive tissue fibrosis [22] Inflammatory biomarkers (IL-6, IL-1β, TNF-α, TNF-β1, MMP-9) [23]	Radiation therapy [21, 24] Number of lymph nodes surgically removed [21] Bilateral neck surgery [21] Chemotherapy [21] Higher stage of disease [21] Location of the tumor [24] Time since treatment completion [24] Greater number of treatment modalities [24]

Abbreviations: *IL* interleukin, *TNF* tumor necrosis factor, *MMP* matrix metalloproteinase

introduce trauma or injury to the at-risk region of the body. Table 4.1 provides an overview of the evidence for modifiable and non-modifiable risk factors associated with developing lymphedema.

Risk Reduction

In the presence of a known cluster of events that introduce risk, there is an opportunity to adapt activities, specifically by addressing modifiable risk factors to reduce the likelihood of triggering lymphedema. Risk-reduction education is advised for all individuals undergoing cancer treatments that disrupt the lymphatic system [4, 25]. Table 4.2 identifies the current evidence for risk-reduction practices.

While non-modifiable risk factors in cancer care cannot be affected by behavioral changes, their presence can be quantified, and risk can be intimated based on their severity. This provides an opportunity for risk stratification [34]. By delineating high- versus low-risk individuals, a healthcare provider can establish a consistent, interval surveillance program to enable repeated assessment for early detection of clinically meaningful tissue changes that may reflect the earliest onset of lymphedema. Furthermore, these interval engagements enable an opportunity to reinforce risk-reduction strategies.

Table 4.2 Secondary lymphedema risk-reduction evidence base

Risk-reduction advice
Maintain healthy weight and a body mass index (BMI) <25 [26]
Reduce risk for skin infection [26, 27]
Reduce inflammatory episodes to the extremity [26]
Minimize extent of lymph node dissection when possible [28, 29]
Consider axillary reverse mapping surgical procedures [28, 29]
Structured education and teaching about the risk of lymphedema, signs and symptoms, and early action for symptoms [30]
Risk stratify patients prior to cancer treatments and establish interval surveillance frequency based on risk [31]
Promote prospective surveillance for early identification and management of swelling [28, 29, 31]
Use of compression garments with early swelling [32, 33]
Inconclusive evidence [27]
Ipsilateral blood draws
Injections into an extremity where nodes were removed
Blood pressure readings
Air travel

Risk stratification and ongoing surveillance monitoring are effective mechanisms to promote early identification of lymphedema and to enable early intervention which may mitigate condition progression. The pathophysiology of lymphedema is a factor that enables risk stratification and monitoring as the condition commonly presents during a relatively distinct time frame after the surgery, treatments, or trauma [12, 20]. The onset of the condition is commonly slow but progressive over time, enabling early detection through astute monitoring.

Prospective Surveillance for Lymphedema Detection

The prospective surveillance model (PSM) is a proactive, standardized method to improve interval surveillance to identify tissue changes consistent with early lymphedema [35, 36]. The model promotes early intervention to reduce the progression of lymphedema to a more chronic condition [33, 37, 38].

The PSM relies on a baseline evaluation of the individual to understand personal and behavioral factors, comorbidities, tissue characteristics, and limb volume prior to the initiation of cancer treatments. This information, combined with an understanding of the oncologic treatment plan, enables a baseline stratification of risk. As the individual moves through cancer treatments, repeated surveillance is conducted to identify clinically meaningful changes in tissue characteristics or limb volume that are associated with early lymphedema. Inherent in this model is the need for patient education regarding risk and risk-reduction advice based on the individual's presentation and their response to treatments. Prospective surveillance is optimally feasible when risk stratification is employed to establish a plan of care and direct the surveillance model.

Individuals who present with a high number of known risk factors, or with more severe involvement across risk factors, should be designated as "high risk" and should receive more frequent monitoring for lymphedema. Those who are deemed lower risk receive less frequent monitoring. Of critical importance is that surveillance findings result in the appropriate clinical pathway for condition management. Referral to a lymphedema specialist is considered the standard of care for condition management. A lymphedema specialist should be consulted for the preoperative education interventions as well as to manage any preexisting swelling or tissue conditions. It is imperative that the lymphedema specialist is consulted at any point in the continuum of cancer care if the patient presents with clinically meaningful changes indicative of the early onset of lymphedema. Figure 4.1 illustrates the model for a PSM clinical pathway.

The PSM requires that valid measurement tools are used to promote early identification of swelling and that standardized diagnostic thresholds for clinically meaningful change are established and provoke intervention. Table 4.3 provides an evidence overview for measuring and identifying early lymphedema.

Implementation into Practice

Leveraging the PSM and engaging clinically valid tests and measures enables optimal clinical integration of risk-reduction practices, monitoring for early onset, and early detection of

Table 4.3 Thresholds for the early diagnosis of lymphedema

Preferred measurement tool	Diagnostic threshold
Perometer	*>3% volume change based on pre-operative measurement* [33]
Bioimpedance spectroscopy	>7.1 L-Dex Score when preoperative measures are not available [39] >10 L-Dex Score above preoperative baseline [39]
Tape measure	Volume change >5% [39] Calculated relative volume change >5–10% [40] >200 ml volume discrepancy between extremities [39] Circumferential measure from upper neck and lower jaw [39, 41]
Symptom report	Heaviness [28] Numbness [28] Tingling Presence of swelling 13-Item self-report Lower Extremity Lymphedema Screening Questionnaire [42] Head and neck facial symptoms [43] Truncal self-reported symptoms [43]
Tissue dielectric constant (TDC)	2–9 TDC units [41, 44]

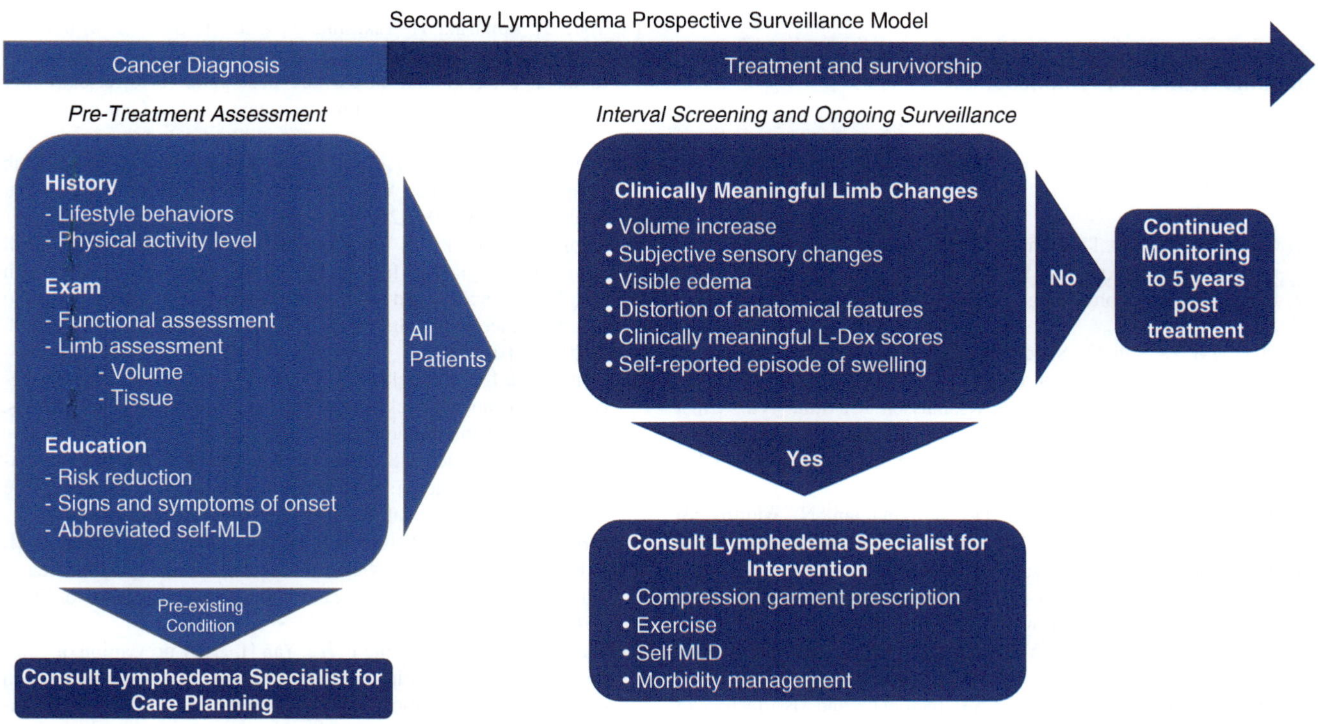

Fig. 4.1 Clinical pathway for lymphedema screening and surveillance using the prospective surveillance model. MLD, manual lymphatic drainage

lymphedema. Clinical practice guidelines for early identification of lymphedema suggest this as an optimal approach [28, 45]. Further, new evidence suggests that risk stratification models using nomograms and other predictive factors can be used to enable more precise prospective follow-up [34]. Clinical practice workflows that can enable risk stratification based on patient report and comorbidities at baseline will best support the establishment of the PSM. Using the electronic health record capabilities, scoring and aggregate risk profiles can be developed, and care pathways established. Conducting baseline limb volume or tissue measures as a part of preoperative workup provides this information for comparison as the patient moves through the trajectory of cancer care. At each follow-up visit, limb volume or tissue measures can be repeated along with review of the risk profile for the individual. When measurable change or self-reported symptoms present, the referral to a lymphedema specialist can be generated to enable early intervention.

Summary

Lymphedema remains a common side effect of cancer treatments. Risk for developing lymphedema can be estimated using individualized risk factor profiles and information from the oncology care plan. Establishing the risk stratification prior to treatment can enable an appropriate frequency of repeated measures and optimize early identification. Preoperative assessment and prospective surveillance are optimal strategies for interval assessment of meaningful tissue changes which can facilitate the earliest identification and intervention for lymphedema.

References

1. Grada AA, Phillips TJ. Lymphedema: pathophysiology and clinical manifestations. J Am Acad Dermatol. 2017;77(6):1009–20.
2. Ridner SH. Pathophysiology of lymphedema. Semin Oncol Nurs. 2013;29(1):4–11.
3. Pfarr KM, Debrah AY, Specht S, Hoerauf A. Filariasis and lymphoedema. Parasite Immunol. 2009;31(11):664–72.
4. Shaitelman SF, Cromwell KD, Rasmussen JC, Stout NL, Armer JM, Lasinski BB, et al. Recent progress in the treatment and prevention of cancer-related lymphedema. CA Cancer J Clin. 2015;65(1):55–81.
5. Anand A, Balasubramanian D, Subramanian N, Murthy S, Limbachiya S, Iyer S, et al. Secondary lymphedema after head and neck cancer therapy: a review. Lymphology. 2018;51(3):109–18.
6. Mendivil AA, Rettenmaier MA, Abaid LN, Brown JV 3rd, Micha JP, Lopez KL, et al. Lower-extremity lymphedema following management for endometrial and cervical cancer. Surg Oncol. 2016;25(3):200–4.
7. Ki EY, Park JS, Lee KH, Hur SY. Incidence and risk factors of lower extremity lymphedema after gynecologic surgery in ovarian cancer. Int J Gynecol Cancer. 2016;26(7):1327–32.
8. Friedman JF, Sunkara B, Jehnsen JS, Durham A, Johnson T, Cohen MS. Risk factors associated with lymphedema after lymph node dissection in melanoma patients. Am J Surg. 2015;210(6):1178–84. discussion 84
9. Siegel RL, Miller KD, Jemal A. Cancer statistics, 2019. CA Cancer J Clin. 2019;69(1):7–34.
10. Rockson SG. The genetic predisposition to breast cancer-associated lymphedema. Mary Ann Liebert, Inc; 2019.
11. Byun HK, Chang JS, Im SH, Kirova YM, Arsene-Henry A, Choi SH, et al. Risk of lymphedema following contemporary treatment for breast cancer: an analysis of 7617 consecutive patients from a multidisciplinary perspective. Ann Surg. 2019;274(1):170–8.
12. McLaughlin SA, Brunelle CL, Taghian A. Breast cancer-related lymphedema: risk factors, screening, management, and the impact of locoregional treatment. J Clin Oncol. 2020;38(20):2341–50.
13. Rupp J, Hadamitzky C, Henkenberens C, Christiansen H, Steinmann D, Bruns F. Frequency and risk factors for arm lymphedema after multimodal breast-conserving treatment of nodal positive breast cancer – a long-term observation. Radiat Oncol. 2019;14(1):39.
14. Warren LE, Miller CL, Horick N, Skolny MN, Jammallo LS, Sadek BT, et al. The impact of radiation therapy on the risk of lymphedema after treatment for breast cancer: a prospective cohort study. Int J Radiat Oncol Biol Phys. 2014;88(3):565–71.
15. Carlson JW, Kauderer J, Hutson A, Carter J, Armer J, Lockwood S, et al. GOG 244-The lymphedema and gynecologic cancer (LEG) study: incidence and risk factors in newly diagnosed patients. Gynecol Oncol. 2020;156(2):467–74.
16. Kuroda K, Yamamoto Y, Yanagisawa M, Kawata A, Akiba N, Suzuki K, et al. Risk factors and a prediction model for lower limb lymphedema following lymphadenectomy in gynecologic cancer: a hospital-based retrospective cohort study. BMC Womens Health. 2017;17(1):50.
17. Hayes SC, Janda M, Ward LC, Reul-Hirche H, Steele ML, Carter J, et al. Lymphedema following gynecological cancer: results from a prospective, longitudinal cohort study on prevalence, incidence and risk factors. Gynecol Oncol. 2017;146(3):623–9.
18. Biglia N, Zanfagnin V, Daniele A, Robba E, Bounous VE. Lower body lymphedema in patients with gynecologic cancer. Anticancer Res. 2017;37(8):4005–15.
19. Todo Y, Yamazaki H, Takeshita S, Ohba Y, Sudo S, Minobe S, et al. Close relationship between removal of circumflex iliac nodes to distal external iliac nodes and postoperative lower-extremity lymphedema in uterine corpus malignant tumors. Gynecol Oncol. 2015;139(1):160–4.
20. Kunitake T, Kakuma T, Ushijima K. Risk factors for lower limb lymphedema in gynecologic cancer patients after initial treatment. Int J Clin Oncol. 2020;25(5):963–71.
21. Tribius S, Pazdyka H, Tennstedt P, Busch C-J, Hanken H, Krüll A, et al. Prognostic factors for lymphedema in patients with locally advanced head and neck cancer after combined radio (chemo) therapy-results of a longitudinal study. Oral Oncol. 2020;109:104856.
22. Deng J, Wulff-Burchfield EM, Murphy BA. Late soft tissue complications of head and neck cancer therapy: lymphedema and fibrosis. J Natl Cancer Inst Monogr. 2019;2019(53):lgz005.
23. Ridner SH, Dietrich MS, Sonis ST, Murphy B. Biomarkers associated with lymphedema and fibrosis in patients with cancer of the head and neck. Lymphat Res Biol. 2018;16(6):516–24.
24. Deng J, Ridner SH, Dietrich MS, Wells N, Wallston KA, Sinard RJ, et al. Factors associated with external and internal lymphedema in patients with head-and-neck cancer. Int J Radiat Oncol Biol Phys. 2012;84(3):e319–28.
25. Wu X, Liu Y, Zhu D, Wang F, Ji J, Yan H. Early prevention of complex decongestive therapy and rehabilitation exercise for prevention of lower extremity lymphedema after operation of gynecologic cancer. Asian J Surg. 2020;44(1):111–5.
26. Asdourian MS, Skolny MN, Brunelle C, Seward CE, Salama L, Taghian AG. Precautions for breast cancer-related lymphoedema: risk from air travel, ipsilateral arm blood pressure measurements,

skin puncture, extreme temperatures, and cellulitis. Lancet Oncol. 2016;17(9):e392–405.
27. Ferguson CM, Swaroop MN, Horick N, Skolny MN, Miller CL, Jammallo LS, et al. Impact of ipsilateral blood draws, injections, blood pressure measurements, and air travel on the risk of lymphedema for patients treated for breast cancer. J Clin Oncol. 2016;34(7):691–8.
28. Armer JM, Hulett JM, Bernas M, Ostby P, Stewart BR, Cormier JN. Best-practice guidelines in assessment, risk reduction, management, and surveillance for post-breast cancer lymphedema. Curr Breast Cancer Rep. 2013;5(2):134–44.
29. McLaughlin SA, Stout NL, Schaverien MV. Avoiding the swell: advances in lymphedema prevention, detection, and management. Am Soc Clin Oncol Educ Book. 2020;40:e17–26.
30. Bland KL, Kosir MA. Improving the quality of life in breast cancer survivors at risk for lymphedema. Surgery. 2019;166(4):686–90.
31. Gillespie TC, Sayegh HE, Brunelle CL, Daniell KM, Taghian AG. Breast cancer-related lymphedema: risk factors, precautionary measures, and treatments. Gland Surg. 2018;7(4):379–403.
32. Hnin YK, Ong LX, Tsai CC, Ong SS, Yee SG, Choo BA, et al. Does initial routine use of a compression garment reduce the risk of lower limb lymphedema after gynecological cancer treatment? A randomized pilot study in an Asian institution and review of the literature. Lymphology. 2018;51(4):174–83.
33. Stout Gergich NL, Pfalzer LA, McGarvey C, Springer B, Gerber LH, Soballe P. Preoperative assessment enables the early diagnosis and successful treatment of lymphedema. Cancer. 2008;112(12):2809–19.
34. Li F, Lu Q, Jin S, Zhao Q, Qin X, Jin S, et al. A scoring system for predicting the risk of breast cancer-related lymphedema. Int J Nurs Sci. 2020;7(1):21–8.
35. Stout NL, Binkley JM, Schmitz KH, Andrews K, Hayes SC, Campbell KL, et al. A prospective surveillance model for rehabilitation for women with breast cancer. Cancer. 2012;118(S8):2191–200.
36. Chance-Hetzler J, Armer J, Van Loo M, Anderson B, Harris R, Ewing R, et al. Prospective lymphedema surveillance in a clinic setting. J Pers Med. 2015;5(3):311–25.
37. Lai L, Binkley J, Jones V, Kirkpatrick S, Furbish C, Stratford P, et al. Implementing the prospective surveillance model (PSM) of rehabilitation for breast cancer patients with 1-year postoperative follow-up, a prospective, observational study. Ann Surg Oncol. 2016;23(10):3379–84.
38. Rafn BS, Hung S, Hoens AM, McNeely ML, Singh CA, Kwan W, et al. Prospective surveillance and targeted physiotherapy for arm morbidity after breast cancer surgery: a pilot randomized controlled trial. Clin Rehabil. 2018;32(6):811–26.
39. Levenhagen K, Davies C, Perdomo M, Ryans K, Gilchrist L. Diagnosis of upper quadrant lymphedema secondary to cancer: clinical practice guideline from the Oncology Section of the American Physical Therapy Association. Phys Ther. 2017;97(7):729–45.
40. Ancukiewicz M, Russell TA, Otoole J, Specht M, Singer M, Kelada A, et al. Standardized method for quantification of developing lymphedema in patients treated for breast cancer. Int J Radiat Oncol Biol Phys. 2011;79(5):1436–43.
41. Purcell A, Nixon J, Fleming J, McCann A, Porceddu S. Measuring head and neck lymphedema: the "ALOHA" trial. Head Neck. 2016;38(1):79–84.
42. Yost KJ, Cheville AL, Weaver AL, Al Hilli M, Dowdy SC. Development and validation of a self-report lower-extremity lymphedema screening questionnaire in women. Phys Ther. 2013;93(5):694–703.
43. Doersam JK, Dietrich MS, Adair MA, Rhoten B, Deng J, Ridner SH. A comparison of symptoms among patients with head and neck or truncal lymphedema and normal controls. Lymphat Res Biol. 2019;17(6):661–70.
44. Mayrovitz HN, Mikulka A, Woody D. Minimum detectable changes associated with tissue dielectric constant measurements as applicable to assessing lymphedema status. Lymphat Res Biol. 2019;17(3):322–8.
45. Shah C, Vicini FA, Arthur D. Bioimpedance spectroscopy for breast cancer related lymphedema assessment: clinical practice guidelines. Breast J. 2016;22(6):645–50.

Key Topic: Multimodal Evaluation of the Lymphedema Patient

5

Mark V. Schaverien and Joseph H. Dayan

Introduction

There are a plethora of etiologies for extremity swelling, each with different treatment algorithms, and around a quarter of patients presenting with suspected lymphedema do not have the condition. Patients with limb swelling present a significant challenge to exclude other causes including lipedema, venous insufficiency, obesity, posttraumatic edema, systemic diseases (including cardiac, renal, hepatic, or rheumatological conditions), lymphovascular malformations, or congenital syndromes [1]. A multimodal structured approach is therefore necessary for accurate diagnosis. Around 90% of patients with lymphedema can be correctly diagnosed by focused clinical history and physical examination [2]; limb measurements and imaging modalities, where indicated, will confirm a lymphedema diagnosis, exclude comorbid conditions, and accurately stage the lymphedema [3–5]. This information informs an algorithmic approach to optimally treat the patient [6]. In patients with acute onset lymphedema (especially if the presentation is delayed) or acute-on-chronic worsening, venous thrombosis or locoregional cancer recurrence must be excluded with appropriate imaging.

Diagnostic modalities can be categorized into objective measurements of volume or extracellular fluid and subjective measures of physiological lymphatic vessel function: these include limb circumference measurements and formulae derived from these, infrared optoelectronic volumetry (perometer), bioimpedance spectroscopy (BIS), lymphoscintigraphy, indocyanine green (ICG) fluorescent lymphography, magnetic resonance imaging/lymphangiography (MRI/MRL), and computed tomographic (CT) imaging [7] (Table 5.1). The use of validated lymphedema-specific patient-reported outcome (PRO) questionnaires and those that evaluate limb function may support a lymphedema diagnosis. A range of consultative services should be available through a multidisciplinary referral framework to manage these complex and diverse presentations, including lymphedema-specialist physical therapy, occupational therapy, radiology, interventional radiology, vascular surgery,

Table 5.1 Assessment tools available for the evaluation of patients presenting with limb swelling

Limb volume measurement	Perometer; tape measure circumference (truncated cone; extremity lymphedema index); water displacement plethysmography; volumetric CT
Extracellular fluid measurement	Bioimpedance spectroscopy (LDex score)
Clinical staging	ISL; Campisi; Cheng Lymphedema Grading; Taiwan Lymphoscintographic Staging
Physiological diagnostic/staging imaging	ICG lymphography (dermal backflow staging scale; MDACC ICG lymphedema staging scale); lymphoscintigraphy (including transport index); MRL
Patient-reported outcomes	LLIS; LYMQOL; ULL-27; LyQLI; FLQA-1; Lymph-ICF-LL; LYMPH-Q.
Limb functional assessment instrument	DASH/ Quick-DASH; LEFS; UEFI; ULDQ.
Assessment of venous system (if suspicion of DVT/venous insufficiency)	Comparative Duplex ultrasound; direct contrast venography; CT venography; MR venography

CT computed tomographic, *ISL* International Society of Lymphology, *ICG* indocyanine green, *MDACC* MD Anderson Cancer Center, *MRL* magnetic resonance lymphangiography, *DVT* deep vein thrombosis, *LLIS* Lymphedema Life Impact Scale, *LYMQOL* Lymphedema Quality of Life, *ULL27* Upper Limb Lymphedema 27, *LyQLI* Lymphedema Quality of Life Inventory, *FLQA-L* Freiburg Life Quality Assessment for Lymphedema, *Lymph-ICF-LL* Lymphedema Functioning, Disability and Health Questionnaire for Lower Limb Lymphedema, *DASH/Quick-DASH* Disabilities of the Arm, Shoulder, and Hand Questionnaire, *LEFS* Lower Extremity Functional Scale, *UEFI* Upper Extremity Functional Index, *ULDQ* Upper Limb Disability Questionnaire

M. V. Schaverien (✉)
Department of Plastic Surgery, The University of Texas MD Anderson Cancer Center, Houston, TX, USA
e-mail: mvschaverien@mdanderson.org

J. H. Dayan (✉)
Division of Plastic and Reconstructive Surgery, Memorial Sloan Kettering Cancer Center, New York, NY, USA
e-mail: dayanj@mskcc.org

M. V. Schaverien, J. H. Dayan (eds.), *Multimodal Management of Upper and Lower Extremity Lymphedema*,
https://doi.org/10.1007/978-3-030-93039-4_5

cardiology, internal medicine, medical and surgical oncology, orthopedics, rheumatology, and nutrition, among others.

At present there is lack of clear consensus regarding how patients presenting with suspected lymphedema should be evaluated, and this complicates comparison of outcomes between different centers performing surgery for lymphedema [8, 9]. This chapter presents an evidence-based practical approach to evaluation of patients with limb swelling suspected to be lymphedema (Table 5.2).

Focused Clinical History

Secondary lymphedema results from injury to a normally developed lymphatic system and accounts for almost all adult cases of lymphedema. A history of axillary or inguinal lymphadenectomy, in particular with regional nodal irradiation, places patients at the highest risk for developing lymphedema. Upper extremity lymphedema following breast cancer treatment is the most common etiology in the United States, and gynecologic/genitourinary malignancies are the most frequent cause of lower extremity lymphedema [10].

There is typically a delay before the onset of symptoms, with the majority developing lymphedema within 3 years [11]. Once clinically evident, lymphedema is usually a chronic condition characterized by progression, and spontaneous intermittent swelling is atypical for lymphedema. The risk is greater in obese patients [12], and severely obese patients can develop obesity-induced lymphedema or massive localized extremity lymphedema, without a history of lymphatic injury [13]. Patients of African-American ethnicity are at higher risk of developing breast cancer-related lymphedema (BCRL). In adults with acquired unilateral lower extremity lymphedema without causative factors, a history of travel to areas where filariasis is prevalent should be sought. The patient population with lymphedema is among the highest risk for cancer recurrence – in those with acute onset lymphedema, especially if the presentation is delayed, or with acute-on-chronic worsening, venous thrombosis (Duplex ultrasonography) and locoregional cancer recurrence (CT or MRI) must be excluded.

In adults presenting with limb swelling, obesity, lipedema, and venous insufficiency are in the differential diagnosis; patients are also queried about systemic diseases, such as congestive heart failure, renal failure, hepatic dysfunction, and rheumatological disorders, as well as a history of extremity trauma. Venous insufficiency is the most common cause of lower extremity swelling in the adult population, predominantly affecting older females and characterized by varicose veins, edema, and trophic skin changes – lymphatic function though is normal. Severe lipedema can create skin folds that result in obstruction of the lymphatic vessels, secondarily resulting in lymphedema.

Primary lymphedema is idiopathic and rare, resulting from an error in lymphatic development. It usually presents prior to adulthood, most commonly during infancy in males and at adolescence in females. Incidence is similar in males and females, and it affects the lower extremities in over 90% of cases, with equal distribution between unilateral and bilateral presentations [14]. Typically, the swelling commences in the distal lower extremity and then progresses proximally. Trauma may precipitate the features of primary lymphedema. A history of parental lymphedema should be sought (although 90% have no family history), and associated con-

Table 5.2 Recommended evidence-based evaluation of the patient presenting with lymphedema

Focused history		History of surgery/radiation therapy to regional lymph node basin; duration; time to onset; history of cellulitis and number of episodes; treatment history/compliance; reversibility; exacerbating factors; fluctuation during day
Lymphedema symptoms		Swelling; heaviness
Lymphedema signs		Pitting edema; Stemmer sign; chronic lymphedema skin changes
Clinical staging		ISL staging
Physiological diagnostic/staging imaging		ICG lymphography (dermal backflow staging scale; MDACC ICG lymphedema staging scale); and/or MRL/MRA
Limb volume measurement		Perometer; or limb circumferential measurements with truncated cone volume.
Extracellular fluid measurement		LDex score
Patient-reported outcome measures		LLIS (version 2); LYMQoL; or ULL-27
Additional investigations as required:	Clinical signs of venous insufficiency	Comparative Duplex ultrasound; direct contrast venography; CTV or MRV
	Recipient site assessment prior to orthotopic VLNT	Lymphoscintigraphy/SPECT
	Donor site assessment prior to inguinal/axillary VLNT	Lymphoscintigraphy/SPECT

ISL International Society of Lymphology, *ICG* indocyanine green, *MRA* magnetic resonance angiography, *MRL* magnetic resonance lymphangiography, *LLIS* Lymphedema Life Impact Scale, *MRV* magnetic resonance venography, *CTV* computed tomographic venography, *VLNT* vascularized lymph node transplant, *SPECT* single-photon emission computerized tomography genital syndromes (in particular Turner or Noonan syndrome) should be excluded. In the pediatric population, the differential diagnosis includes capillary/venous/lymphatic malformations, infantile hemangioma, kaposiform hemangioendothelioma, CLOVES (Congenital Lipomatosis, Overgrowth, Vascular malformations, Epidermal nevi, and Scoliosis/Skeletal/Spinal anomalies) syndrome, Klippel–Trenaunay syndrome, and Parkes Weber syndrome. Where primary lymphedema is suspected, patients should be referred to a specialist genetic clinic for testing and counseling, and patients with combined vascular malformations should be managed in a specialist center.

It is important to record an accurate history of the lymphedema duration, which relates to severity, as well as a detailed treatment history including complete decongestive therapy (CDT), noting the time between onset and instituting these, and most importantly compliance with these treatments. A history of cellulitis episodes in the affected extremity and whether intravenous antibiotics were required should be sought, together with frequency and timing; infectious episodes are related to more severe lymphedema pathologies. Improvement of the lymphedema when instituting compression or elevation, or overnight, should be ascertained to indicate physiological reversibility, as well as aggravating factors and fluctuations during the day.

Extremity Lymphedema Symptoms

Regardless of whether the lymphedema is congenital or acquired, the subsequent pathophysiology of the condition is similar. Symptoms include limb swelling, truncal swelling, heaviness, tightness, numbness, tenderness, pain, aching, tingling (paresthesia), and impaired limb mobility [15]. The most common of these symptoms reported in patients presenting with lymphedema are swelling and heaviness, and a self-report of arm swelling is sensitive for diagnosing lymphedema [8]. Reporting of multiple symptoms improves the accuracy in diagnosis, with a diagnostic cutoff of three symptoms found to discriminate breast cancer survivors with lymphedema from healthy women with a sensitivity of 94% and a specificity of 97% [16]. A history of time of day and activities that cause/exacerbate or alleviate swelling should also be sought. While pain is not an unusual symptom, a complaint of significant pain is atypical and should prompt further investigation to exclude recurrence, etc.

Physical Examination Findings

The presence of pitting edema comparing the affected with the unaffected extremity is assessed by pressing the examiner's thumb into consistent locations for 60 s; the degree of pitting edema can be expressed using the Pitting Edema Scale [17]. Significant pitting signifies a fluid dominant limb and its presence corresponds to dermal backflow on lymphatic imaging [18]; the degree of pitting edema correlates with the LDex score but not the limb volume difference (LVD)/excess, likely due to the associated fibrosis that characterizes advanced lymphedema [4]. The presence of significant pitting edema should prompt timely referral to lymphedema therapy for reductive CDT. Significant reversibility of pitting edema may indicate suitability for a physiological surgical procedure; patients with minimal or no pitting and significant adipose soft tissue excess may be candidates for a debulking procedure. The degree of fibrosis of the tissues should also be evaluated, as well as the presence of other skin stigmata of chronic advanced stage lymphedema, including dermal lymphedema, hyperkeratosis, and lymphorrhea. The (Kaposi-)Stemmer sign is a sign of distal fibrosis, and therefore advanced stage lymphedema, and is positive if the examiner is unable to pinch the skin on the dorsum of the hand or foot [19, 20].

The degree of fibrosis and skin tethering at the lymphadenectomy surgical site should also be assessed to determine the need for surgical intervention, as well as signs of venous insufficiency distally such as skin color changes and varicose veins. Venous insufficiency may be a contraindication to a physiological surgical procedure. New onset varicosities may indicate deep vein thrombosis, such as prominent chest wall veins in axillary vein thrombosis. It is important to note that in patients with positive clinic signs but normal lymphatic imaging, venous insufficiency is the most common cause of swelling and work-up should include evaluation of cardiac function [19]. Body mass index (BMI) should be evaluated at each clinic visit.

Lymphedema Clinical Staging Scales

The clinical history and physical examination findings inform the International Society of Lymphology (ISL) staging scale [21]. This is the most commonly used system to classify the severity of the lymphedema, describing progression through four stages:

Stage 0 describes latent or subclinical lymphedema without swelling but with impaired lymph transport, subtle alterations in tissue fluid/composition, and changes in subjective symptoms; Stage I lymphedema is characterized by swelling which subsides with limb elevation, and pitting edema may occur. Stage II lymphedema is characterized by subcutaneous fat accumulation – limb elevation alone rarely reduces tissue swelling, and pitting edema is evident – later on the limb may not pit as soft tissue fibrosis develops. Stage III is advanced lymphedema where pitting can be absent and there are trophic skin changes such as hyperkeratosis and acanthosis. A limb may exhibit more than one stage. Several studies however have found that the ISL stage correlates poorly with other lymphedema measures, including LVD and the LDex score [8], likely due to the highly subjective nature of the staging system, with each stage representing a broad spectrum of phenotypes (majority Stage II), and it does not link with surgical treatment decisions. The Campisi lymphedema staging expanded this scale to six stages: Stage I includes latent (A) and initial (B) lymphedema; Stage II includes increasing lymphedema (A) and column-shaped limb fibrolymphedema (B); and Stage III is elephantiasis [22]. The Cheng Lymphedema Grading scale and the Taiwan Lymphoscintographic Staging system utilize lymphoscintigraphy and/or limb circumferential difference to provide additional objective measures of lymphedema for staging [23]. Physiological staging scales utilizing ICG lymphography (see below) allow for surgical decision-making and are the current mainstay for lymphedema staging.

Limb Volume Measurements

Limb measurements are the most commonly used modality for diagnosis and evaluation of lymphedema and can be used to define severity; these include circumferential measurements, volumetry using a perometer, or water displacement.

Tape measurements are well-established and may be used to derive limb volumes using truncated cone formulae from measurements taken at 4 cm intervals for the length of the extremity, or to calculate the upper or lower extremity lymphedema indices [24]. There is significant inter- and intra-rater variability due to difficulty replicating both the exact reference points and the tension applied to the tape measure. Information regarding the localization of the swelling is provided, though the hand and foot volumes cannot be calculated. An increase of ≥2 cm in circumference measurements has been used as a simple means of diagnosis [15]. For limb volume, diagnostic thresholds include limb volume change (LVC) ≥5% or ≥200 ml absolute difference [25]. When compared with limb volume measurements, circumferential measurements have a relatively low sensitivity, specificity, and positive predictive value, suggesting that the use of circumference measurements alone results in underdiagnosis and underestimation of the degree of lymphedema [8, 26].

The perometer, which uses mobile infrared optoelectronic volumetry, is fast, valid, and reliable for limb volume measurements [5, 27]; however, it is expensive and portability can be problematic. Perometer measurements correlate closely with volume measures derived from circumferential measurements using the truncated cone formula, although manual measurements underestimate the total limb volume. Horizontally configured perometers are specifically designed for the upper extremity (Fig. 5.1a), and upright perometers are used for measurement of lower extremity volumes (Fig. 5.1b); it may be possible to use these interchangeably with adaptations. To decrease variance, it is important that the device is regularly recalibrated, operated by consistent trained staff, and that measurements are taken from defined and reproducible points with the same limb length used for each measurement and for each limb. Multiple bilateral measurements may improve the reliability, and variance, particularly of the unaffected limb, should be a benchmark – ideally less than 1% – while accounting for variations in BMI, etc.

The differences between the affected and unaffected limbs are expressed as relative and absolute limb volume excess ratios; in bilateral lymphedema, the excess volume cannot be determined and so the percentage change in volume for each limb is reported. LVC ≥3% based on the preoperative measurement is a diagnostic threshold [28], with LVC ≥5% classified as mild lymphedema, and ≥10% as moderate to severe [29]. As limb volume excess is a significant feature of lymphedema that surgery aims to improve, limb volume measurements, preferably using a perometer to reduce variability, should be used for diagnosis and in longitudinal assessment [4].

Although limb volume measurement using water displacement plethysmography is highly accurate, there are significant practical limitations to its use in the clinical setting, particularly as the water needs to be changed for successive patients, and it is rarely used.

Bioimpedance Spectroscopy (BIS)

BIS provides rapid and reliable noninvasive measurement of extracellular water in an extremity by calculating the resistance at 0 Hz frequency (R0), at which the cell membrane acts as an insulator [5, 27, 30]. The LDex® U400 (Impedimed, Carlsbad, CA), a portable adhesive electrode and lead-based system, has been the most studied BIS device for lymphedema; however, both a significant amount of training and standardization are required for consistent results. The SOZO® can be used in the office setting where the contact electrode pads are built into a fixed system to improve usability and reliability by standardizing palm, sole, and patient positioning (Fig. 5.2). The ratio of the impedance values between the affected and unaffected limb is calculated after adjusting for sex, upper/lower limb, and right/left dominance, to give the LDex score [31]. An LDex score of −10 to +10 has been considered normal (LDex score of 0 represents the mean impedance ratio, and 10 is equal to a linear change of approximately three standard deviations), and above 10 is diagnostic for lymphedema [30, 32]. A growing evidence-base supports the use of an LDex score of ≥7 to be a more accurate diagnostic threshold for lymphedema of the upper

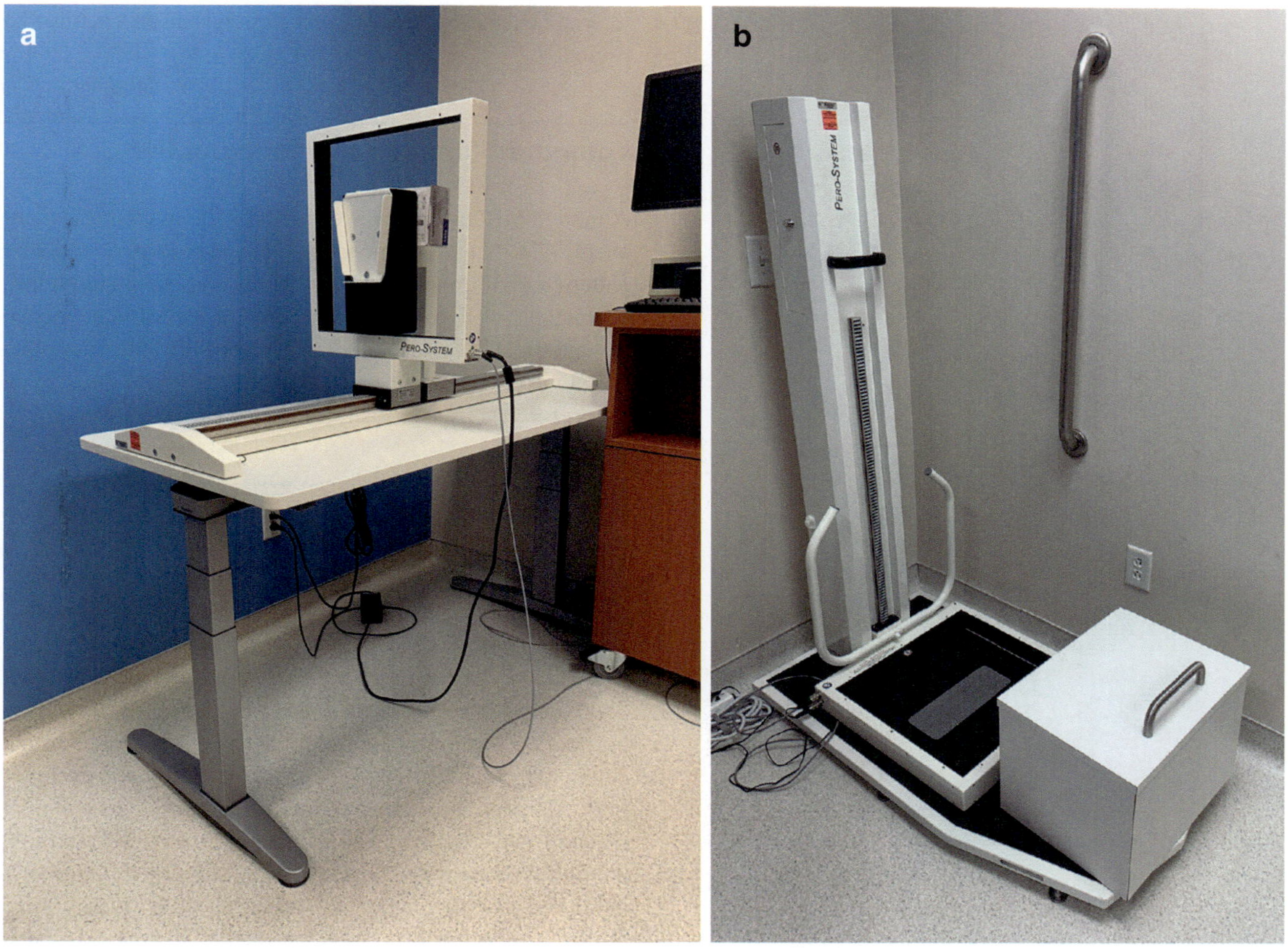

Fig. 5.1 (**a**) Limb volumetric measurements can be taken using a perometer, a mobile infrared optoelectronic volumeter, that is fast, valid, and reliable. A horizontally configured perometer, as shown here, is specifically designed for measurement of the upper extremity. (**b**) The upright perometer shown here is used for measurement of lower extremity limb volume, although it may also be used for measurement of the upper extremity with adaptations. A standardized technique should be used to reduce variance as well as the use of the mean value of multiple bilateral measurements

extremity (≥6.5 for subclinical lymphedema) [30, 33]. Using a cutoff of LDex ratio ≥+7.1 has an 80% sensitivity and 90% specificity to discriminate between at-risk breast cancer survivors and those with lymphedema, and it is therefore important for clinicians to integrate the LDex score with other assessment methods to ensure accurate diagnosis [30]. For patients with preoperative measurements, a change in the LDex score of >10 units is diagnostic [25]. The LDex score is sensitive for the early detection of lymphedema [33], and significantly correlates with lymphedema severity stage and limb volume excess [4, 34]; it is also highly responsive to nonsurgical and surgical interventions [4, 8].

When compared with limb circumference measurements for the upper extremity, one study found that the LDex score was more sensitive in diagnosing lymphedema and had a higher positive predictive value when using an LVD of >10% as the diagnostic threshold [8]. A significant limitation of BIS remains the ability to independently and reliably measure bilateral extremity lymphedema.

Magnetic Resonance Imaging/Angiography

MRI enables high-resolution imaging of the soft tissues which can be used to assess the relative fluid and lymphedema-related fat hypertrophy compositions of an extremity using T1-weighted imaging with and without fat saturation gradient echo images. Gadolinium contrast-enhanced imaging with delayed-phase vascular imaging can be used to evaluate for venous stenosis or thrombosis. Alternatively, T2-weighted fast spin-echo sequences can also visualize the lymphatic vessels without the need for contrast [35].

MRI has a similar sensitivity to ICG lymphography in diagnosing lymphedema, and is superior to lymphoscintigra-

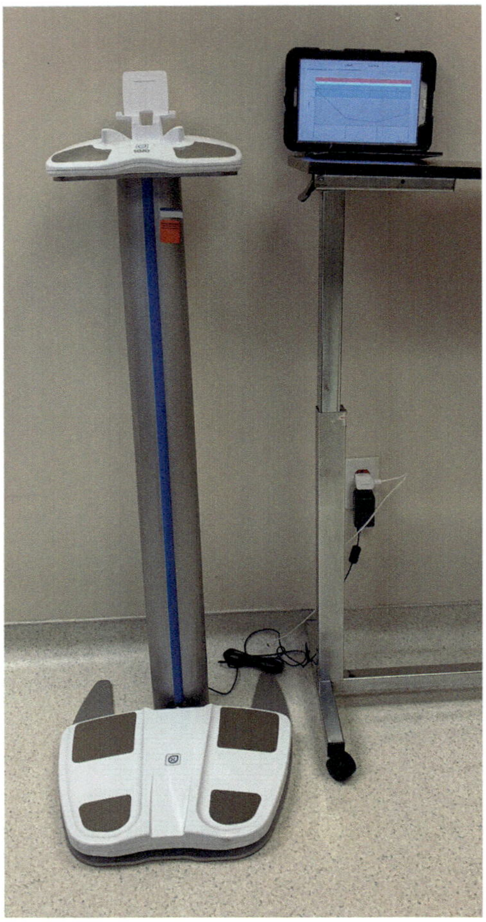

Fig. 5.2 Bioimpedance spectroscopy (BIS) provides rapid and reliable noninvasive measurement of extracellular water in an extremity. The SOZO® device shown here can be used in the office setting where the contact electrode pads are built into a fixed system to standardize palm, sole, and patient positioning, and improve reliability

phy [36]. Fluid accumulation or fat hypertrophy on MRI is highly sensitive for the diagnosis of lymphedema as defined by a limb volume excess ≥10%, with both high negative and positive predictive values for evidence of fluid accumulation. MRI is not only helpful in confirming the diagnosis of lymphedema but also in excluding other etiologies of limb swelling; in lipedema, for example, the fat accumulation typically occurs without signs of fluid accumulation, or there is subcutaneous infiltration of soft tissue with a classical reticular appearance [37]. MRA has the added advantage of imaging of the venous system; one study found that evidence of narrowing or stenosis in the axillary vein was found in around 15% of patients, which may result in venous insufficiency and contribute to the lymphedema pathology, as well as reducing the effectiveness of physiological lymphedema surgeries [8]. Where concordant venous insufficiency is suspected, additional venous investigations, including comparative duplex ultrasonography, CT venography, or direct contrast venography, may be indicated. Occult metastatic disease contributing to lymphedema by venous compression/stenosis can also be excluded.

Computed Tomography/Venography

Although MRI is the preferred modality for assessing lymphedema, CT imaging demonstrates the characteristic reticular pattern and thickening of the subcutaneous tissue in lymphedema, as well as anatomic localization of the edema. Volumetric CT measurements also significantly correlate with limb circumference measures [38]. CT venography can assess for venous stenosis/thrombosis.

Lymphoscintigraphy

Radionuclide lymphoscintigraphy has been extensively studied for the investigation of lymphatic physiological function, allowing for evaluation of both the deep and superficial lymphatic systems and their draining lymph nodes, lymphatic collateralization, and dermal backflow, as well as lymphatic transport using transit times [39]. It may also assist in the adjunctive classification of the degree of lymphatic dysfunction. Intradermal injection of technetium-99m-colloidal albumin into the digit webspaces of both the affected and unaffected extremities is performed, with serial hemi-body radioscintigraphic imaging of the transit of the radioisotope through the lymphatic system typically at 10 min and then at 30-min intervals up to 3 h post-injection [39]. Asymmetric lymphatic drainage with delayed transit time to the regional lymph nodes and visualization of collateral lymphatic channels is suggestive of lymphedema, and the presence of dermal backflow is diagnostic.

The transport index (TI) evaluates several parameters in serial scans, including lymphatic transport kinetics, radiocontrast distribution pattern, time to appearance of lymph nodes, and assessment of lymph nodes and lymph vessels. It is valid for measuring dynamic lymphatic function with high interobserver reliability [40], and staging scales using the dermal backflow pattern and severity have been described and validated [39]. The Taiwan Lymphoscintigraphy Staging system evaluates the lymph nodes, lymphatic ducts, and presence and distribution of dermal backflow [23].

Studies are inconsistent regarding the reliability of lymphoscintigraphy for the diagnosis of lymphedema [39, 41], and results are likely affected by the definitions used, as well as the experience of the radiologist and interpreter. One study found that the sensitivity and specificity with a minimum limb volume excess of 10% were 88% and 41.4%, respectively, and the positive and negative predictive values were 72.1% and 66.7%, respectively [8].

Lymphoscintigraphy enables evaluation of the presence of residual functional axillary lymph nodes, which may imply a better prognosis, in those planned for orthotopic vascularized lymph node transplantation (VLNT) so that they can be preserved during axillary scar release. It also has great utility in reverse lymphatic mapping [8], and can be combined with CT imaging to produce a SPECT/CT for three-dimensional localizations of the sentinel lymph nodes in the superficial inguinal or axillary regional lymphatic basins to reduce the risk of donor-extremity lymphedema after groin or lateral thoracic VLN flap harvest, respectively [42, 43]. It can also be used for follow-up to determine the function of transplanted lymph nodes, although in proximal lymph node transfer the contrast needs to transit from the webspaces to the transplant to be visualized on lymphoscintigraphy.

Indocyanine Green (ICG) Fluorescent Lymphography

ICG fluorescent lymphography is the primary tool for physiological lymphedema staging and enables decision-making between the available surgical options. It allows for detailed visualization of the superficial lymphatic system and is primarily used for intraoperative lymphatic mapping for lymphovenous bypass (LVB). It enables sites of dermal backflow and their "feeding" vessels to be identified, assessment of lymphatic valvular competence by anterograde or retrograde "milking" of the lymphatics to help determine the optimal lymphatic-venous anastomosis configuration, and localization of venules as "shadows" over the lymphatic vessels (Fig. 5.3) – adjunctive use of a vein imager allows identification of nearby venules and assessment of their valvular competence for selection for anastomosis (Fig. 5.4). The comparative transit time between affected and unaffected extremities can also be measured. Dermal backflow severity

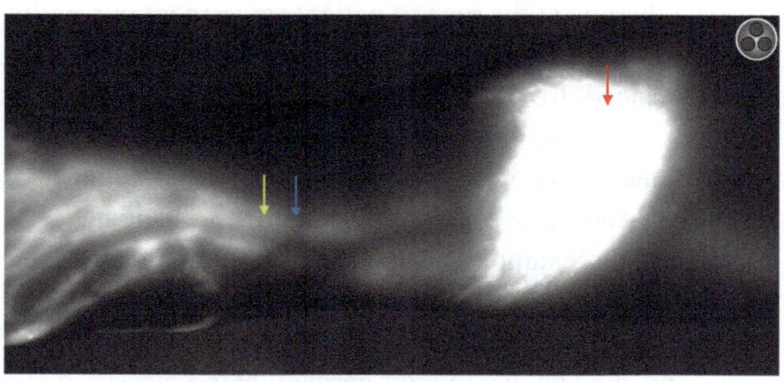

Fig. 5.3 Indocyanine green (ICG) fluorescent lymphography allows for detailed visualization of the superficial lymphatic system and is used for staging and surgical planning. Sites of dermal backflow (*red arrow*) and their linear lymphatic "feeding" vessels (*yellow arrow*) can be identified, as well as localization of venules as "shadows" over the lymphatic vessels (*blue arrow*)

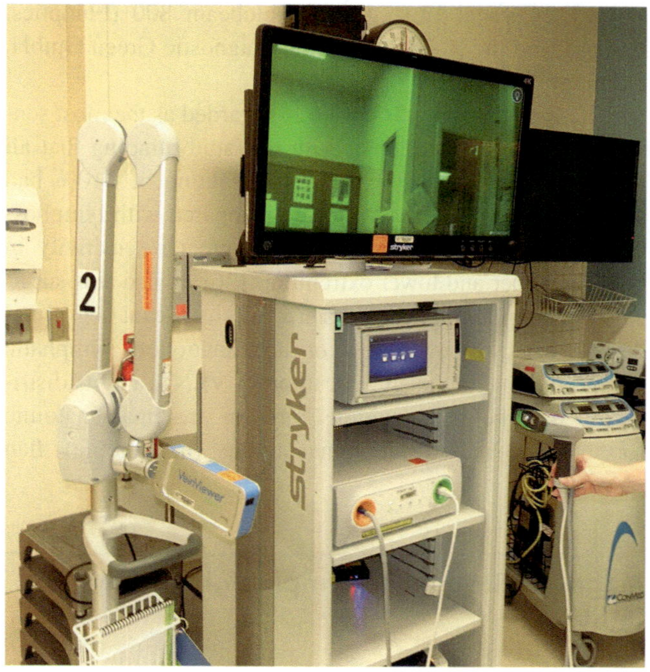

Fig. 5.4 Commercial devices for indocyanine green (ICG) fluorescent lymphography include the PhotoDynamic Eye (PDE, Hamamatsu Inc., Japan) and the SPY Phi (Stryker Inc., USA) (*right*). For surgical planning, the adjunctive use of a vein imager can aid in identification of nearby venules and assessment of their valvular competence for selection for anastomosis (*left*)

and distribution correlate closely with the pathological condition of the lymphatic vessels [44].

Physiological staging systems utilizing ICG lymphography evaluate the following: lymphatic transport, presence of functional lymphatic vessels, and pattern and distribution of dermal backflow. These include the dermal backflow staging scale, a 12-subtype scale, and the MD Anderson Cancer Centre (MDACC) ICG lymphedema staging scale, a five-stage scale [45, 46]. The dermal backflow pattern is additionally characterized as splash, stardust, or diffuse pattern representing increasing levels of fibrosis/sclerosis of the lymphatic vessels, ranging from normal to ectatic, then contraction, and finally sclerosis with obliteration of the lymphatic vessel lumen [46]. These physiological staging systems aid in surgical decision-making – for example, the presence of advanced dermal backflow patterns without visualization of linear lymphatic vessels may be an indication for VLNT.

Approximately 0.05–0.1 mL of ICG (0.25–0.5 mg) is injected intradermally into each webspace, in particular the first and the third [8]. Lidocaine (1%) preinjection is helpful in preventing the local discomfort. Images are acquired using a near-infrared (NIR) fluorescent imager, and several commercial systems are available, including the PhotoDynamic Eye (PDE, Hamamatsu Inc., Japan), the SPY systems including the SPY Elite and Phi (Stryker Inc., USA) (Fig. 5.4),

FLARE (Curadel LLC, USA), Fluobeam 800 (Fluoptics, France), and the IC-Flow system (Diagnostic Green GmbH, Germany).

ICG lymphography is currently regarded as the most sensitive test for lymphedema, with one study finding that all abnormal upper limbs with a limb volume of >10% had abnormal ICG patterns [8]. When compared with lymphoscintigraphy, ICG lymphography has greater sensitivity in both the upper and lower extremities [36]. It also aids surgical decision-making: the presence of significant segmental dermal backflow with few or no functioning lymphatic vessels on imaging is an indication for VLNT, and its distribution may help in deciding between proximal anatomic (orthotopic) and distal nonanatomic (heterotopic) flap placement.

Magnetic Resonance Lymphangiography (MRL)

MRL is a relatively noninvasive technique in which a gadolinium-based MRI contrast agent (e.g., gadobenate dimeglumine) is injected intradermally into the interdigital webspaces of the hand or foot. This allows the visualization of the anatomical and functional status of lymphatic vessels, lymph nodes, and dermal backflow in patients with lymphedema, in addition to the inherent ability of MR to image interstitial fluid and subcutaneous adipose tissue [47, 48]. Subtraction venography can be used additionally to discriminate between lymphatic vessels and veins, for example, by intravenous administration of gadobenate dimeglumine contrast [48].

Staging scales using MRL are specific for stratifying patients for surgical intervention [35, 48]. In one study, MRL was found to have greater sensitivity and specificity than lymphoscintigraphy across a range of measures [49]. The main disadvantages of this modality are the operator dependence and necessity for a radiologist with expertise in post-processing and in evaluation of patients with lymphedema.

Patient-Reported Outcome Measures (PROMs) and Limb Functional Assessment Instruments

Patient-reported outcomes (PROs) are important for evaluation of the lymphedema patient as well as for longitudinal assessment in response to nonsurgical or surgical intervention. Several scales have been validated for the measurement of PROs specific for lymphedema and are increasingly being used in the routine clinical setting. These scales include the Lymphedema Life Impact Scale (LLIS), the Lymphedema Quality of Life (LYMQoL) questionnaire, and the Upper Limb Lymphedema 27 (ULL-27). Others include the Lymphedema Quality of Life Inventory (LyQLI), the Freiburg Life Quality Assessment for Lymphedema (FLQA-L), the Lymphedema Functioning, Disability and Health Questionnaire for Lower Limb Lymphedema (Lymph-ICF-LL), and most recently the LYMPH-Q. The LLIS (version 2), which includes 18 questions about the past week distributed across physical, functional, and psychological domains [50], was found to correlate highly with the ULL-27 and was more sensitive in measuring physical and functional disability. There was a weak correlation between the physical and functional domains of the LLIS and limb volume excess, suggesting that even minor increases in limb volume can have a significant impact on quality of life measures, with no correlation found for psychological impairment [8]. A study using the LYMQOL found no correlation with the ISL stage or the LDex score for both upper and lower extremity lymphedema [51].

Limb functional assessment instruments validated in other domains can provide complementary information regarding the physical disability resulting from lymphedema. These tools include the Disabilities of the Arm, Shoulder, and Hand Questionnaire (DASH/Quick-DASH), Lower Extremity Functional Scale (LEFS), Upper Extremity Functional Index (UEFI), and Upper Limb Disability Questionnaire (ULDQ). One study found no correlation between the DASH and LEFS scores and ISL stage or the LDex score for upper and lower extremities, respectively [51].

Lymphedema Physical Therapy

The availability of lymphedema therapy delivered by certified lymphedema therapists (CLT) is of central importance for the management of patients with lymphedema, as well as for other causes of edema such as venous insufficiency. Consideration should be made to incorporate lymphedema physical therapy at the time of patient assessment in a multidisciplinary clinic for patient education, to enable therapy to be commenced, for patients to be measured for compression garments, for pneumatic compression pumps to be prescribed, and for coordination of care. If noncompliance is diagnosed, then reasons for it need to be elucidated and addressed: for example, patients may complain that their garment is too tight at the upper arm or wrist, that they feel it is not making a difference, or that it causes their hand to swell. This may be due to their garment being measured at a garment shop without the necessary specialist expertise – custom garments should ideally be measured by an experienced lymphedema therapist or manufacturer representative. During periods of reduced compliance, the limb may become more edematous which adversely affects the garment fitment, and a short course of bandaging may be required, in particular if a new compression garment has been ordered.

Multidisciplinary Lymphedema Team

A comprehensive range of consultative services is important through a multidisciplinary referral framework for the combined management of complex patients with non-lymphedema etiologies or comorbid conditions. In addition to lymphedema-specialist plastic surgery and lymphedema-specialist physical therapy, these include occupational therapy, vascular surgery, diagnostic/interventional radiology with capability for venoplasty/stenting for management of concomitant venous insufficiency, medical and surgical oncology, dieticians/nutritionists (for management of obesity), internal medicine, bariatric specialists, dermatology, orthopedics, rheumatology, physical medicine and rehabilitation, researchers, and geneticists (for primary lymphedema) [52].

References

1. Maclellan RA, Couto RA, Sullivan JE, Grant FD, Slavin SA, Greene AK. Management of primary and secondary lymphedema: analysis of 225 referrals to a center. Ann Plast Surg. 2015;75:197–200.
2. Greene AK, Goss JA. Diagnosis and staging of lymphedema. Semin Plast Surg. 2018;32:12–6.
3. Dylke ES, Schembri GP, Bailey DL, Bailey E, Ward LC, Refshauge K, Beith J, Black D, Kilbreath SL. Diagnosis of upper limb lymphoedema: development of an evidence based approach. Acta Oncol. 2016;55:1477–83.
4. Coroneos CJ, Wong FC, DeSnyder SM, Shaitelman SF, Schaverien MV. Correlation of l-dex bioimpedance spectroscopy with limb volume and lymphatic function in lymphedema. Lymphat Res Biol. 2019;17:301–7.
5. Jain MS, Danoff JV, Paul SM. Correlation between bioelectrical spectroscopy and perometry in assessment of upper extremity swelling. Lymphology. 2010;43:85–94.
6. Schaverien MV, Coroneos CJ. Surgical treatment of lymphedema. Plast Reconstr Surg. 2019;144(3):738–58.
7. Hidding JT, Viehoff PB, Beurskens CH, van Laarhoven HW, et al. Measurement properties of instruments for measuring of lymphedema: systematic. Review. 2016;96:1965–81.
8. Wiser I, Mehrara BJ, Coriddi M, Kenworthy E, Cavalli M, Encarnacion E, Dayan JH. Preoperative assessment of upper extremity secondary lymphedema. Cancers (Basel). 2020;12:135.
9. Pappalardo M, Patel K, Cheng MH. Vascularized lymph node transfer for treatment of extremity lymphedema: an overview of current controversies regarding donor sites, recipient sites and outcomes. J Surg Oncol. 2018;117:1420–31.
10. Cormier JN, Askew RL, Mungovan KS, Xing Y, Ross MI, Armer JM. Lymphedema beyond breast cancer: a systematic review and meta-analysis of cancer-related secondary lymphedema. Cancer. 2010;116:5138–49.
11. Petrek JA, Senie RT, Peters M, Rosen PP. Lymphedema in a cohort of breast carcinoma survivors 20 years after diagnosis. Cancer. 2001;92:1368–77.
12. Helyer LK, Varnic M, Le LW, Leong W, McCready D. Obesity is a risk factor for developing postoperative lymphedema in breast cancer patients. Breast J. 2010;16:48–54.
13. Greene AK, Grant FD, Slavin SA, Maclellan RA. Obesity-induced lymphedema: clinical and lymphoscintigraphic features. Plast Reconstr Surg. 2015;135:1715–9.
14. Schook CC, Mulliken JB, Fishman SJ, Grant F, Zurakowski D, Greene AK. Primary lymphedema: clinical features and management in 138 pediatric patients. Plast Reconstr Surg. 2011;127:2419–31.
15. Armer JM, Hulett JM, Bernas M, Ostby P, Stewart BR, Cormier JN. Best-practice guidelines in assessment, risk reduction, management, and surveillance for post-breast cancer lymphedema. Curr Breast Cancer Rep. 2013;5:134–44.
16. Fu MR, Axelrod D, Cleland CM, Qiu Z, Guth AA, Kleinman R, Scagliola J, Haber J. Symptom report in detecting breast cancer-related lymphedema. Breast Cancer (Dove Med Press). 2015;7:345–52.
17. Brodovicz KG, McNaughton K, Uemura N, Meininger G, Girman CJ, Yale SH. Reliability and feasibility of methods to quantitatively assess peripheral edema. Clin Med Res. 2009;7(1-2):21–31.
18. Thomis S, Dams L, Fourneau I, De Vrieze T, Nevelsteen I, Neven P, Gebruers N, Devoogdt N. Correlation between clinical assessment and lymphofluoroscopy in patients with breast cancer-related lymphedema: a study of concurrent validity. Lymphat Res Biol. 2020;18(6):539–48.
19. Jayaraj A, Raju S, May C, Pace N. The diagnostic unreliability of classic physical signs of lymphedema. J Vasc Surg Venous Lymphat Disord. 2019;7:890–7.
20. Goss JA, Greene AK. Sensitivity and specificity of the stemmer sign for lymphedema: a clinical lymphoscintigraphic study. Plast Reconstr Surg Glob Open. 2019;7:e2295.
21. Executive Committee. The diagnosis and treatment of peripheral lymphedema: 2016 consensus document of the international society of lymphology. Lymphology. 2016;49:170–84.
22. Campisi C. Lymphoedema: modern diagnostic and therapeutic aspects. Int Angiol. 1999;18:14–24.
23. Cheng MH, Pappalardo M, Lin C, Kuo CF, Lin CY, Chung KC. Validity of the novel Taiwan lymphoscintigraphy staging and correlation of Cheng lymphedema grading for unilateral extremity lymphedema. Ann Surg. 2018;268:513–25.
24. Yamamoto N, Yamamoto T, Hayashi N, et al. Arm volumetry versus upper extremity lymphedema index: validity of upper extremity lymphedema index for body-type corrected arm volume evaluation. Ann Plast Surg. 2016;76:697–9.
25. Levenhagen K, Davies C, Perdomo M, Ryans K, Gilchrist L. Diagnosis of upper quadrant lymphedema secondary to cancer: clinical practice guideline from the Oncology Section of the American Physical Therapy Association. Phys Ther. 2017;97:729–45.
26. Sun F, Hall A, Tighe MP, Brunelle CL, Sayegh HE, Gillespie TC, Daniell KM, Taghian AG. Perometry versus simulated circumferential tape measurement for the detection of breast cancer-related lymphedema. Breast Cancer Res Treat. 2018;172:83–91.
27. Adriaenssens N, Buyl R, Lievens P, Fontaine C, Lamote J. Comparative study between mobile infrared optoelectronic volumetry with a Perometer and two commonly used methods for the evaluation of arm volume in patients with breast cancer related lymphedema of the arm. Lymphology. 2013;46:132–43.
28. Stout Gergich NL, Pfalzer LA, McGarvey C, Springer B, Gerber LH, Soballe P. Preoperative assessment enables the early diagnosis and successful treatment of lymphedema. Cancer. 2008;112:2809–19.
29. Specht MC, Miller CL, Russell TA, et al. Defining a threshold for intervention in breast cancer-related lymphedema: what level of arm volume increase predicts progression? Breast Cancer Res Treat. 2013;140:485–94.
30. Fu MR, Cleland CM, Guth AA, Kayal M, Haber J, Cartwright F, Kleinman R, Kang Y, Scagliola J, Axelrod D. L-dex ratio in detecting breast cancer-related lymphedema: reliability, sensitivity, and specificity. Lymphology. 2013;46:85–96.

31. Czerniec SA, Ward LC, Refshauge KM, Beith J, Lee MJ, York S, Kilbreath SL. Assessment of breast cancer-related arm lymphedema-comparison of physical measurement methods and self-report. Cancer Investig. 2010;28:54–62.
32. Barrio AV, Eaton A, Frazier TG. A prospective validation study of bioimpedance with volume displacement in early-stage breast cancer patients at risk for lymphedema. Ann Surg Oncol. 2015;22:S370–5.
33. Ridner SH, Dietrich MS, Spotanski K, Doersam JK, Cowher MS, Taback B, McLaughlin S, Ajkay N, Boyages J, Koelmeyer L, DeSnyder S, Shah C, Vicini F. A prospective study of l-dex values in breast cancer patients pretreatment and through 12 months post-operatively. Lymphat Res Biol. 2018;16:435–41.
34. Szuba A, Strauss W, Sirsikar SP, Rockson SG. Quantitative radionuclide lymphoscintigraphy predicts outcome of manual lymphatic therapy in breast cancer-related lymphedema of the upper extremity. Nucl Med Commun. 2002;23:1171–5.
35. Arrivé L, Derhy S, El Mouhadi S, Monnier-Cholley L, Menu Y, Becker C. Noncontrast magnetic resonance Lymphography. J Reconstr Microsurg. 2016;32:80–6.
36. Mihara M, Hara H, Araki J, Kikuchi K, Narushima M, Yamamoto T, Iida T, Yoshimatsu H, Murai N, Mitsui K, Okitsu T, Koshima I. Indocyanine green (ICG) lymphography is superior to lymphoscintigraphy for diagnostic imaging of early lymphedema of the upper limbs. PLoS One. 2012;7:e38182.
37. Haaverstad R, Nilsen G, Rinck PA, Myhre HO. The use of MRI in the diagnosis of chronic lymphedema of the lower extremity. Int Angiol. 1994;13:115–8.
38. Ho OA, Chu SY, Huang YL, Chen WH, Lin CY, Cheng MH. Effectiveness of vascularized lymph node transfer for extremity lymphedema using volumetric and circumferential differences. Plast Reconstr Surg Glob Open. 2019;7:e2003.
39. Maclellan RA, Zurakowski D, Voss S, Greene AK. Correlation between lymphedema disease severity and lymphoscintigraphic findings: a clinical-radiologic study. J Am Coll Surg. 2017;225:366–70.
40. Kleinhans E, Baumeister RG, Hahn D, et al. Evaluation of transport kinetics in lymphoscintigraphy: follow-up study in patients with transplanted lymphatic vessels. Eur J Nucl Med. 1985;10: 349–52.
41. Hassanein AH, Maclellan RA, Grant FD, Greene AK. Diagnostic accuracy of lymphoscintigraphy for lymphedema and analysis of false-negative tests. Plast Reconstr Surg Glob Open. 2017;5:e1396.
42. Dayan JH, Dayan E, Smith ML. Reverse lymphatic mapping: a new technique for maximizing safety in vascularized lymph node transfer. Plast Reconstr Surg. 2015;135:277–85.
43. Giżewska A, Witkowska-Patena E, Osiecki S, Mazurek A, Stembrowicz-Nowakowska Z, Dziuk M. Utility of single-photon emission tomography/computed tomography for sentinel lymph node localization in breast cancer patients. Nucl Med Commun. 2017;38(6):493–9.
44. Hara H, Mihara M, Seki Y, Todokoro T, Iida T, Koshima I. Comparison of indocyanine green lymphographic findings with the conditions of collecting lymphatic vessels of limbs in patients with lymphedema. Plast Reconstr Surg. 2013;132:1612–8.
45. Chang DW, Suami H, Skoracki R. A prospective analysis of 100 consecutive lymphovenous bypass cases for treatment of extremity lymphedema. Plast Reconstr Surg. 2013;132:1305–14.
46. Yamamoto T, Yamamoto N, Doi K, et al. Indocyanine green-enhanced lymphography for upper extremity lymphedema: a novel severity staging system using dermal backflow patterns. Plast Reconstr Surg. 2011;128:941–7.
47. Miseré RML, Wolfs JAGN, Lobbes MBI, van der Hulst RRWJ, Qiu SS. A systematic review of magnetic resonance lymphography for the evaluation of peripheral lymphedema. J Vasc Surg Venous Lymphat Disord. 2020;8(5):882–92.
48. Neligan PC, Kung TA, Maki JH. MR lymphangiography in the treatment of lymphedema. J Surg Oncol. 2017;115:18–22.
49. Bae JS, Yoo RE, Choi SH, Park SO, Chang H, Suh M, Cheon GJ. Evaluation of lymphedema in upper extremities by MR lymphangiography: comparison with lymphoscintigraphy. Magn Reson Imaging. 2018;49:63–70.
50. Weiss J, Daniel T. Validation of the lymphedema life impact scale version 2: a condition specific measurement tool for persons with lymphedema. Lymphology. 2015;48:128–38.
51. Lee TS, Morris CM, Czerniec SA, Mangion AJ. Does lymphedema severity affect quality of life? Simple question. Challenging answers. Lymphat Res Biol. 2018;16:85–91.
52. Raju S, Furrh JB 4th, Neglén P. Diagnosis and treatment of venous lymphedema. J Vasc Surg. 2012;55:141–9.

6 Nonsurgical Management of the Lymphedema Patient

Marc A. Miller, Mark V. Schaverien, and Dawn N. Chen

Conservative lymphedema physical therapy is the mainstay of lymphedema management. The current gold standard for this is complete decongestive therapy (CDT), also termed complex decongestive therapy. It consists of two phases – a reduction phase to achieve rapid reduction in the pitting edema, followed by a maintenance phase to stabilize the limb volume. The reduction phase typically consists of low-stretch bandages, although specialized reduction garments may also be used [1–3]. Once the limb volume reduction has plateaued, there is a transition to the maintenance phase. This consists predominantly of the use of a compression garment during the day, and, dependent on severity, either daily manual lymphatic drainage (MLD) or self-lymphatic drainage (SLD) and/or use of a sequential gradient pump (also termed a pneumatic compression device, PCD). This may be supplemented by the use of nighttime bandaging or the use of a specialized night garment. Optimal conservative therapy is effective at preventing or reducing the rate of progression of the lymphedema and reducing the risk of cellulitis. Lymphedema-specific exercises are strongly recommended for lymphedema patients when progressive in intensity and under the supervision of a trained lymphedema therapist, ideally performed while wearing their compression (Table 6.1).

There is increasing recognition of the importance of conservative therapy in improving outcomes of lymphedema surgery. This has resulted in the introduction of nonsurgical lymphedema physical therapy as the principal component of *prehabilitation* to optimize patients *before* lymphedema surgery where it is most effective, rather than the traditional approach of delivering this lymphedema therapy mainly postoperatively. Herein we review the techniques for conservative management of upper and lower extremity lymphedema, and the process for optimization prior to lymphedema surgery.

Table 6.1 Phases of complete/complex decongestive therapy (CDT)

Intensive reduction phase	Maintenance phase
Low-stretch bandages (or adjustable reduction garment)	Compression garments (custom compression/nighttime bandaging or specialist nighttime garment)
Manual lymphatic drainage (MLD)	Manual Lymphatic Drainage (MLD) or Self-Lymphatic Drainage (SLD)
Pneumatic compression device (PCD)	Pneumatic compression device (PCD)
Lymphedema-specific exercises	Lymphedema-specific exercises
Skin care and risk-reduction precautions	Skin care and risk-reduction precautions

Complete/Complex Decongestive Physical Therapy (CDT)

Lymphedema occurs due to dysfunction of the lymphatic system, which results in reflux of lymphatic fluid into the interstitial space – its stasis incites a localized chronic inflammatory process. The inflammatory cell infiltrate then further impairs lymphatic vessel contractility and hence lymphatic fluid transport [4]. This inflammatory process leads to extracellular matrix remodeling and fibrosis, hypoxia-mediated adipose tissue hypertrophy, and progressive sclerosis of the lymphatic vessel wall resulting eventually in obliteration of the lymphatic lumen [5, 6] (see Chap. 3).

M. A. Miller (✉)
MD Anderson Cancer Center, Rehabilitation Services, Houston, TX, USA
e-mail: MAMiller1@mdanderson.org

M. V. Schaverien (✉)
Department of Plastic Surgery, The University of Texas MD Anderson Cancer Center, Houston, TX, USA
e-mail: mvschaverien@mdanderson.org

D. N. Chen (✉)
MD Anderson Cancer Center – West Houston, Rehabilitation Services, Houston, TX, USA
e-mail: DNophsker@mdanderson.org

M. V. Schaverien, J. H. Dayan (eds.), *Multimodal Management of Upper and Lower Extremity Lymphedema*,
https://doi.org/10.1007/978-3-030-93039-4_6

The International Society of Lymphology (ISL) recommends the use of CDT as the standard of care for lymphedema treatment [7]. The aim of CDT is to reduce the proteinaceous lymphatic fluid accumulation in the interstitial space, decreasing the limb volume and slowing the rate of progression of the lymphedema including adipose tissue hypertrophy by reducing the inflammatory response. The application of extrinsic compression increases the interstitial pressure, which in turn decreases the capillary filtration to reduce or prevent the accumulation of extracellular fluid, and this is the basis for compressive treatment regimens. The application of MLD and/or use of a PCD supports this process by increasing lymph transport including opening collapsed lymphatic vessels.

CDT consists of an intensive volume reduction phase to reduce the pitting edema until the limb volume plateaus, followed by a maintenance phase to stabilize the limb volume [1] (Table 6.1). The reduction phase predominantly consists of compressive therapy using low-stretch bandaging, although reduction garments are an alternative. This is supplemented by MLD, skin and nail care, and specialist exercises [2, 3]. Once a stable maximal lymph volume reduction is achieved with minimal or no pitting edema, typically after 2–4 weeks of intensive therapy, maintenance therapy is then instituted using compression garments, specialist exercises, and skin and nail care. Patient education to reduce the risk of developing cellulitis is also important [7]. This includes moisturizing the limb to prevent desiccation and subsequent skin breakdown that can cause cellulitis. Protective clothing should also be worn to prevent incidental trauma that can lead to cellulitis. Patients elevate the affected extremity when able. Exercise is encouraged and patients are allowed to participate in all activities. Exercise improves lymphedema by stimulating muscle contraction and proximal lymph flow. Patients should maintain a normal body mass index (BMI) because obesity can worsen lymphatic dysfunction; although there are no dietary restrictions, many patients find a low-salt diet beneficial.

The effectiveness of CDT at reducing the volume of the affected limb and improving quality of life has been demonstrated in several studies [8–11]. A recent systematic review of outcomes of CDT including eight randomized controlled trials and ten prospective cohort studies demonstrated that CDT is effective at reducing limb volume [12]. Many of these studies though combined CDT with other interventions, making it difficult to determine effectiveness of the single components of CDT.

The individual components of CDT include the following:

Wrapping with Low-Stretch Bandages

Wrapping with low-stretch bandages is a major part of the volume reduction phase. Low-stretch bandages are woven with cotton fibers and stretch to around 30–60% of their length, applying a low pressure that increases with muscular contracture during exercises to promote flow of excess interstitial fluid out of the extremity. The bandages are typically worn for 23 h and reapplied daily as they tend to slip as the limb circumference reduces.

The low-stretch bandage is wrapped in multiple layers (typically two to four) after covering the affected limb with padding composed of foam or cotton batting (Fig. 6.1). "Chip bags" or dense foam can be used for areas of fibrosis. Kinesio tape can be also be used under the bandaging as an adjunct to improve the lymph fluid drainage with limb movement. The bandages exert a high pressure during activity, and a low but even pressure during rest, and are worn on a 23-h basis during active treatment. The PCD can be used once the bandages are removed. The bandaging should initially be applied and taught by a lymphedema therapist, applying the bandage without undue pressure or tightness that can cause pain. The bandages are applied progressively from distal (hand or foot, including the fingers or toes if affected) to proximal (axilla or groin, respectively). Therapist-directed bandaging is continued until the patient and/or carers learn to perform it self-directed. An alternative to low-stretch bandaging in selected patients is the use of a made-to-measure Circaid redux garment [13].

The aim during the maintenance phase is to achieve stable limb volume without recurrence of the edema, and patient compliance is key to achieving a stable volume reduction [14]. Overnight bandaging is recommended during the long-term maintenance phase while a compression garment is worn during the day; an alternative in the chronic maintenance phase is use of a Circaid device or JoViPak. During this phase, follow-up visits are scheduled every 6 months, and then annually thereafter to ensure stable volume and reinforce technique. Wrapping supplies need to be replaced every 3–6 months to maintain correct compression.

Prior to lower extremity wrapping, Ankle- or Toe-Brachial Index (ABI/TBI) measurements are performed. The use of compression should be avoided in those diagnosed with arterial insufficiency, active cellulitis, or uncontrolled congestive cardiac failure, and used with caution in diabetics with peripheral neuropathy. The effectiveness of compression bandaging in treating lymphedema during the reduction phase is supported by the results of several randomized control trials; in one study of women with arm lymphedema, an average limb volume reduction of 53% at 1 month was achieved [15].

Manual Lymphatic Drainage (MLD)

MLD is a specialist lymphatic drainage technique practiced and taught by lymphedema therapists. It is indicated in patients with pitting edema of the extremity, trunk, or chest wall, with fibrotic or sclerotic tissue changes, and in those

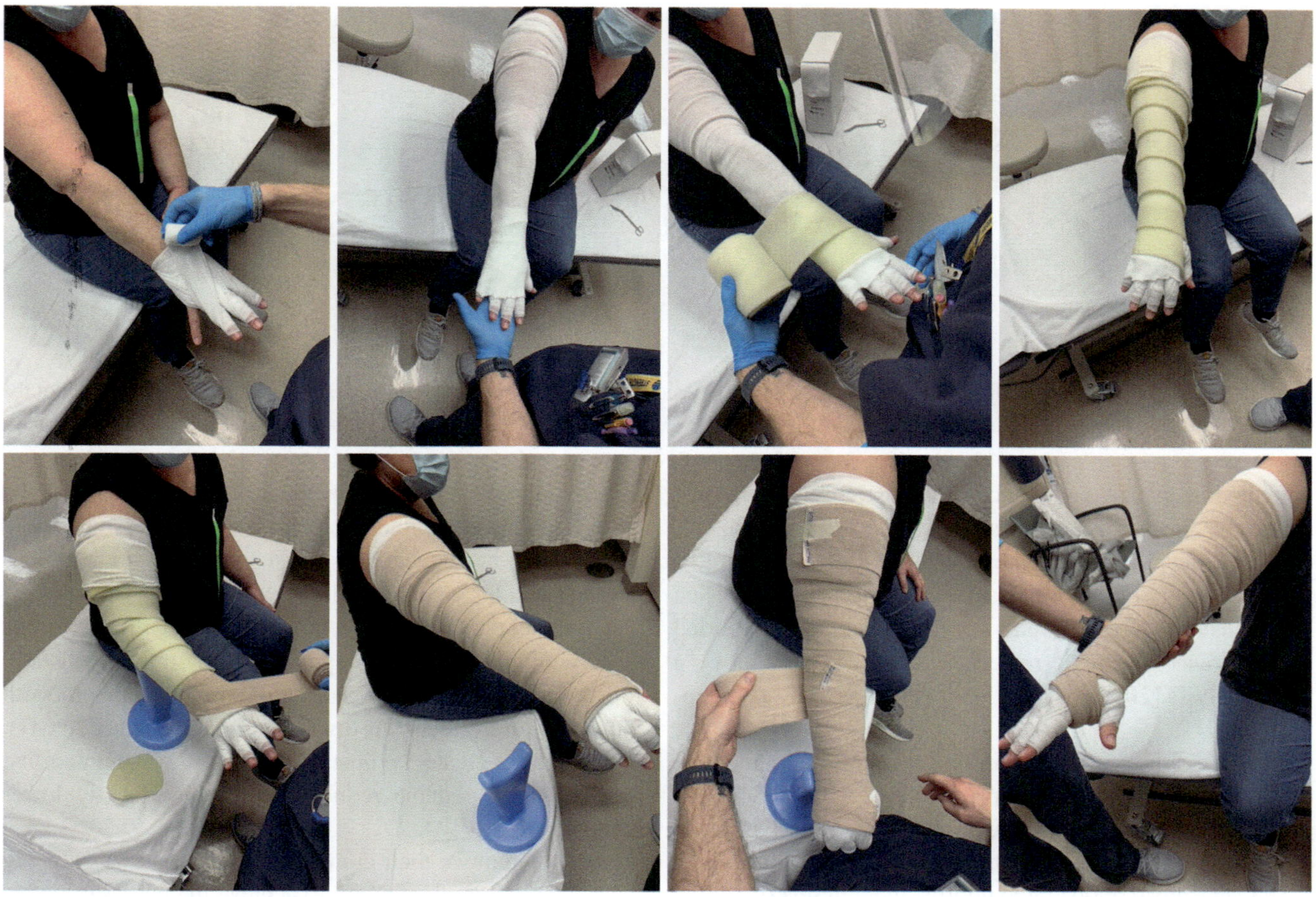

Fig. 6.1 Technique of wrapping with low-stretch bandages. The low-stretch bandage is wrapped in multiple layers (typically two to four layers) after covering the affected limb with padding composed of foam (or cotton batting). The bandaging should initially be applied and taught by a lymphedema therapist, applying the bandage without undue pressure or tightness that can cause pain. Here the bandages are applied progressively from the hand distally, including the fingers, to the axilla proximally. Therapist-directed bandaging is continued until the patient and/or carers learn to perform it self-directed

with lymphedema symptoms including heaviness or tightness. The purpose of MLD is to increase the transit of lymphatic fluid through directional gentle manual pressure from areas of congestion to adjacent lymphatics in non-edematous regions by developing new lymphatic channels and inducing lymphatic vessel wall contractility.

There are several technical variations of MLD, including the Földi, Vodder, Leduc, or Casley-Smith methods, among others, that share common processes [11]. Typically, manual decongestion is performed in sequence from proximal to the distal, starting with the non-edematous quadrant of the trunk, then the edematous trunk quadrant, next the proximal aspect of the edematous extremity, and lastly the distal part of the edematous extremity (Fig. 6.2). Soft tissue release is performed before commencing MLD if adhesions are present that are impeding lymph fluid flow, and treatment can be directed to treat localized fibrotic tissue deposits. Each session typically lasts around 30–60 min, and the sessions are performed at least three times a week for 2–6 weeks as necessary.

To be effective, MLD is performed as an adjunctive treatment in combination regimens during the intensive reduction phase of CDT, immediately prior to applying bandaging [16, 17], and is particularly useful for treating edematous regions that are not easily amenable to compression, including the breast, trunk, inguinal region, and head and neck [11]. It can also be a component of the maintenance phase where it is performed in a self-directed fashion (SLD). Like bandaging, regular follow-up with a lymphedema therapist is advised to check compliance, reinforce technique, and maintain motivation. Disadvantages of MLD include substantial time burden for patients, reliance on a provider for treatment, and cost. The techniques are most helpful in managing early/mild disease and are less effective in chronic lymphedema characterized by fibroadipose tissue predominance. MLD is contraindicated or relatively contraindicated in patients with

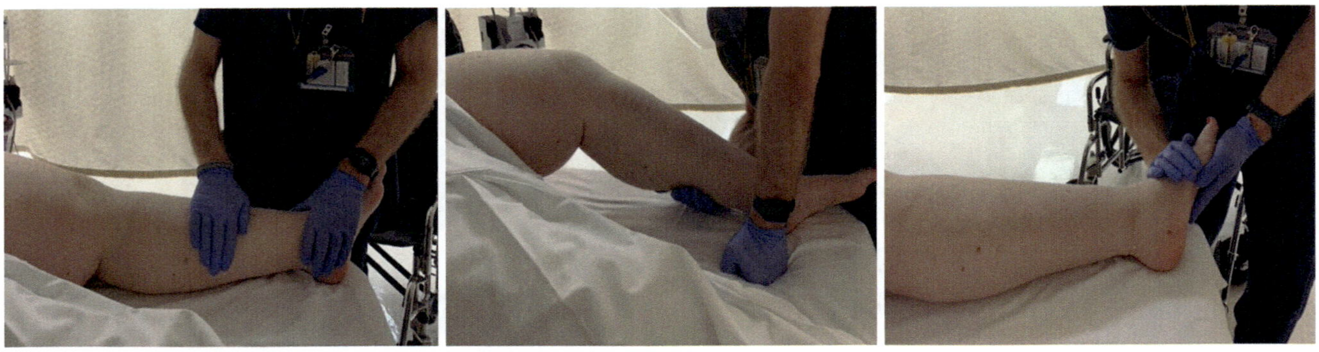

Fig. 6.2 Technique of manual lymphatic drainage (MLD). Manual decongestion is performed in sequence, starting at the proximal aspect of the edematous extremity, and finishing at the distal part of the edematous extremity

untreated neoplasia/malignancy of the extremity or regional lymphatic basin, decompensated right-sided heart failure, untreated deep vein thrombosis of the affected extremity, active cellulitis of the limb, acute asthma, or uncontrolled hypertension. The effectiveness of the technique is supported by Cochrane systematic reviews [18, 19], as well as by a meta-analysis [20], provided that it is delivered as a component of CDT.

A recent advance has been the use of indocyanine green (ICG) fluorescent lymphography to guide MLD. ICG fluorescent lymphography enables visualization of lymphatic fluid localization in the interstitial space as dermal backflow [21]. One study demonstrated improvement in severity of the pathological pattern of the lymphedema in 42% of patients studied following ICG-guided MLD [22], and another study demonstrated a 23% mean increase in lymph vessel contraction speed immediately following MLD [23].

Pneumatic Compression Device (PCD)

Intermittent pneumatic compression increases the transport of lymph by mechanically directing the flow of the lymph fluid to functional lymphatics and may help to open lymphatics considered to be obstructed or fibrosed. It may be used adjunctively with bandaging during the intensive reduction phase to reduce the pitting edema, as well as for maintenance in conjunction with compression garments to prevent its recurrence [7, 24]. The effectiveness of the addition of pneumatic compression using a PCD (also termed as pneumatic sequential gradient pump) to CDT for lymphedema of the upper or lower extremities in reducing limb volume is well-established, with extremity volume reduced by up to two-thirds using daily pneumatic compression [24–29]. Intermittent pneumatic compression therapy can be performed unaided by the patient at home, and treatment is not dependent on a therapist; it is particularly useful for lower extremity lymphedema where effective SLD is difficult to perform. PCDs deliver intermittent pressure through an inflatable sleeve consisting of multiple chambers, sequential inflation of which propagates directional flow [30]. They vary by manufacturer in the amount of pressure applied, the pattern of delivery, and the total time of compression. These devices may be sequential/nonsequential and gradient/non-gradient and have single/multiple compartments. A sequential, gradient device with multiple compartments most closely mimics physiologic lymph flow by inflating distally followed by the expansion of more proximal chambers, with more force delivered in the distal chambers. Advanced PCDs, which have greater adjustability and programmability, achieve greater edema reduction and consequently lower rates of cellulitis [24, 29].

Patients remove their compression garments when using the sequential gradient pump to achieve the necessary interstitial pressure. The upper extremity is typically treated at 30 mmHg pressure and the lower extremity at 35–40 mmHg pressure. In advanced lymphedema with a significant fibrotic component, MLD can be a useful adjunct to improve the soft tissue compliance and therefore increase the effectiveness of the PCD [30]. Devices are usually set for around 50–60 min of treatment and patients are encouraged to use them daily [31, 32]; patients can increase the treatment duration to up to 2 h if necessary. Pneumatic compression therapy is contraindicated in patients with an active infection or deep vein thrombosis in the limb, local malignancy, or that are receiving scheduled anticoagulant therapy [33].

Exercises

Exercises involving the affected extremity are an important component of CDT, in particular for upper extremity lymphedema [2]. These include range of motion exercises, dynamic or isometric exercises against resistance, and also aerobic exercises. Progression of the repetitions and load is performed under the supervision of a trained lymphedema therapist to avoid limb fatigue or injury which may exacerbate the edema. Exercise of any intensity is recommended for patients with lymphedema as it does not cause worsening and may improve or prevent it [34, 35]. Significant reductions in arm volume and subjective patient measures have been demonstrated for aquatic therapy, swimming, resistance exercises, yoga, aerobic, and gravity-resistive exercise; swimming, in particular, is helpful because it avoids dependency of both the upper and lower extremities. Additionally, weightbearing exercises can be performed safely under a supervised program in patients with lymphedema or those at risk of developing it [34]. These exercises have been shown to increase the rate of transport of the lymphatic fluid to the venous circulation by up to three- to fourfold. When performed while wearing low-stretch bandaging or a compression garment, muscular contraction against the compression further facilitates lymph transit [33, 36]. The Strength After Breast Cancer program is an evidence-based rehabilitative exercise program for breast cancer survivors in which therapists can be certified. Self-directed lymphedema-specific regular daily exercises are recommended both during the reduction phase and in particular during the maintenance phase.

Skin Care and Cellulitis Risk Reduction

All patients need to be educated in the importance of skin and nail care, as well as other risk-reducing precautions, to lower the risk of cellulitis that patients with lymphedema are more susceptible to. Cellulitis can necessitate inpatient treatment, and recurrent episodes exacerbate the fibrosis of the lymphatic vessels and lead to a more advanced lymphedema stage. Daily skin cleansing and moisturizer application should be performed to avoid drying and cracking of the skin under the compression garments. Patients should inspect their affected arm or leg daily and seek medical help right away if they develop any signs of infection. They need to avoid any injury to the affected limb and treat injuries immediately to avoid infection. Sensible precautions include wearing long oven mitts when cooking, gloves when gardening or doing yard work, and high-factor sunblock or long-sleeved clothing to avoid sunburn. Patients should use insect repellant spray when outside, avoid using a razor and instead use an electric shaver or cream for hair removal, avoid moving or carrying very heavy objects or fatiguing the limb, and avoid sauna use. General risk-reducing behavior includes maintaining an active lifestyle and healthy weight, and beginning a weight-loss program if overweight [37]. Blood pressure readings and blood draws (following appropriate skin asepsis) from the affected arm can be performed safely although patients may prefer to use their unaffected arm where practical to do so [38].

Patients that develop an episode of cellulitis should immediately contact their medical provider and will likely need antibiotics; they typically should discontinue compression and elevate the extremity until cleared by their doctor, typically until after 72 h of being on antibiotics once there is resolution of the cellulitis. If there is significant resultant pitting edema, then these patients may benefit from a return to bandaging for reduction. Patients experiencing three or more episodes of cellulitis each year may benefit from chronic suppressive antibiotic therapy active against *Streptococcus pyogenes*.

Compression Garments

Elastic compression garments form the mainstay of lymphedema maintenance, and in some patients may substitute multilayer compression bandaging in the reductive phase [39]. Lifelong compliance with a compression garment of suitable fitment and compression is essential to control the edema and prevent progression of lymphedema. Patients typically wear compression garments throughout the day, and either perform wrapping at night or use a specialized garment such as a Circaid device or JoViPak.

Compression garments deliver pressures of 20–60 mmHg, with grading differing between manufacturers and garment types, aiming to achieve minimal or no pitting edema. The compression requirements may differ between patients and need to be individualized, guided by a trained lymphedema therapist, including the necessary frequency of ordering of new garments and the degree of compression required. Patients need to be fitted by a trained lymphedema therapist for a garment of sufficient compression class to maintain the limb volume with minimal or no pitting edema, and that they can tolerate and will maintain compliance with.

Compression garments differ between manufacturers and are woven either as flat-knitted with a seam or circular-knitted garments without a seam, and may be custom-made or "off-the-shelf." The higher compression class (CCL) garments are typically flat-knitted. Compression garments for the arm and hand are usually ordered in CCL 1 (15–21 mmHg) or more commonly CCL 2 (23–32 mmHg). Compression garments for the leg are typically CCL 3 (34–46 mmHg), although CCL 4 (49+ mmHg) may occasionally be required, or alternatively the use of double-layered compression garments. Flat knit is preferable to circular knit in patients with deep folds to avoid skin breakdown.

The advantages of "off-the-shelf" compression garments are their greater availability, ease of measurement, and range of colors and designs. Although these may be suitable for early-stage mild lymphedema [40], the elastic material used may result in compromised durability of compression; for more advanced-stage lymphedema phenotypes, custom garments conform better to the limb and provide more homogenous compression throughout the limb. Custom garments may be progressively tightened (controlled compression therapy, CCT), and extremity volume may be reduced by almost 50% over 1 year. The disadvantage is that their measurement requires a skilled lymphedema therapist or manufacturer representative, and they need to be constructed and delivered from the manufacturer. If fitment of the garment is not ideal, then manufacturers offer a return time window for necessary adjustments although these may again need to be made by the lymphedema therapist. For the arm, garments may include the hand or fingers, or a separate glove or gauntlet can be worn, and may incorporate a silicon band or shoulder strap to prevent slippage. For legs, garments can include the whole leg, may include the foot or have a separate toe cap, or can be only below the knee, or thigh-only; the top of the garment may differ, such as having a silicon band or belt for around the waist to reduce slippage. Adjunctive devices can be used to facilitate donning of the garment, and undergarments can be used to improve comfort.

Compression garments need to be replaced on a regular basis to maintain sufficient compression. Each garment should ideally be washed every 1–2 days to restore the compression and replaced after 3 months of continuous daily use – very active patients though may require these to be replaced more often. For custom garments, it is therefore prudent that after good fitment of a newly measured garment is confirmed, a second is ordered so that the garments can be alternated. During the first 12 months, patients should be seen frequently by a lymphedema therapist and remeasured until a plateau is reached, then around once every 12 months. Occasionally, patients will experience significant recurrence of pitting edema during the maintenance phase necessitating return to the reductive phase of CDT.

Ultimately, it must be remembered that the best compression garment is one that the patient will be compliant with wearing: wearing an off-the-shelf compression sleeve may therefore be better suited to selected patients over custom medical grade garments. This is particularly an issue with adolescents/young adults where the appearance of a custom garment and its impact on clothing selection may adversely affect compliance, and off-the-shelf garments can be used if it is the only option to achieve compliance.

Other Therapies

Nonsurgical treatments other than CDT can be considered for the treatment of lymphedema. A systematic review of complementary, alternative, and other non-CDT lymphedema treatments found that use of these treatments is widespread [41]. The lymphedema modalities evaluated included ultrasound therapy, electrically stimulated lymphatic drainage, high-voltage electrical stimulation, diathermy, low-level laser therapy, hyperbaric oxygen therapy, elastic taping, and acupuncture. The review concluded that the evidence supporting the use of any of these therapies remains limited. There is also insufficient evidence to support the use of Kinesio tape alone [42]. Diuretics are no longer indicated as they are ineffective in lymphedema and may exacerbate the disease by increasing the concentration of the interstitial proteins. Coumarin, a benzopyrone immunomodulator, is also not recommended as it has minimal efficacy and may cause hepatotoxicity.

Maintaining a stable normal body weight is important and weight loss should be undertaken if necessary. Although evidence for superiority between differed weight-loss methods and diets is limited, a small study found that a ketogenic diet reduced limb volume and improved quality of life in obese patients with limb lymphedema, however further evidence is needed [43].

Prehabilitation for Lymphedema Surgery

There is increasing recognition of the importance of the role of *prehabilitation* to optimize patients *before* lymphedema surgery, rather than the traditional approach of delivering this lymphedema therapy mainly postoperatively. Although prehabilitation is a multifaceted approach, the mainstay is completion of a full course of optimized conservative lymphedema physical therapy as above, with demonstration of continuous compliance with this optimal conservative therapy for a minimum of 3 months preoperatively. This principally aids in patient selection as unanticipated noncompliance can adversely affect surgical outcomes, ensures good fitment of a compression garment of the necessary compression class that will be required during the postoperative rehabilitative phase, and in addition optimizes conditions for surgery by transition toward the maintenance phase with a reduction in inflammation [44].

References

1. Cheville AL, McGarvey CL, Petrek JA, Russo SA, Taylor ME, Thiadens SR. Lymphedema management. Semin Radiat Oncol. 2003;13:290–301.
2. Ko DS, Lerner R, Klose G, Cosimi AB. Effective treatment of lymphedema of the extremities. Arch Surg. 1998;133:452–8.
3. Szuba A, Cooke JP, Yousuf S, Rockson SG. Decongestive lymphatic therapy for patients with cancer-related or primary lymphedema. Am J Med. 2000;109:296–300.
4. Avraham T, Zampell JC, Yan A, et al. Th2 differentiation is necessary for soft tissue fibrosis and lymphatic dysfunction resulting from lymphedema. FASEB J. 2013;27:1114–26.
5. Mihara M, Hara H, Hayashi Y, et al. Pathological steps of cancer-related lymphedema: histological changes in the collecting lymphatic vessels after lymphadenectomy. PLoS One. 2012;7:e41126.
6. Zampell JC, Yan A, Elhadad S, Avraham T, Weitman E, Mehrara BJ. CD4(+) cells regulate fibrosis and lymphangiogenesis in response to lymphatic fluid stasis. PLoS One. 2012;7:e49940.
7. International Society of Lymphology. The diagnosis and treatment of peripheral lymphedema: 2013 consensus document of the International Society of Lymphology. Lymphology. 2013;46:1–11.
8. Smile TD, Tendulkar R, Schwarz G, Arthur D, Grobmyer S, Valente S, Vicini F, Shah C. A review of treatment for breast cancer-related lymphedema: paradigms for clinical practice. Am J Clin Oncol. 2018 Feb;41(2):178–90.

9. Haghighat S, Lotfi-Tokaldany M, Maboudi AA, et al. Predictive factors of response to phase I complete decongestive therapy in upper extremity lymphedema following breast carcinoma in Iran. Lymphology. 2013;46:97–104.
10. Vignes S, Blanchard M, Arrault M, et al. Intensive complete decongestive physiotherapy for cancer-related upper-limb lymphedema: 11 days achieved greater volume reduction than 4. Gynecol Oncol. 2013;131:127–30.
11. Atalay OT, Özkir A, Çalik BB, Baskan E, Taşkin H. Effects of phase I complex decongestive physiotherapy on physical functions and depression levels in breast cancer related lymphedema. J Phys Ther Sci. 2015;27:865–70.
12. Lasinski BB, McKillip Thrift K, Squire D, et al. A systematic review of the evidence for complete decongestive therapy in the treatment of lymphedema from 2004 to 2011. PM R. 2012;4:580–601.
13. Borman P, Koyuncu EG, Yaman A, Calp E, Koç F, Sargut R, Karahan S. The comparative efficacy of conventional short-stretch multilayer bandages and velcro adjustable compression wraps in active treatment phase of patients with lower limb lymphedema. Lymphat Res Biol. 2020;19(3):286–94.
14. Vignes S, Porcher R, Arrault M, Dupuy A. Factors influencing breast cancer-related lymphedema volume after intensive decongestive physiotherapy. Support Care Cancer. 2011;19:935–40.
15. Smykla A, Walewicz K, Trybulski R, et al. Effect of kinesiology taping on breast cancer-related lymphedema: a randomized single blind controlled pilot study. Biomed Res Int. 2013;2013:767106.
16. McNeely ML, Magee DJ, Lees AW, Bagnall KM, Haykowsky M, Hanson J. The addition of manual lymph drainage to compression therapy for breast cancer related lymphedema: a randomized controlled trial. Breast Cancer Res Treat. 2004;86:95–106.
17. Ezzo J, Manheimer E, McNeely ML, et al. Manual lymphatic drainage for lymphedema following breast cancer treatment. Cochrane Database Syst Rev. 2015;5:CD003475.
18. Stuiver MM, Ten Tusscher MR, Agasi-Idenburg CS, et al. Conservative interventions for preventing clinically detectable upper-limb lymphoedema in patients who are at risk of developing lymphoedema after breast cancer therapy. Cochrane Database Syst Rev. 2015;2:CD009765.
19. Shao Y, Zhong DS. Manual lymphatic drainage for breast cancer-related lymphoedema. Eur J Cancer Care (Engl). 2017;26(5) https://doi.org/10.1111/ecc.12517.
20. Koelmeyer LA, Thompson BM, Mackie H, et al. Personalizing conservative lymphedema management using indocyanine green-guided manual lymphatic drainage. Lymphat Res Biol. 2020;19(1):56–65.
21. Medina-Rodríguez ME, de-la-Casa-Almeida M, González Martín J, et al. Changes in indocyanine green lymphography patterns after physical treatment in secondary upper limb lymphedema. J Clin Med. 2020;22:9.
22. Tan IC, Maus EA, Rasmussen JC, Marshall MV, Adams KE, Fife CE, Smith LA, Chan W, Sevick-Muraca EM. Assessment of lymphatic contractile function after manual lymphatic drainage using near-infrared fluorescence imaging. Arch Phys Med Rehabil. 2011;92:756–64.
23. Fife CE, Davey S, Maus EA, Guilliod R, Mayrovitz HN. A randomized controlled trial comparing two types of pneumatic compression for breast cancer-related lymphedema treatment in the home. Support Care Cancer. 2012;20:3279–86.
24. Harris SR, Schmitz KH, Campbell KL, McNeely ML. Clinical practice guidelines for breast cancer rehabilitation: syntheses of guideline recommendations and qualitative appraisals. Cancer. 2012;118:2312–24.
25. Szolnoky G, Lakatos B, Keskeny T, et al. Intermittent pneumatic compression acts synergistically with manual lymphatic drainage in complex decongestive physiotherapy for breast cancer treatment-related lymphedema. Lymphology. 2009;42:188–94.
26. Johansson K, Lie E, Ekdahl C, Lindfeldt J. A randomized study comparing manual lymph drainage with sequential pneumatic compression for treatment of postoperative arm lymphedema. Lymphology. 1998;31:56–64.
27. Szuba A, Achalu R, Rockson SG. Decongestive lymphatic therapy for patients with breast carcinoma associated lymphedema. A randomized, prospective study of a role for adjunctive intermittent pneumatic compression. Cancer. 2002;95:2260–7.
28. Muluk SC, Hirsch AT, Taffe EC. Pneumatic compression device treatment of lower extremity lymphedema elicits improved limb volume and patient-reported outcomes. Eur J Vasc Endovasc Surg. 2013;46:480–7.
29. Feldman JL, Stout NL, Wanchai A, Stewart BR, Cormier JN, Armer JM. Intermittent pneumatic compression therapy: a systematic review. Lymphology. 2012;45:13–25.
30. Raines JK, O'Donnell TF Jr, Kalisher L, Darling RC. Selection of patients with lymphedema for compression therapy. Am J Surg. 1977;133:430–7.
31. Ridner SH, McMahon E, Dietrich MS, Hoy S. Home based lymphedema treatment in patients with cancer related lymphedema or non cancer-related lymphedema. Oncol Nurs Forum. 2008;35:671–80.
32. Zaleska M, Olszewski WL, Durlik M. The effectiveness of intermittent pneumatic compression in long term therapy of lymphedema of lower limbs. Lymphat Res Biol. 2014;12:103–9.
33. Brennan MJ, Miller LT. Overview of treatment options and review of the current role and use of compression garments, intermittent pumps, and exercise in the management of lymphedema. Cancer. 1998;83:2821–7.
34. Schmitz KH, Ahmed RL, Troxel A, et al. Weight lifting in women with breast-cancer-related lymphedema. N Engl J Med. 2009;361(07):664–73.
35. Baumann FT, Reike A, Reimer V, Schumann M, Hallek M, Taaffe DR, Newton RU, Galvao DA. Effects of physical exercise on breast cancer-related secondary lymphedema: a systematic review. Breast Cancer Res Treat. 2018;170:1–13.
36. Johansson K, Tibe K, Weibull A, Newton RC. Low intensity resistance exercise for breast cancer patients with arm lymphedema with or without compression sleeve. Lymphology. 2005;38:167–80.
37. Ridner SH, Dietrich MS, Stewart BR, Armer JM. Body mass index and breast cancer treatment- related lymphedema. Support Care Cancer. 2011;19:853–7.
38. Asdourian MS, Skolny MN, Brunelle C, Seward CE, Salama L, Taghian AG. Precautions for breast cancer-related lymphoedema: risk from air travel, ipsilateral arm blood pressure measurements, skin puncture, extreme temperatures, and cellulitis. Lancet Oncol. 2016;17:392–405.
39. Dayes IS, Whelan TJ, Julian JA, et al. Randomized trial of decongestive lymphatic therapy for the treatment of lymphedema in women with breast cancer. J Clin Oncol. 2013;31:3758–63.
40. Stout Gergich NL, Pfalzer LA, McGarvey C, et al. Preoperative assessment enables the early diagnosis and successful treatment of lymphedema. Cancer. 2008;112:2809–19.
41. Rodrick JR, Poage E, Wanchai A, Stewart BR, Cormier JN, Armer JM. Complementary, alternative, and other non complete decongestive therapy treatment methods in the management of lymphedema: a systematic search and review. PM R. 2014;6:250–74.
42. Torres-Lacomba M, Navarro-Brazález B, Prieto-Gómez V, Ferrandez JC, Bouchet JY, Romay-Barrero H. Effectiveness of four types of bandages and kinesio-tape for treating breast-cancer-related lymphoedema: a randomized, single-blind, clinical trial. Clin Rehabil. 2020;34:1230–41.
43. Keith L, Rowsemitt C, Richards LG. Lifestyle modification group for lymphedema and obesity results in significant health outcomes. Am J Lifestyle Med. 2017;14(4):420–8.
44. Yamamoto R, Yamamoto T. Effectiveness of the treatment-phase of two-phase complex decongestive physiotherapy for the treatment of extremity lymphedema. Int J Clin Oncol. 2007;12:463–8.

7 Key Topic: Patient Selection and Evidence-Based Algorithmic Approach to Surgical Management of Lymphedema

Mark V. Schaverien and Joseph H. Dayan

Introduction

The multimodal evaluation of patients presenting with limb swelling is essential for correct diagnosis, to exclude other causes of swelling, and to accurately stage their lymphedema to direct the optimal nonsurgical and surgical treatment. There are certain situations where surgery to treat lymphedema is not indicated, and treatment decisions may be made within a multidisciplinary team. Several studies have demonstrated that surgery for lymphedema results in better outcomes than for conservative therapy alone [1–4]. Comorbid conditions, such as obesity and venous insufficiency, which are diagnosed during work-up, may require management before lymphedema surgery is indicated. Outcomes of surgery may be improved if patients are optimized *prior* to surgery through *prehabilitation*, predominantly involving optimizing the delivery and effectiveness of their conservative therapy. To be eligible for surgery, patients must have completed a course of complete decongestive therapy (CDT) and maintained continuous compliance with optimal conservative therapy for at least 3 months.

The current evidence and published algorithms for lymphedema surgeries support that lymphovenous bypass (LVB) is indicated for early stage lymphedema and vascularized lymph node transplant (VLNT) for advanced lymphedema. Debulking surgeries including minimally invasive suction-assisted lipectomy (SAL) with controlled compression therapy (CCT), or rarely direct excisional procedures, are indicated for advanced chronic lymphedema characterized by significant soft tissue excess [3–11]. Combination approaches, including performing LVB synchronously with VLNT, and performing SAL either following [12–15], or in preparation for [16], physiological surgeries (LVB and/or VLNT), have demonstrated improved outcomes by extending the indications for physiological surgery to those with significant soft tissue excess.

Monitoring for lymphedema in patients at risk following breast cancer surgery through a prospective lymphedema screening program is recommended, including preoperative baseline measurements, to diagnose patients at the earliest stages of lymphedema when their condition is most amenable to treatment. In this chapter, we present criteria for patient selection and an evidenced-based algorithmic approach to surgery for patients presenting with lymphedema (Fig. 7.1).

Diagnosis and Staging

Diagnosis is conducted as previously outlined by a focused clinical history (including duration, previous treatments and compliance, reversibility, and cellulitis episodes) and evaluation of symptoms (in particular swelling and heaviness), physical examination (presence, severity, and localization of pitting edema; Stemmer sign; severity and distribution of fibroadipose soft tissue excess; evaluation of comorbid venous insufficiency), limb volume measurements, and LDex score [17–26].

The presence of dermal backflow on contrast-enhanced imaging of the lymphatic system is diagnostic for lymphedema, with the severity and distribution of this backflow correlating closely with the pathological condition of the lymphatic vessels [20, 27, 28]. Indocyanine green (ICG) fluorescent lymphography enables detailed dynamic functional evaluation of the superficial lymphatic system [29], and is the most commonly used modality for lymphedema diagnosis and staging, evaluating the lymphatic transport, identifying functional lymphatic vessels, and evaluating the

M. V. Schaverien (✉)
Department of Plastic Surgery, The University of Texas MD Anderson Cancer Center, Houston, TX, USA
e-mail: mvschaverien@mdanderson.org

J. H. Dayan (✉)
Division of Plastic and Reconstructive Surgery, Memorial Sloan Kettering Cancer Center, New York, NY, USA
e-mail: dayanj@mskcc.org

M. V. Schaverien, J. H. Dayan (eds.), *Multimodal Management of Upper and Lower Extremity Lymphedema*,
https://doi.org/10.1007/978-3-030-93039-4_7

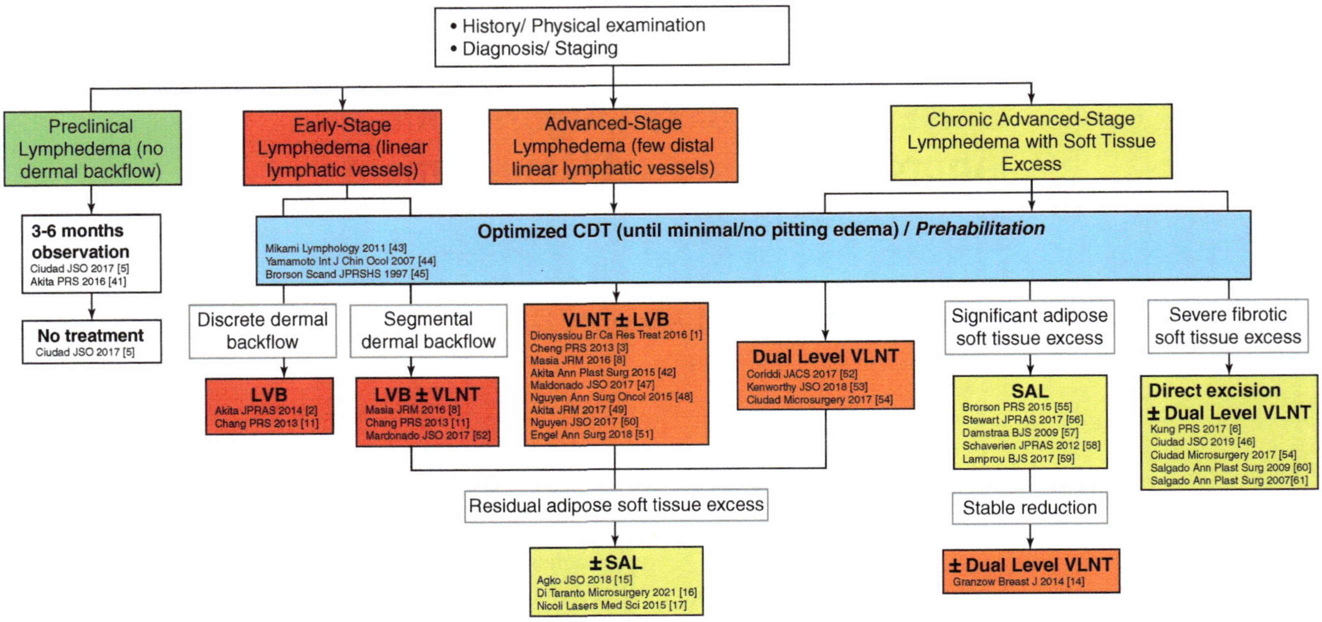

Fig. 7.1 An evidenced-based algorithm for patients presenting with lymphedema. ICG indocyanine green, MR magnetic resonance, UE upper extremity, LE lower extremity, CDT complete decongestive therapy, LVB lymphovenous bypass, VLNT vascularized lymph node transplant, SAL suction-assisted lipectomy

pattern and distribution of the dermal backflow [20, 27–31]. It is an important tool for surgical decision-making in determining suitability for LVB by the presence of obstructed linear lymphatic vessels, and the optimal recipient site for VLNT (orthotopic versus heterotopic/dual-level). Validated lymphedema staging systems using ICG fluorescent lymphography include the MD Anderson Cancer Center (MDACC) Lymphedema Staging Scale [10–12] and the Dermal Backflow Staging System [29, 30]. Other imaging modalities include magnetic resonance lymphangiography (MRL), which enables global detailed visualization of individual lymphatic vessels and lymph nodes and can be used both for diagnosis of lymphedema and for surgical planning [31], and radioisotope lymphoscintigraphy, which allows for the global serial assessment of lymphatic physiological function and lymphatic fluid transit, as well as of the draining lymph nodes [32, 33].

Several clinical staging systems for lymphedema derived from these imaging modalities have been reported [8, 9, 20, 27, 28, 33–36], which may aid in informing treatment algorithms and in evaluating the outcomes of surgery, and all are in general agreement regarding the indications for LVB, VLNT, and SAL.

Patient Selection for Surgical Intervention

Patients with a diagnosis of lymphedema confirmed on lymphatic imaging, and where other causes of limb swelling have been excluded, are potentially candidates for surgery. Patients with untreated or uncontrolled primary cancer or locoregional recurrence, or those medically unfit to undergo surgery, should receive optimized nonsurgical management only. Cardiopulmonary considerations are typically the main determinants for microsurgical candidacy – optimizing these systems will help to minimize the risks associated with long operative interventions and anesthesia-related morbidity. Those that experience frequent episodes of cellulitis (three or more a year) despite compliance with optimized conservative therapy may require perioperative prophylactic antibiotics active against *Streptococcus pyogenes*, as the presence of an active infection is a contraindication to lymphedema surgery.

Patients that are planned for lymphadenectomy, in particular those at high risk of developing lymphedema (risk factors including anticipated or delivered radiation therapy, taxane-based chemotherapy, and body mass index >30), are receiving bilateral lymphadenectomy, or are undergoing lymphadenectomy and have lymphedema of the contralateral extremity, may be candidates for immediate lymphatic reconstruction under reverse lymphatic mapping [37].

Preclinical Lymphedema

Patients presenting with symptoms of lymphedema but without meeting objective criteria by limb volume measurements and LDex score, and with normal lymphatic function without dermal backflow visualized on lymphatic imaging, are diagnosed with *preclinical* lymphedema and can be observed for 3–6 months followed by repeat lymphatic imaging [5].

If patients develop dermal backflow on lymphatic imaging, then in selected patients with upper extremity lymphedema a 3–6 month course of CDT is instituted [2–6, 38, 39]. This should be combined with general risk-reduction behaviors, including achieving a stable normal weight, achieving a full range of active motion of the upper extremity, and engaging purposefully in physical exercise of the arm. In these selected low-risk patients with upper extremity lymphedema, treatment with 3–6 months of CDT and engaging in risk-reduction measures may result in downstaging of the lymphedema to the *preclinical* stage without the need for ongoing treatment; it is imperative that these patients are regularly reevaluated, with ICG lymphography imaging performed where indicated, to ensure that recurrence of their lymphedema does not occur [38].

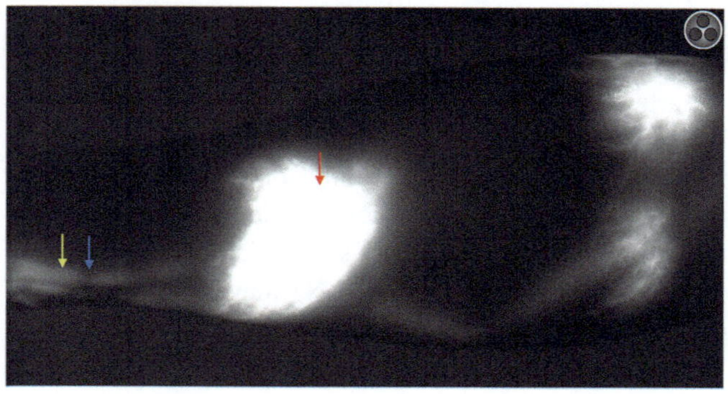

Fig. 7.2 Indocyanine green (ICG) lymphography of the upper extremity demonstrating the presence of many linear patent lymphatic vessels (*yellow arrow*) with discrete areas of dermal backflow visualized (*red arrow*). Venules crossing the lymphatic vessels can be visualized as "shadows" (*blue arrow*)

Prehabilitation

Prehabilitation has an important role in optimizing patients prior to lymphedema surgery (see Chap. 6). Although prehabilitation is a multifaceted approach, the mainstay is completion of a course of optimized conservative lymphedema physical therapy preoperatively, rather than the traditional approach of only delivering this postoperatively. Patients must have completed a full course of CDT and have demonstrated continuous compliance with optimal conservative therapy for a minimum of 3 months until there is minimal or no pitting edema. This principally aids in patient selection as unanticipated noncompliance can adversely affect surgical outcomes [4]. Another advantage of this approach is ensuring good fitment of, and hence ability to maintain compliance with, a compression garment of the required compression class that will be necessary during the postoperative rehabilitative phase. Moreover, conditions for surgery are optimized by transition toward the maintenance phase [9, 40], decreasing the inflammatory response by reducing the extracellular proteinaceous lymph fluid.

Comorbid obesity exacerbates lymphatic dysfunction which is reversible, and therefore another key component of prehabilitation is preoperative weight management toward a stable normal weight range. This may be achieved by referral to a dietician/nutritionist, or a bariatric surgeon, as indicated.

Early-Stage Lymphedema

For patients presenting soon after developing upper extremity lymphedema, where their lymphedema is at an early stage on ICG imaging, characterized by the presence of many linear patent lymphatic vessels with discrete or segmental areas of splash-pattern dermal backflow visualized (Fig. 7.2), a 3-month course of CDT is completed [2–6, 9, 38, 40]. Surgical intervention with the LVB procedure may be indicated following prehabilitation including optimization with CDT [2–4, 6, 10, 38]. Where ICG imaging demonstrates a single linear lymphatic channel reaching the axilla or inguinal region, supplemental imaging with lymphoscintigraphy or MRL is necessary to determine if the channel is draining into a lymph node within the regional lymphatic basin, in which case the lymphatic vessel continuity should be preserved.

For patients with long-term chronic lymphedema that is early-stage based on lymphatic imaging with segmental areas of dermal backflow, the lymphatic vessels available for bypass may be more fibrotic/sclerotic than is apparent from the dermal backflow pattern visualized on their imaging. Prehabilitation including optimization with CDT is performed, with reduction if required until there is minimal or no pitting edema, and the patient has been continuously complaint with custom compression garments for at least 3 months. Patients who are overweight should be encouraged to achieve a stable normal weight with referral to a dietician/nutritionist, or bariatric surgeon, as indicated. The fibrosis/sclerosis of the lymphatic vessels may adversely affect the long-term patency of the LVB procedure – therefore, for selected patients in this group, VLNT may be indicated at the time of LVB [7, 10].

In the upper extremity, the dermal backflow distribution is typically most severe proximally, and therefore orthotopic VLNT is typically indicated, with the use of reverse lymphatic mapping for intraoperative guidance to preserve any functioning lymphatic vessels/lymph nodes. Proximal transfer (including dual-level VLNT) is additionally indicated when there is tethered axillary scaring that may be impairing shoulder range of motion; lysis of scar adhesions can be performed, including those causing static or dynamic compression of the axillary vein, and the lymph node flap prevents scar recurrence. In postmastectomy lymphedema syndrome, this is typically achieved by combined deep inferior epigastric artery perforator flap breast reconstruction with composite groin VLNT. In the lower extremity, following deep inguinal/pelvic lymphadenectomy, or in primary lymphedema, care must be taken in orthotopic VLNT to avoid disruption to the otherwise intact superficial lymphatic system and lymph nodes; heterotopic VLNT may be indicated if the dermal backflow is most severe distally.

Advanced-Stage Lymphedema

For patients with advanced-stage lymphedema, characterized by few or no patent linear lymphatic vessels visualized distally and confluent splash or stardust pattern dermal backflow, prehabilitation including reductive CDT is performed until there is minimal or no pitting edema and the patient has been continuously complaint with custom compression garments for at least 3 months [9, 40, 41]. Patients that are overweight should be encouraged to achieve a stable normal weight with dietician/nutritionist, or bariatric surgical, support if necessary. In advanced-stage lymphedema, the VLNT procedure is indicated, and where obstructed lymphatic vessels are visualized, LVB is performed synchronously [1, 3, 7, 39, 42–47]. For early advanced lymphedema where the swelling and dermal backflow is localized proximally, orthotopic VLNT is indicated. In long-term chronic advanced lymphedema, the swelling is gravity dependent and therefore distally localized within the extremity, and heterotopic VLNT may be indicated. Where the whole extremity is uniformly affected, dual-level transfer (simultaneous orthotopic and heterotopic VLNT) [48–50] and synchronous LVB may be indicated [4, 11].

In primary lymphedema where the majority of patients have hypoplasia/aplasia of their lymphatics, heterotopic VLNT distally within the limb is typically indicated over orthotopic transplantation; operating in the axillary or inguinal region of a patient with primary lymphedema risks injuring functioning lymphatics and/or lymph nodes and worsening the lymphedema and localization of the lymphatic fluid is typically distally within the most gravity-dependent parts of the limb. It is important to recognize that patients with primary lymphedema are at increased risk for developing lymphedema at other sites and may be at higher risk of donor site lymphedema from the harvest of lymph nodes – omental VLNT is therefore preferred to VLN flaps harvested from the axillary or inguinal regional lymphatic basins.

Approximately 6–12 months following VLNT surgery, focused SAL can be performed if indicated, typically proximally to the upper arm/thigh, with continuation of compression garments until the postsurgical edema has resolved as appropriate [12–15].

Advanced-Stage Lymphedema with Fibroadipose Soft Tissue Excess

For patients with advanced-stage lymphedema characterized by severe stardust or diffuse pattern dermal backflow affecting the entire extremity with significant fibroadipose soft tissue excess, prehabilitation including reductive CDT is performed until there is minimal or no pitting edema and the patient has been continuously complaint with custom compression garments for at least 3 months. Patients that are overweight should be encouraged/supported to achieve a stable normal weight.

Where the limb volume excess is predominantly adipose as assessed clinically, with adjunctive MR imaging as necessary, this can be removed by SAL followed by CCT [51–55]. This is best indicated for patients experiencing significant morbidity despite maximal conservative therapy, including functional limitations, cosmetic appearance, interference with clothing fitment, or recurrent cellulitis episodes. The volume reduction achieved by SAL with CCT is typically complete for the upper extremity unless there is a significant fibrous component, and the volume reduction is usually less than this in the lower extremity due to soft tissue fibrosis. Once stable reduction has been achieved with minimal pitting edema, typically at around 6–12 months postoperatively, the patient may be a candidate for dual-level VLNT (± synchronous LVB), where indicated, to reduce their reliance on continuous compression garment use [13, 48–50].

In the most severe lymphedema cases where the soft tissue excess is predominantly fibrous, this can only be removed by direct excision [56]. Rarely the upper extremity is affected, where a modified brachioplasty excision of the upper arm is typically utilized with preservation of the draining lymphatics using ICG lymphography guidance. For the lower extremity, excision is preferentially performed using a modified Homans perforator-sparing procedure to avoid the use of skin grafts and the ensuing morbidity and scarring, with staging of the medial and lateral excisions, and, if necessary, a posterior excision. The patient may be a candidate for synchronous dual-level VLNT if indicated [6, 43, 46, 47, 57].

Summary

An evidence-based algorithmic approach to the nonsurgical and surgical management of lymphedema is essential to optimize outcomes of surgery and standardize approaches to enable pooled analysis of results. Results from future comparative outcomes studies are awaited to better define surgical treatment algorithms, in particular for newer and combination therapies.

References

1. Dionyssiou D, Demiri E, Tsimponis A, et al. A randomized control study of treating secondary stage II breast cancer-related lymphoedema with free lymph node transfer. Breast Cancer Res Treat. 2016;156:73–9.
2. Akita S, Mitsukawa N, Kuriyama M, et al. Suitable therapy options for sub-clinical and early-stage lymphoedema patients. J Plast Reconstr Aesthet Surg. 2014;67:520–5.
3. Cheng MH, Chen SC, Henry SL, et al. Vascularized groin lymph node flap transfer for postmastectomy upper limb lymphedema: flap anatomy, recipient sites, and outcomes. Plast Reconstr Surg. 2013;131:1286.
4. Schaverien MV, Asaad M, Selber JC, Liu J, Chen DN, Hall MS, Butler CE. Outcomes of vascularized lymph node transplantation for the treatment of lymphedema. J Am Coll Surg. 2021;232(6):982–94.
5. Ciudad P, Agko M, Perez Coca JJ, et al. Comparison of long-term clinical outcomes among different vascularized lymph node transfers: 6-year experience of a single center's approach to the treatment of lymphedema. J Surg Oncol. 2017;116:671–82.
6. Kung TA, Champaneria MC, Maki JH, Neligan PC. Current concepts in the surgical management of lymphedema. Plast Reconstr Surg. 2017;139:1003–13.
7. Masià J, Pons G, Rodríguez-Bauzà E. Barcelona lymphedema algorithm for surgical treatment in breast cancer-related lymphedema. J Reconstr Microsurg. 2016;32:329–35.
8. Campisi C, Bellini C, Campisi C, Accogli S, Bonioli E, Boccardo F. Microsurgery for lymphedema: clinical research and long-term results. Microsurgery. 2010;30:256–60.
9. Mikami T, Hosono M, Yabuki Y, et al. Classification of lymphoscintigraphy and relevance to surgical indication for lymphaticovenous anastomosis in upper limb lymphedema. Lymphology. 2011;44:155–67.
10. Chang DW, Suami H, Skoracki R. A prospective analysis of 100 consecutive lymphovenous bypass cases for treatment of extremity lymphedema. Plast Reconstr Surg. 2013;132:1305–14.
11. Beederman M, Garza RM, Agarwal S, Chang DW. Outcomes for physiologic microsurgical treatment of secondary lymphedema involving the extremity. Ann Surg. 2020; https://doi.org/10.1097/SLA.0000000000004457.
12. Granzow JW, Soderberg JM, Kaji AH, Dauphine C. An effective system of surgical treatment of lymphedema. Ann Surg Oncol. 2014;21:1189–94.
13. Granzow JW, Soderberg JM, Dauphine C. A novel two-stage surgical approach to treat chronic lymphedema. Breast J. 2014;20:420–2.
14. Agko M, Ciudad P, Chen HC. Staged surgical treatment of extremity lymphedema with dual gastroepiploic vascularized lymph node transfers followed by suction-assisted lipectomy-A prospective study. J Surg Oncol. 2018;117:1148–56.
15. Di Taranto G, Bolletta A, Chen SH, Losco L, Elia R, Cigna E, Rubino C, Ribuffo D, Chen HC. A prospective study on combined lymphedema surgery: gastroepiploic vascularized lymph nodes transfer and lymphaticovenous anastomosis followed by suction lipectomy. Microsurgery. 2021;41(1):34–43.
16. Nicoli F, Constantinides J, Ciudad P, et al. Free lymph node flap transfer and laser-assisted liposuction: a combined technique for the treatment of moderate upper limb lymphedema. Lasers Med Sci. 2015;30:1377–85.
17. Coroneos CJ, Wong FC, DeSnyder SM, Shaitelman SF, Schaverien MV. Correlation of L-Dex bioimpedance spectroscopy with limb volume and lymphatic function in lymphedema. Lymphat Res Biol. 2019;17:301–7.
18. Wiser I, Mehrara BJ, Coriddi M, Kenworthy E, Cavalli M, Encarnacion E, Dayan JH. Preoperative assessment of upper extremity secondary lymphedema. Cancers (Basel). 2020;12:135.
19. Thomis S, Dams L, Fourneau I, De Vrieze T, Nevelsteen I, Neven P, Gebruers N, Devoogdt N. Correlation between clinical assessment and lymphofluoroscopy in patients with breast cancer-related lymphedema: a study of concurrent validity. Lymphat Res Biol. 2020;18(6):539–48.
20. Narushima M, Yamamoto T, Ogata F, Yoshimatsu H, Mihara M, Koshima I. Indocyanine green lymphography findings in limb lymphedema. J Reconstr Microsurg. 2016;32:72–9.
21. Levenhagen K, Davies C, Perdomo M, Ryans K, Gilchrist L. Diagnosis of upper quadrant lymphedema secondary to cancer: clinical practice guideline from the Oncology Section of the American Physical Therapy Association. Phys Ther. 2017;97:729–45.
22. Stout Gergich NL, Pfalzer LA, McGarvey C, Springer B, Gerber LH, Soballe P. Preoperative assessment enables the early diagnosis and successful treatment of lymphedema. Cancer. 2008;112:2809–19.
23. Specht MC, Miller CL, Russell TA, et al. Defining a threshold for intervention in breast cancer-related lymphedema: what level of arm volume increase predicts progression? Breast Cancer Res Treat. 2013;140:485–94.
24. Fu MR, Cleland CM, Guth AA, Kayal M, Haber J, Cartwright F, Kleinman R, Kang Y, Scagliola J, Axelrod D. L-dex ratio in detecting breast cancer-related lymphedema: reliability, sensitivity, and specificity. Lymphology. 2013;46:85–96.
25. Barrio AV, Eaton A, Frazier TG. A prospective validation study of bioimpedance with volume displacement in early-stage breast cancer patients at risk for lymphedema. Ann Surg Oncol. 2015;22:S370–5.
26. Ridner SH, Dietrich MS, Spotanski K, Doersam JK, Cowher MS, Taback B, McLaughlin S, Ajkay N, Boyages J, Koelmeyer L, DeSnyder S, Shah C, Vicini F. A prospective study of L-Dex values in breast cancer patients pretreatment and through 12 months postoperatively. Lymphat Res Biol. 2018;16:435–41.
27. Hara H, Mihara M, Seki Y, Todokoro T, Iida T, Koshima I. Comparison of indocyanine green lymphographic findings with the conditions of collecting lymphatic vessels of limbs in patients with lymphedema. Plast Reconstr Surg. 2013;132:1612–8.
28. Suami H, Chang DW, Yamada K, Kimata Y. Use of indocyanine green fluorescent lymphography for evaluating dynamic lymphatic status. Plast Reconstr Surg. 2011;127:74–6.
29. Yamamoto T, Yamamoto N, Doi K, et al. Indocyanine green-enhanced lymphography for upper extremity lymphedema: a novel severity staging system using dermal backflow patterns. Plast Reconstr Surg. 2011;128:941–7.
30. Yamamoto T, Matsuda N, Doi K, et al. The earliest finding of indocyanine green lymphography in asymptomatic limbs of lower extremity lymphedema patients secondary to cancer treatment: the modified dermal backflow stage and concept of subclinical lymphedema. Plast Reconstr Surg. 2011;128:314–21.
31. Neligan PC, Kung TA, Maki JH. MR lymphangiography in the treatment of lymphedema. J Surg Oncol. 2017;115:18–22.
32. Kleinhans E, Baumeister RG, Hahn D, et al. Evaluation of transport kinetics in lymphoscintigraphy: follow-up study in patients with transplanted lymphatic vessels. Eur J Nucl Med. 1985;10:349–52.
33. Cheng MH, Pappalardo M, Lin C, Kuo CF, Lin CY, Chung KC. Validity of the novel Taiwan lymphoscintigraphy staging and correlation of Cheng lymphedema grading for unilateral extremity lymphedema. Ann Surg. 2018;268:513–25.
34. Executive Committee. The diagnosis and treatment of peripheral lymphedema: 2016 consensus document of the International Society of Lymphology. Lymphology. 2016;49:170–84.

35. Patel KM, Lin CY, Cheng MH. A prospective evaluation of lymphedema-specific quality-of-life outcomes following vascularized lymph node transfer. Ann Surg Oncol. 2015;22:2424–30.
36. Arrivé L, Derhy S, Dlimi C, El Mouhadi S, Monnier-Cholley L, Becker C. Noncontrast magnetic resonance lymphography for evaluation of lymph node transfer for secondary upper limb lymphedema. Plast Reconstr Surg. 2017;140:806–11.
37. Johnson AR, Kimball S, Epstein S, Recht A, Lin SJ, Lee BT, James TA, Singhal D. Lymphedema incidence after axillary lymph node dissection: quantifying the impact of radiation and the lymphatic microsurgical preventive healing approach. Ann Plast Surg. 2019;82(4S Suppl 3):S234–41.
38. Akita S, Nakamura R, Yamamoto N, et al. Early detection of lymphatic disorder and treatment for lymphedema following breast cancer. Plast Reconstr Surg. 2016;138:192–202.
39. Akita S, Mitsukawa N, Kuriyama M, et al. Comparison of vascularized supraclavicular lymph node transfer and lymphaticovenular anastomosis for advanced stage lower extremity lymphedema. Ann Plast Surg. 2015;74:573–9.
40. Yamamoto R, Yamamoto T. Effectiveness of the treatment- phase of two-phase complex decongestive physiotherapy for the treatment of extremity lymphoedema. Int J Clin Oncol. 2007;12:463–8.
41. Brorson H, Svensson H. Complete reduction of lymphoedema of the arm by liposuction after breast cancer. Scand J Plast Reconstr Surg Hand Surg. 1997;31:137–43.
42. Ciudad P, Manrique OJ, Adabi K, Huang TC, Agko M, Trignano E, Chang WL, Chen TW, Salgado CJ, Chen HC. Combined double vascularized lymph node transfers and modified radical reduction with preservation of perforators for advanced stages of lymphedema. J Surg Oncol. 2019;119:439–48.
43. Maldonado AA, Chen R, Chang DW. The use of supraclavicular free flap with vascularized lymph node transfer for treatment of lymphedema: a prospective study of 100 consecutive cases. J Surg Oncol. 2017;115:68–71.
44. Nguyen AT, Chang EI, Suami H, Chang DW. An algorithmic approach to simultaneous vascularized lymph node transfer with microvascular breast reconstruction. Ann Surg Oncol. 2015;22:2919–24.
45. Akita S, Tokumoto H, Yamaji Y, et al. Contribution of simultaneous breast reconstruction by deep inferior epigastric artery perforator flap to the efficacy of vascularized lymph node transfer in patients with breast cancer-related lymphedema. J Reconstr Microsurg. 2017;33:571–8.
46. Nguyen AT, Suami H, Hanasono MM, Womack VA, Wong FC, Chang EI. Long-term outcomes of the minimally invasive free vascularized omental lymphatic flap for the treatment of lymphedema. J Surg Oncol. 2017;115:84–9.
47. Engel H, Lin CY, Huang JJ, Cheng MH. Outcomes of lymphedema microsurgery for breast cancer-related lymphedema with or without microvascular breast reconstruction. Ann Surg. 2018;268:1076–83.
48. Coriddi M, Wee C, Meyerson J, Eiferman D, Skoracki R. Vascularized Jejunal mesenteric lymph node transfer: a novel surgical treatment for extremity lymphedema. J Am Coll Surg. 2017;225:650–7.
49. Kenworthy EO, Nelson JA, Verma R, Mbabuike J, Mehrara BJ, Dayan JH. Double vascularized omentum lymphatic transplant (VOLT) for the treatment of lymphedema. J Surg Oncol. 2018;117:1413–9.
50. Ciudad P, Manrique OJ, Date S, Agko M, Perez Coca JJ, Chang WL, Lo Torto F, Nicoli F, Maruccia M, López Mendoza J, Chen HC. Double gastroepiploic vascularized lymph node transfers to middle and distal limb for the treatment of lymphedema. Microsurgery. 2017;37:771–9.
51. Brorson H. Complete reduction of arm lymphedema following breast cancer – a prospective twenty-one years' study. Plast Reconstr Surg. 2015;136:134–5.
52. Stewart CJ, Munnoch DA. Liposuction as an effective treatment for lower extremity lymphoedema: a single surgeon's experience over nine years. J Plast Reconstr Aesthet Surg. 2017;71(2):239–45.
53. Damstra RJ, Voesten HG, Klinkert P, Brorson H. Circumferential suction-assisted lipectomy for lymphoedema after surgery for breast cancer. Br J Surg. 2009;96:859–64.
54. Schaverien MV, Munro KJ, Baker PA, Munnoch DA. Liposuction for chronic lymphoedema of the upper limb: 5 years of experience. J Plast Reconstr Aesthet Surg. 2012;65:935–42.
55. Lamprou DA, Voesten HG, Damstra RJ, Wikkeling OR. Circumferential suction-assisted lipectomy in the treatment of primary and secondary end-stage lymphoedema of the leg. Br J Surg. 2017;104:84–9.
56. Salgado CJ, Mardini S, Spanio S, Tang WR, Sassu P, Chen HC. Radical reduction of lymphedema with preservation of perforators. Ann Plast Surg. 2007;59:173–9.
57. Salgado CJ, Sassu P, Gharb BB, Spanio di Spilimbergo S, Mardini S, Chen HC. Radical reduction of upper extremity lymphedema with preservation of perforators. Ann Plast Surg. 2009;63:302–6.

Step-by-Step Instruction: Lymphaticovenular Anastomosis (LVA) Assessment and Planning

8

Akitatsu Hayashi

Introduction

When performing the lymphaticovenular anastomosis (LVA) procedure, the surgical strategy should be planned based on the patients' lymphedema severity including the locations of the edema and symptoms. In secondary lymphedema, following the lymph node dissection that produces a surgical break in the lymphatic drainage pattern, individuals have different capabilities of restoring the lymph drainage of the limbs, based on their intrinsic anatomical features, regenerative processes, and extrinsic factors. When lymphedema affects the extremities, both clinical and subclinical, the restored lymphatic drainage is overloaded and low outflow failure is already present. Residual or restored functioning lymphatic channels that exhibit dermal backflow are already suffering from lymphatic hypertension and will degenerate over time, losing their function to drain lymph out of the affected limb. On the other hand, lymphatic channels that do not show dermal backflow are acting as a precious compensation. Therefore, as the human extremities cannot restore perfectly what nature created, only the lymph channels that show sufferance should be addressed by LVA – to obtain clinical improvement, prevent their degeneration, and protect the compensation pathways. As lymphedema is a chronic and progressive disease, compensatory lymph channels may suffer over time, and thus during the follow-up, other LVAs can be performed if and when necessary.

A. Hayashi (✉)
Lymphedema Center, Kameda General Hospital, Kamogawa, Chiba, Japan
e-mail: hayashi.akitatsu@kameda.jp

Assessment of Where to Perform the Lymphaticovenular Anastomosis (LVA)

LVA for Primary Lower Extremity Lymphedema

Primary lower extremity lymphedema (LEL) typically progresses proximally from the distal regions of the foot and the ankle [1, 2]. Lymphatic vessels at the distal areas tend to show degeneration with reduced function. Although the basic LVA strategy for LEL is creating LVAs at the lymphedematous areas to reduce stagnation of lymphatic fluid at the corresponding areas, LVA at the proximal areas can also lead to improvement in primary LEL patients who only display distal lymphedema. LVA for primary LEL may not only reduce stagnation of the lymphatic fluid at the lymphedematous area but may also reduce the total amount of the lymphatic fluid, which is a possible burden for less functional lymphatic valves and vessels. For this reason, multiple site LVAs at the foot, ankle, lower leg, and thigh can be the treatment of choice for primary LEL patients.

A small population of primary lymphedema patients display aplasia or severe hypoplasia in their superficial lymphatic system with no enhancement of any lymphatic vessels on lymphoscintigraphy or indocyanine green (ICG) lymphography. Most of these aplasia or severe hypoplasia cases are not candidates for LVA [1–3].

LVA for Secondary Lower Extremity Lymphedema

Very early stage secondary LEL only exhibits localized lymphedema at the lower abdomen and the groin areas. While these early lymphedema patients have functional superficial inguinal lymph nodes at the affected limbs, just a single LVA using the efferent lymphatic vessel at the superficial inguinal lymph node may prevent progression of the lymphedema [4]. However, lymphedema symptoms including swelling and

M. V. Schaverien, J. H. Dayan (eds.), *Multimodal Management of Upper and Lower Extremity Lymphedema*,
https://doi.org/10.1007/978-3-030-93039-4_8

stiffness gradually spread from the groin area to the thigh, lower leg, and foot [5]. In this circumstance, the LVA procedure should be added to reduce stagnation of lymphatic fluid at the corresponding areas of the edema.

LVA for Upper Extremity Lymphedema

Patients affected by upper extremity lymphedema (UEL) usually complain about heaviness and swelling mainly at the forearm and eventually the hand – it is quite uncommon that patients complain about upper arm swelling. Even patients without clinically evident swelling but that complain of itching/stinging demonstrate areas of spotty dermal backflow in the forearm with a linear pattern in the background on ICG lymphography.

With the progression of edema, the forearm becomes worse and eventually the hand becomes swollen. Even if the arm also shows an increase in circumference, it is usually soft and the patient usually complains more about excess tissue rather than a sense of heaviness as in the forearm. This scenario is typical for patients with International Society of Lymphology (ISL) Stage 1 to Stage 2b UEL in our clinical experience. Patients with ISL Stage 3 UEL complain about the entire arm.

There could be different reasons why secondary UEL patients differ from secondary LEL in the locoregional expression of swelling. Previous research has reported two different effects of LVA for LEL and UEL [6]. Horizontal improvement was shown in LEL, whereas longitudinal improvement was shown in UEL. These findings support this theory as the greatest net blockage effect is seen in LEL, which explains why the LVA can improve a "horizontal" portion of the limb, below or above which another bypass would be needed. In UEL, the arm is able to compensate totally or partially, thus the forearm and hand lymphatics compensate with greater difficulty.

Planning Where to Make the Incisions for the Lymphaticovenular Anastomosis (LVA)

In order to successfully perform the LVA, it is important to identify functional lymphatic vessels and determine the location of lymphatic vessels and venules preoperatively. ICG lymphography is particularly useful as a minimally invasive imaging modality that can be used not only to evaluate the severity of the lymphedema but also to determine where the incisions should be placed for the LVA by visualizing lymphatic vessels and lymphatic fluid stagnations preoperatively. However, ICG lymphography cannot visualize lymphatic flow that is masked beneath immediate dermal backflow patterns, particularly in stardust and diffuse patterns, in extremities affected with severe lymphedema [7] (Fig. 8.1). ICG lymphography also requires ICG injection before the examination, which cannot be performed in patients that are allergic to iodine.

To detect lymphatic vessels in a region masked by immediate dermal backflow pattern or in patients with allergic reactions to ICG, conventional high-frequency ultrasound (CHFUS) and ultrahigh-frequency ultrasound (UHFUS) have been reported to be useful as a substitute for ICG lymphography even in extremities severely affected by lymphedema [8–11]. Ultrasonography has greater utility for preoperative planning of LVA, and ultrasound-guided detection of lymphatic vessels for lymphedema results in more effective LVA surgery.

Detection and Selection of the Lymphatic Vessels Using Conventional High-Frequency Ultrasound (CHFUS)

The most important aspect for detection of lymphatic vessels is distinguishing them from blood vessels and nerves. Each has characteristic shapes, echogenic textures, and color Doppler modes (Fig. 8.2). It is desirable to use a linear probe in color Doppler mode at a frequency of more than 15 MHz to precisely distinguish between these. Lymphatic vessels are identified as intermittent homogeneous, hypoechoic, and specular misshapen images using CHFUS. However, when lymphatic vessels are too small (smaller than 0.3 mm), they may be mistaken for subcutaneous veins and nerves, because it is hard to judge the shape of small vessels even if the color Doppler mode is used.

ICG lymphography has a depth limit, and is only capable of detecting lymphatic vessels within 1.5–2 cm of the body surface. Some lymphatic vessels in the thigh and upper arm region are located 2–3 cm from the skin surface. Thus, detection of lymphatic vessels in these regions is difficult

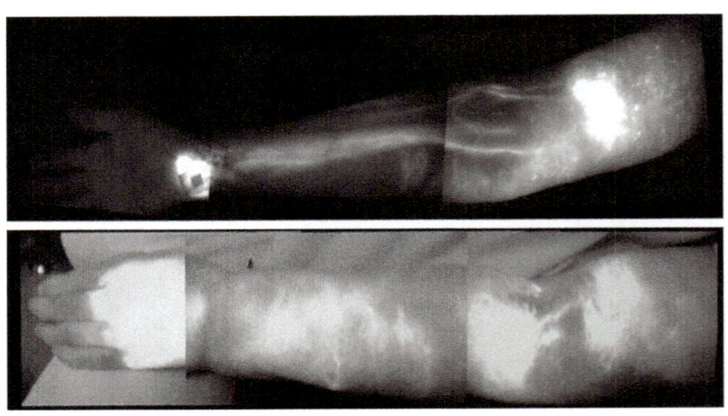

Fig. 8.1 Indocyanine green (ICG) lymphography is useful to determine where incisions should be placed in the case above, but is not useful in the case below

using ICG lymphography. Lymphatic vessels in these areas sometimes reside in rich fatty tissue in the deep layer, making their detection consistently challenging for surgeons. Because LVA incisions in these areas are placed mainly according to the experience of surgeons, non-detection of lymphatic vessels in some incisions is a common occurrence. Preoperative ultrasound detection of lymphatic vessels resolves this uncertainty, revealing the exact location of the lymphatic vessels even in the deep layer residing in rich fatty tissue (Fig. 8.3).

The presence of large lymphatic vessels with abundant lymph flow is an important factor determining the therapeutic effect of LVA in patients with extremity lymphedema. By using CHFUS, surgeons can detect and select the lymphatic vessels that have expanded lumens using ultrasound preoperatively. Lymphatic vessels that have expanded lumens on ultrasound still have valve function and high flow.

	Shape	Echogenic texture	Color Doppler mode
Lymphatic vessel 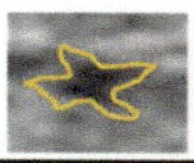	spicular misshapen	hypoechoic	–
Blood vessel 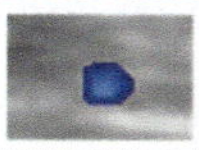	round	hypoechoic	+/–
Nerve 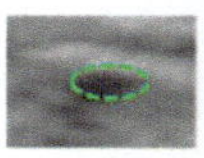	honey comb oval (superficial N.)	bright echogenic texture with hypoechoic fascicle one hypoechoic fascicle (Superficial N.)	–

Fig. 8.2 Characteristic findings of lymphatic vessels, blood vessels, and nerves on ultrasonographic imaging. N., nerve

Detection and Selection of the Lymphatic Vessels Using Ultrahigh-Frequency Ultrasound (UHFUS)

Disadvantages of the CHFUS system with an upper frequency of 15–20 MHz are that it is highly operator dependent and that it is difficult to distinguish the lymphatic vessels from the subcutaneous veins or the nerves when the lymphatic vessels are smaller than 0.3 mm. Precise imaging of small anatomical structures is often difficult with CHFUS. Recent developments in ultrahigh-resolution ultrasound systems provide frequencies as high as 70 MHz and a resolution capability as fine as 30 μm, which can allow more precise imaging of small anatomical structures (Fig. 8.4). UHFUS allows for more accurate imaging of the lymphatic vessels and provides valuable and new information for the detection of the lymphatic vessels. UHFUS shows clearer images for detecting lymphatic vessels and surrounding tissues than CHFUS. The veins are collapsed when the transducer is pushed against the skin of the examined sites, while the lymphatic vessels are less likely to collapse under the same conditions. Lymphatic fluid moving inside the lumen, as well as functioning valves, is visualized. Also, from the recent studies comparing imaging findings with histological analysis, a high echoic region around a low echoic region demonstrated a degenerative status of smooth muscle cells and hyperplasia of collagenous fibers in the lymphatic vessels (Fig. 8.5). The surgeon can therefore select the best lymphatic vessels at each point preoperatively using UHFUS.

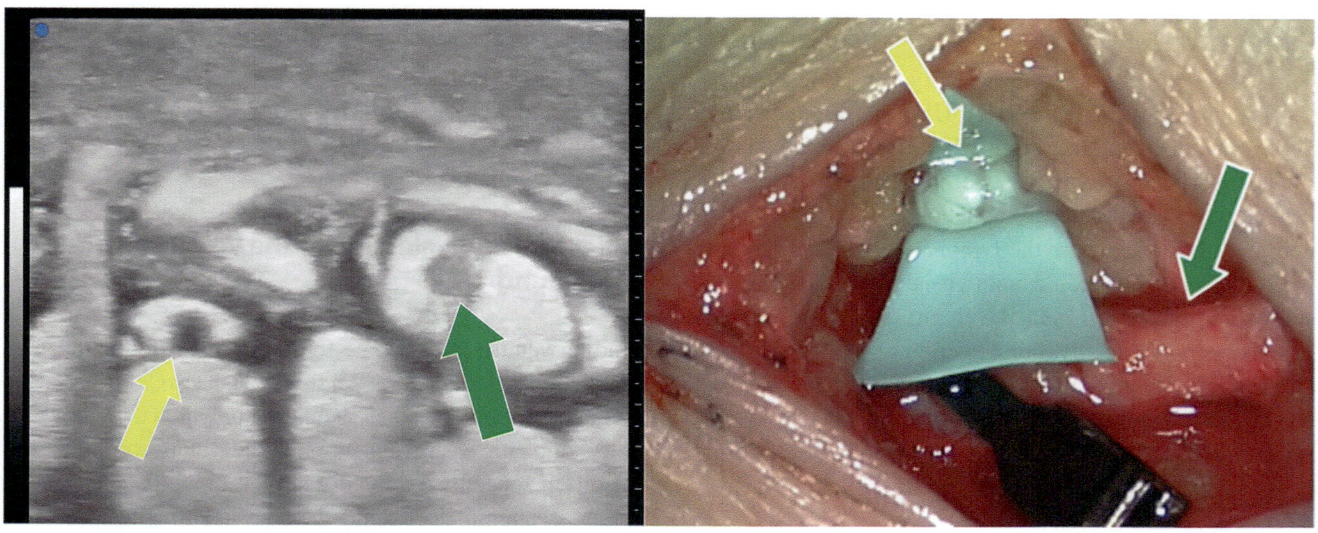

Fig. 8.3 (Left) Conventional high-frequency ultrasound (CHFUS) detection of a lymphatic vessel (yellow arrow) and vein (green arrow) in the knee was performed. The lymphatic vessel in the knee resided in rich fatty tissue in the deep layer. (Right) The lymphatic vessel (yellow arrow) and vein (green arrow) in the rich fatty tissue were dissected as CHFUS had indicated in the incision site of the knee

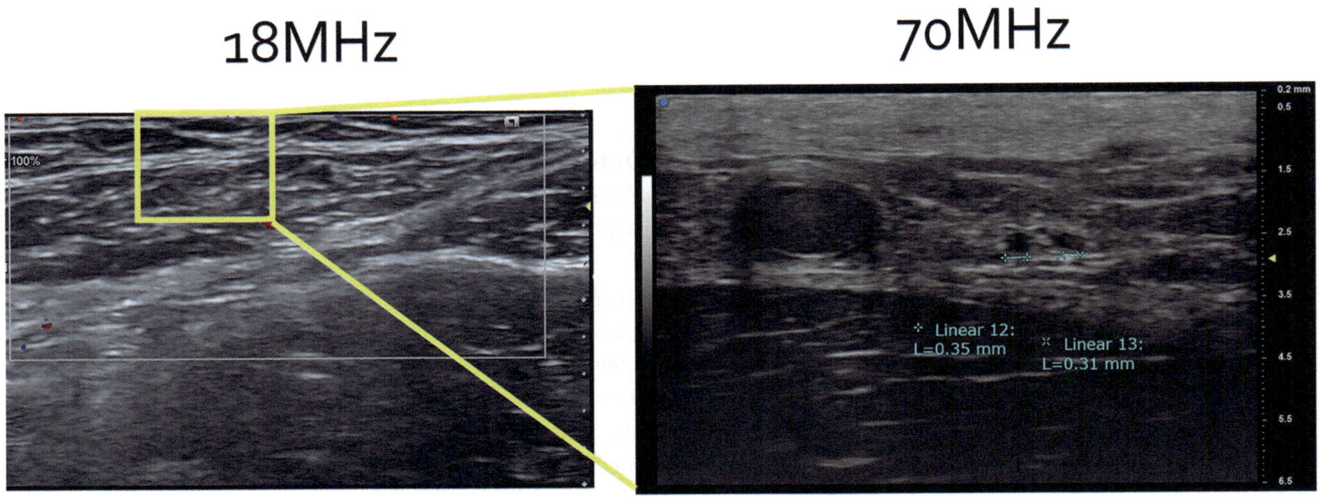

Fig. 8.4 Comparison of ultrasonographic images between conventional high-frequency ultrasound (CHFUS) and ultrahigh-frequency ultrasound (UHFUS)

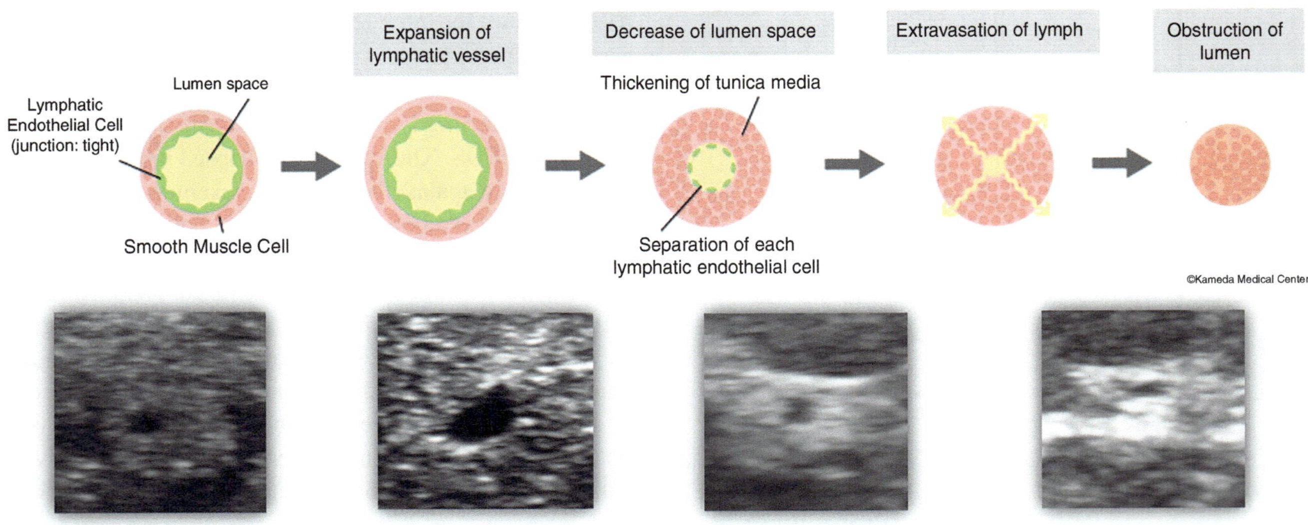

Fig. 8.5 Evaluation of the degenerative status of the lymphatic vessels using ultrahigh-frequency ultrasound (UHFUS)

One of disadvantages of UHFUS is its limited imaging depth. The deepest layer from which the device can obtain images is 10 mm from the superficial surface. Although it can clearly visualize the lymphatic vessels in the forearm and the lower leg, where the lymphatic vessels lie in a relatively superficial layer, it cannot visualize the lymphatic vessels in the upper arm and the thigh, where the lymphatic vessels run more deeply. For detection of the lymphatic vessels running deeper than 10 mm from the skin surface, use of a transducer with 48 MHz (max image depth: 23.5 mm) is recommended. The recommended protocol of UHFUS is as follows:

- Hand and forearm: 70 MHz
- Upper arm: 70 MHz → 48 MHz
- Foot and lower leg: 70 MHz → 48 MHz
- Thigh: 48 MHz → CHFUS

Detection and Selection of the Venules Using Ultrasound

Finding venules appropriate for anastomosis to the detected lymphatic vessels intraoperatively is also difficult and demanding. Surgeons face a situation in which there is a suitable lymphatic vessel but no suitable venule for LVA frequently, especially in the forearm region. In such cases, surgeons attempt to extend the incision to find a suitable vein, and this leaves a long scar with no contribution to the therapeutic outcome. Ultrasound can detect not only lymphatic vessels but also venules. Surgeons can select the venule with suitable size for the diameter of lymphatic vessels easily and also know the location of the venules. Surgeons can also select the venule which has less backflow using the push and release technique in ultrasound color Doppler mode for prevention of venous reflux at the lymphaticovenular shunt preoperatively. These advantages of the preoperative ultrasound detection technique reduce the time required for dissecting vessels to use for LVA, and also increase the postoperative limb volume reduction rate.

The strategy of vein selection for LVA differs between patients with UEL and those with LEL. In UEL patients, selecting the pumping vein for LVA is essential for high therapeutic effect [12]. However, selecting the ideal vein in LVA for LEL patients seems to be different from that for UEL; just selecting the pumping vein in LVA for LEL might have no clinical advantages. The gravity effect is considered stronger than the effect of venous pumping power alone in LEL patients. The good valve function of the vein, which could prevent regurgitation of the blood to the anastomosed lymphatic vessel against the gravity effect on standing position or sitting position, is more important in LVA for LEL [13, 14].

References

1. Yamamoto T, Yoshimatsu H, Narushima M, et al. Indocyanine green lymphography findings in primary leg lymphedema. Eur J Vasc Endovasc Surg. 2015;49:95–102.
2. Mangialardi ML, Lorenzano V, Pagliara D, et al. Indocyanine green lymphography, lymphoscintigraphy, and genetic analysis in nonsyndromic primary lymphedema: the distal dermal backflow grading system and the print sign. J Reconstr Microsurg. 2019;36(3):157–64. https://doi.org/10.1055/s-0039-1698748.
3. Hara H, Mihara M, Ohtsu H, et al. Indication of lymphaticovenous anastomosis for lower limb primary lymphedema. Plast Reconstr Surg. 2015;136:883–93.
4. Yamamoto T, Yamamoto N, Yamashita M, et al. Efferent lymphatic vessel anastomosis: supermicrosurgical efferent lymphatic vessel-to-venous anastomosis for the prophylactic treatment of subclinical lymphedema. Ann Plast Surg. 2016;76:424–7.
5. Yamamoto T, Matsuda N, Doi K, et al. The earliest finding of indocyanine green lymphography in asymptomatic limbs of lower extremity lymphedema patients secondary to cancer treatment: the modified dermal backflow stage and concept of subclinical lymphedema. Plast Reconstr Surg. 2011;128:314e–21e.
6. Seki Y, Yamamoto T, Kajikawa A. Lymphaticovenular anastomosis for breast cancer treatment-related lymphedema: three-line strategy for optimal outcome. J Plast Reconstr Aesthet Surg. 2018;71(6):e13–4.
7. Ogata F, Narushima M, Mihara M, et al. Intraoperative lymphography using indocyanine green dye for near-infrared fluorescence labeling in lymphedema. Ann Plast Surg. 2007;59:180–4.
8. Hayashi A, Yamamoto T, Yoshimatsu H, et al. Ultrasound visualization of the lymphatic vessels in the lower leg. Microsurgery. 2016;36:397–401.
9. Hayashi A, Hayashi N, Yoshimatsu H, et al. Effective and efficient lymphaticovenular anastomosis using preoperative ultrasound detection technique of lymphatic vessels in lower extremity lymphedema. J Surg Oncol. 2018;117:290–8.
10. Hayashi A, Giacalone G, Yamamoto T, et al. Comparative study of ultra high-frequency ultrasonographic imaging with 70 MHz scanner for visualization of the superficial lymphatic vessels in extremities. Plast Reconstr Surg Glob Open. 2019;7(1):e2086. https://doi.org/10.1097/GOX.0000000000002086.
11. Visconti G, Yamamoto T, Hayashi N, et al. Ultrasound-assisted lymphaticovenular anastomosis for the treatment of peripheral lymphedema. Plast Reconstr Surg. 2017;139:1380e–1e.
12. Seki Y, Kajikawa A, Yamamoto T, et al. The dynamic-lymphaticovenular anastomosis method for breast cancer treatment-related lymphedema: creation of functional lymphaticovenular anastomoses with use of preoperative dynamic ultrasonography. J Plast Reconstr Aesthet Surg. 2019;72:62–70.
13. Yang JC, Wu SC, Chiang MH, Lin WC. Targeting reflux-free veins with a vein visualizer to identify the ideal recipient vein preoperatively for optimal lymphaticovenous anastomosis in treating lymphedema. Plast Reconstr Surg. 2018;141:793–7.
14. Visconti G, Salgarello M, Hayashi A. The recipient venule in supermicrosurgical lymphaticovenular anastomosis: flow dynamic classification and correlation with surgical outcomes. J Reconstr Microsurg. 2018;34:581–9.

Step-by-Step Instruction: Lymphaticovenular Anastomosis (LVA) Techniques

9

Takumi Yamamoto and Jose Ramon Rodriguez

Introduction

Lymphaticovenular anastomosis (LVA) is one of the lymphovenous shunt operations. Historically, various lymphovenous shunt operations have been performed for the treatment of obstructive lymphedema, including lymph node-to-venous shunt, microsurgical lymphovenous implantation or classical lymphovenous anastomosis, and supermicrosurgical LVA [1–7]. As lymph originally flows into the venous circulation at the venous angle, lymphovenous shunt operations, which bypass congested lymph into the venous circulation, address the pathophysiology of obstructive lymphedema [1–3, 6–10]. Unlike other lymphovenous shunts in which a lymph node or a lymph vessel is inserted into a relatively large vein, in an LVA a lymph vessel is anastomosed to a venule or a small vein in an intima-to-intima coaptation manner (Fig. 9.1) [1, 3–6, 11–13]. Since the anastomosis site of supermicrosurgical LVA is covered intraluminally with the endothelium, whereas adventitia or other tissues are exposed at the anastomosis site when the other lymphovenous shunt techniques are performed, there is a lower risk of anastomosis site thrombosis and no serious complication has been reported after supermicrosurgical LVA [4, 12–14].

Supplementary Information The online version of this chapter (https://doi.org/10.1007/978-3-030-93039-4_9) contains supplementary material, which is available to authorized users.

T. Yamamoto (✉)
Department of Plastic and Reconstructive Surgery, Center Hospital of National Center for Global Health and Medicine, Tokyo, Japan
e-mail: tyamamoto-tky@umin.ac.jp

J. R. Rodriguez
Department of Plastic and Reconstructive Surgery, Center Hospital of National Center for Global Health and Medicine, Tokyo, Japan

Department of Plastic and Reconstructive Surgery, Clinica Las Condes, Santiago, Chile

Patient Selection and Preoperative Evaluation

LVA is a bypass surgery and is indicated for obstructive lymphedema, as well as for chylous disorders due to lymph flow obstruction such as chylothorax and chyloabdomen [3–9, 14–16]. In obstructive lymphedema, it is indicated in cases refractory to conservative treatments; all patients receive conservative therapy, such as compression therapy with an elastic stocking, lymph drainage, or elastic bandage compression, for at least 3 months with no significant clinical improvement. LVA is not effective for some types of primary lymphedema [5, 17–19]. Lymph vessels become sclerotic and have reduced lymph flow with progression of lymphedema; LVA is therefore barely effective in advanced lymphedema with severe lymphosclerosis (Table 9.1) [4, 7, 20–23]. To maximize the therapeutic efficacy of LVA, thorough preoperative evaluation and appropriate patient selection are important; a slightly sclerotic "S1" lymph vessel is the best for LVA [3, 6, 10, 14, 19]. As immediate postoperative compression is critical after LVA, a patient should be compliant with compression therapy using a compression garment: Class 3 compression for the lower extremity and Class 2 for upper extremity cases [13, 14, 19].

Lymph flow imaging is the most important facet of lymphedema evaluation. Among various evaluations, such as lymphoscintigraphy and magnetic resonance lymphangiography (MRL), indocyanine green (ICG) lymphography has the strongest evidence base for its utility in severity staging of lymphedema, allowing prognosis prediction, preoperative lymphatic mapping, intraoperative navigation, and postoperative follow-up for LVA surgery [6, 10, 13–16, 24–30]. Dual-phase observation ICG lymphography, known as dynamic ICG lymphography, allows evaluation of pathophysiological severity and localization of lymph vessels suitable for LVA with one ICG injection [19, 29, 30]. The first observation is done immediately after the ICG injection at an early transient phase, when Linear pattern (linear fluorescent

M. V. Schaverien, J. H. Dayan (eds.), *Multimodal Management of Upper and Lower Extremity Lymphedema*,
https://doi.org/10.1007/978-3-030-93039-4_9

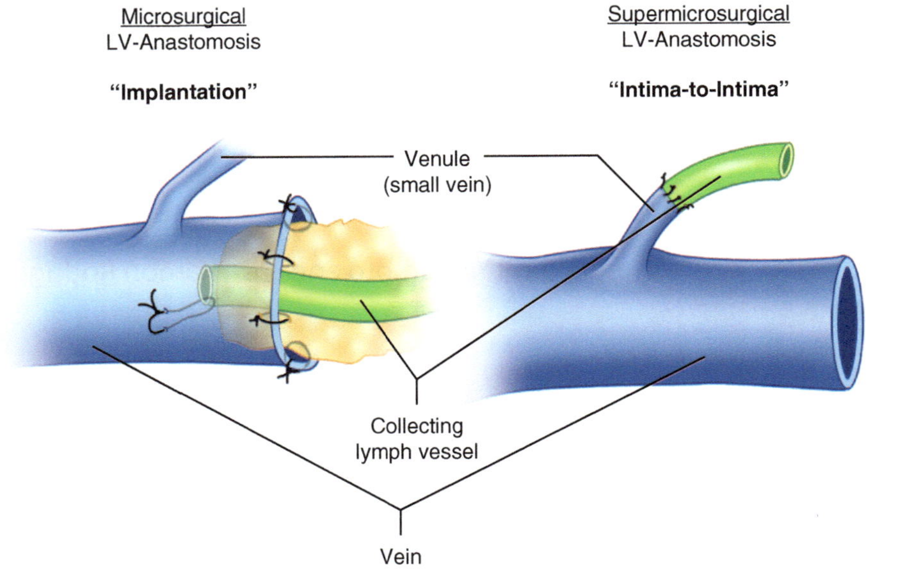

Fig. 9.1 Microsurgical lymphovenous anastomosis or implantation and supermicrosurgical lymphaticovenular anastomosis (LVA). When venous reflux occurs, thrombosis formation is inevitable in microsurgical implantation, whereas thrombosis can be prevented in supermicrosurgical LVA

Table 9.1 Severity grading of lymphosclerosis

Severity	Intraoperative findings of lymph vessel[a]			
	Wall thickness	Appearance	Wall expandability	Lumen
s0	Very thin	Translucent	Expandable	Identifiable
s1	Thin	White	Expandable	Identifiable
s2	Thick	White	Not expandable	Identifiable
s3	Very thick	White	Not expandable	Not identifiable

Yamamoto et al. [20], with permission from Wolters Kluwer Health, Inc
[a]Evaluated under an operating microscope

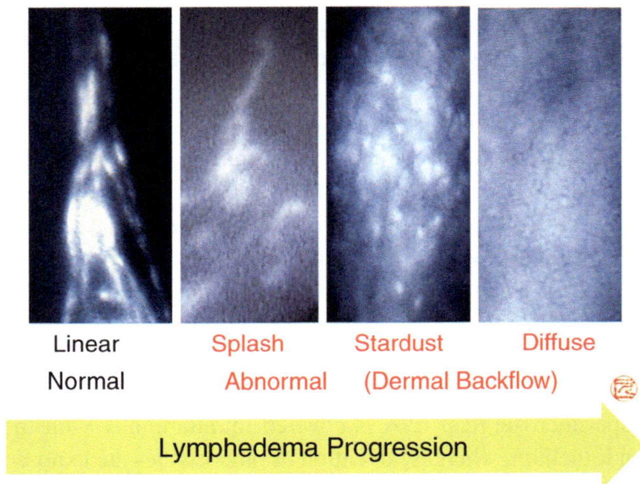

Fig. 9.2 Typical indocyanine green (ICG) lymphography findings at a late plateau phase observation. Normal Linear pattern and abnormal dermal backflow (DB) patterns (Splash, Stardust, and Diffuse pattern)

image) is marked to localize collecting lymphatic vessels. The second observation is done 2 or more hours after the ICG injection at a late plateau phase, when extension of dermal backflow (DB) patterns (Splash, Stardust, and Diffuse patterns) is evaluated (Fig. 9.2) [19, 29, 30].

For secondary lymphedema, ICG stage is determined based on dynamic ICG lymphography findings (Table 9.2; Fig. 9.3) [20–25]. LVA is best indicated for ICG Stage II–IV lymphedema where ICG lymphography shows both Linear pattern and DB pattern (usually Stardust pattern). ICG Stage I represents subclinical lymphedema, and prophylactic LVA may be performed. In ICG Stage V, no Linear pattern is present and LVA is barely effective because of severe lymphosclerosis; therefore, vascularized lymph node transfer (VLNT) is better indicated for ICG Stage V cases [6, 18, 20].

For primary lymphedema, the ICG classification is determined based on ICG lymphographic findings – these include the proximal DB (PDB), distal DB (DDB), less enhancement (LE), and no enhancement (NE) types (Table 9.3; Fig. 9.4) [17, 19]. The PDB type and DDB type represent obstructive lymphedema, and LVA is indicated; VLNT is considered when LVA is ineffective [17, 19]. The LE type is usually associated with deteriorated lymphatic pump function or a hypoplastic superficial lymphatic system, and strict compression therapy is recommended. The NE type represents localized aplasia or severe hypoplasia of the lymphatics, and LVA is not recommended; usually only fibrotic cords are found without any collecting lymphatic vessels suitable for LVA; VLNT or liposuction is thus better indicated for NE type primary lymphedema.

Incision Site Design

Incision sites for LVA should be designed where pitting edema is evident and there are pathologic but functional lymph vessels suitable for anastomosis. Although many microsurgeons misunderstand that LVA is performed where

ICG lymphography shows Linear pattern representing intact lymph vessels, therapeutic efficacy of LVA is maximized when it is performed where there are slightly sclerotic "S1" lymph vessels [3–11, 18, 20, 23] as shown in Table 9.1. LVA using intact "S0" lymph vessels can even be harmful because every anastomosis has a risk of obstruction, leading to additional lymph flow obstruction and further lymphedema progression; intact lymph vessels, shown as Linear pattern on ICG lymphography, should be preserved. Rather, lymph vessels in DB pattern can be better for LVA; LVA works to improve lymph circulation by salvaging affected but still functional lymph vessels [19–21, 23].

To localize such salvageable lymph vessels most suitable for LVA, dynamic ICG lymphography is the most useful imaging modality [19, 29, 30]. With dual-phase observation, "overlapping" regions are identified and targeted for LVA; these regions are where ICG lymphography shows Linear pattern at an early transient phase and DB pattern, usually Stardust pattern, at a late plateau phase (Fig. 9.5) [19, 24–30]. The overlapping regions represent slightly pathologic and still functional lymph vessels, where a surgeon can easily find lymph vessels as ICG lymphography transiently shows Linear pattern. More importantly, the lymph vessels are somewhat sclerotic and mostly have high lymph flows [19, 20, 23]. Lymph vessels with Diffuse pattern are usually severely sclerotic and unsuitable for LVA.

The upper/lower extremity is divided into three regions: upper arm/thigh, forearm/lower leg, and hand/foot [14, 19–23]. At least one incision is designed in one region where dynamic

Table 9.2 Indocyanine green (ICG) staging for secondary lymphedema

ICG stage	ICG lymphography findings
Stage 0	Linear pattern only (no dermal backflow pattern)
Stage I	Linear pattern + Splash pattern[a]
Stage II	Linear pattern + Stardust/Diffuse pattern (1 region)[b]
Stage III	Linear pattern + Stardust/Diffuse pattern (2 regions)[b]
Stage IV	Linear pattern + Stardust/Diffuse pattern (3 regions)[b]
Stage V	Stardust/Diffuse pattern only (no Linear pattern)

ICG indocyanine green
[a]Splash pattern is usually seen around the axilla/groin
[b]Upper/lower extremity is divided into three regions: the upper arm/thigh, the forearm/lower leg, and the hand/foot

Table 9.3 Indocyanine green (ICG) classification for primary lymphedema

ICG classification	ICG lymphography findings
PDB type	DB pattern mainly in the proximal region
DDB type	DB pattern mainly in the distal region
LE type	Linear pattern only in the distal region (no DB pattern)
NE type	No enhancement (no Linear or DB pattern)

ICG indocyanine green, *DB* dermal backflow, *PDB* proximal DB, *DDB* distal DB, *LE* less enhancement, *NE* no enhancement

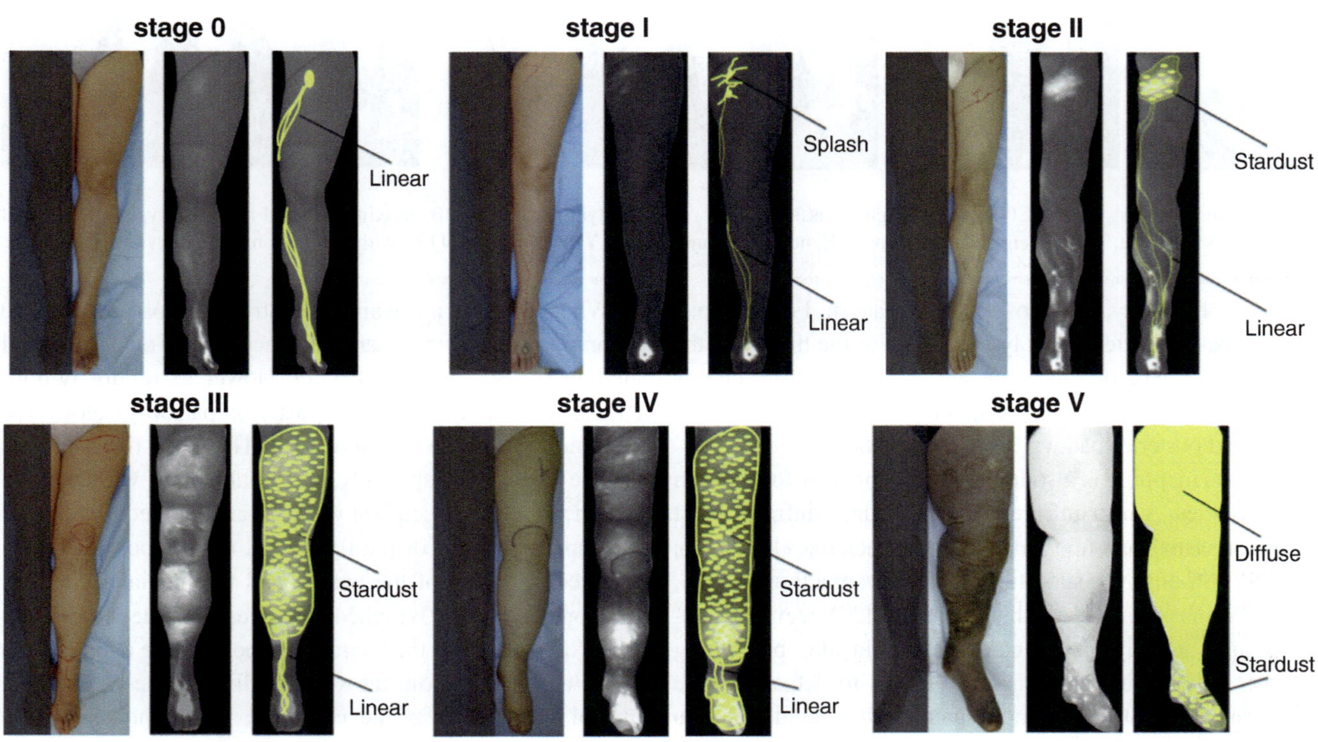

Fig. 9.3 Indocyanine green (ICG) lymphography stage for secondary lymphedema. (Yamamoto et al. [22], with permission from Elsevier)

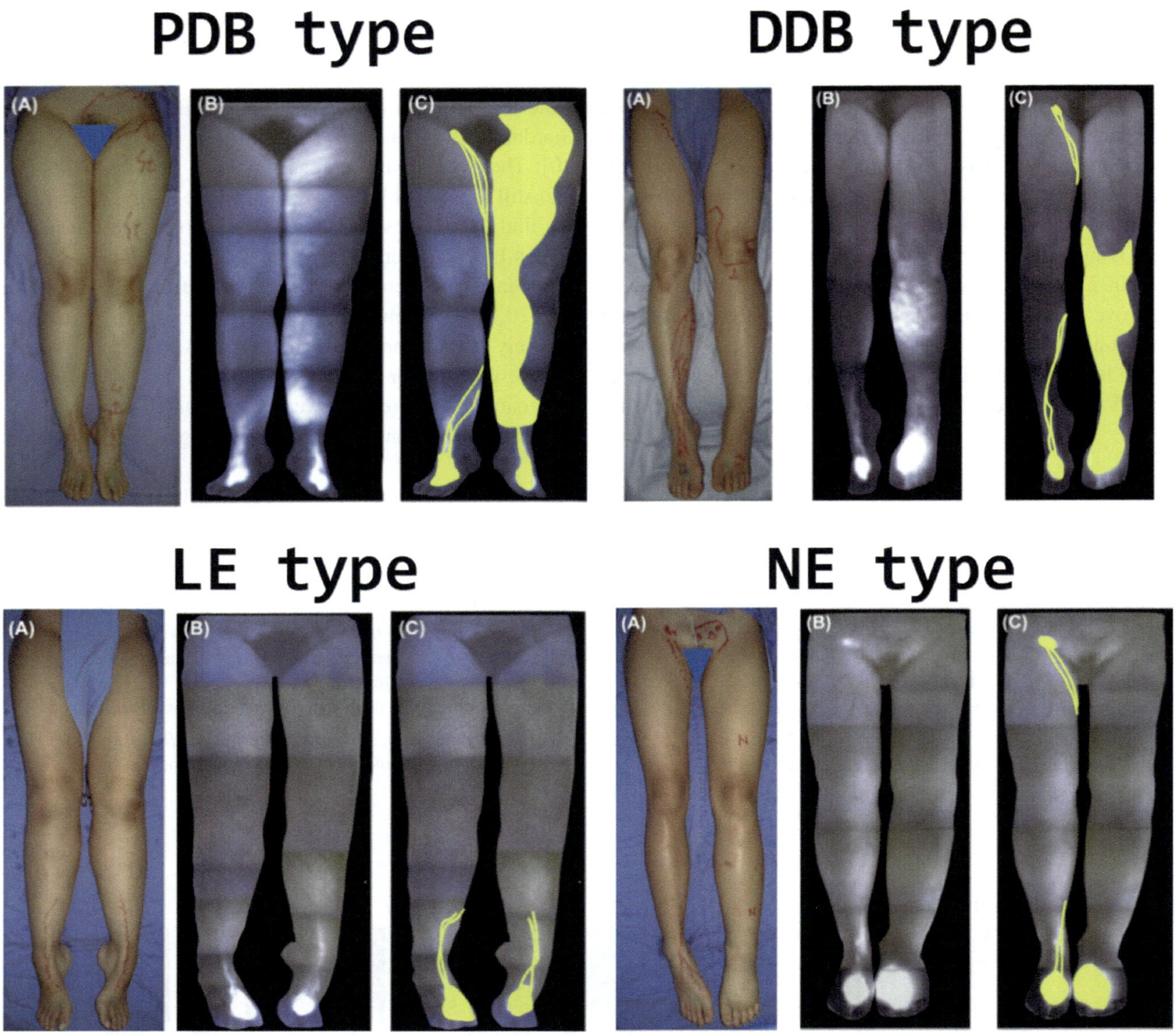

Fig. 9.4 Indocyanine green (ICG) lymphography classification for primary lymphedema. PDB, proximal dermal backflow type; DDB, distal dermal backflow type; LE, less enhancement type; NE, no enhancement type. (Yamamoto et al. [17], with permission from Elsevier)

ICG lymphography shows overlapping pattern. For example, when a patient suffers from lymphedema of the thigh and the lower leg, at least two incisions are designed. When there is significant circumferential edema, minor pathways, such as the lateral and posterior pathways, should also be addressed.

Venous mapping is also important to consider for the skin incision sites. A near-infrared camera without infrared light emission visualizes superficial veins as black lines [6, 15, 16, 24–28]. Although the superficial veins are sometimes useful, deeper veins are more suitable for use as LVA recipient vessels; they usually have intact valves inside, preventing venous reflux. Ultrasound is more useful to detect suitable recipient veins. In experienced hands, ultrasound can also localize lymph vessels suitable for LVA [13, 14, 19].

When there is no available instrument for preoperative mapping, incision sites are designed based on anatomical landmarks [3, 4, 8, 10, 19]. For lower extremity lymphedema, the anterior and the posterior pathways along the saphenous veins are recommended. The distal thigh and the middle lower leg, especially, are reliable sites with suitable lymph vessels and recipient veins, as are the medial aspect at the superior border of the thigh, and the midpoint between the medial border of the patella and the medial malleolus. For upper extremity lymphedema, lines from the second web space of the hand to the lateral third point at the cubital fossa to the axilla, and from the volar midline at the wrist to the medial third point at the cubital fossa to the axilla, are recommended.

Consideration of Anastomotic Configuration

There are four basic anastomotic configurations: end-to-end (EE), end-to-side (ES), side-to-end (SE), and side-to-side (SS) anastomoses (Fig. 9.6) [4, 7–9, 19]. From a lymphodynamic point of view, SE and SS anastomoses are better; they divert bidirectional lymph flow via one anastomosis [7–9]. However, SE and SS anastomoses require technically demanding lymphotomy, which is especially difficult when a lymph vessel is sclerotic [7, 9, 20]. Long-term patency is the most important factor to consider in anastomotic configurations. Among the four basic anastomoses, EE anastomosis has the highest patency, whereas ES anastomosis has the lowest [13, 14, 19]. EE anastomosis is the most basic and technically least demanding. Therefore, EE anastomosis is recommended in most cases [4, 8, 19]. The ideal anastomotic configurations for one lymph vessel is double EE anastomoses; a lymph vessel is transected and then both stumps are anastomosed to two veins in an EE manner [4, 19]. In this chapter, the LVA technique for single EE anastomosis is described.

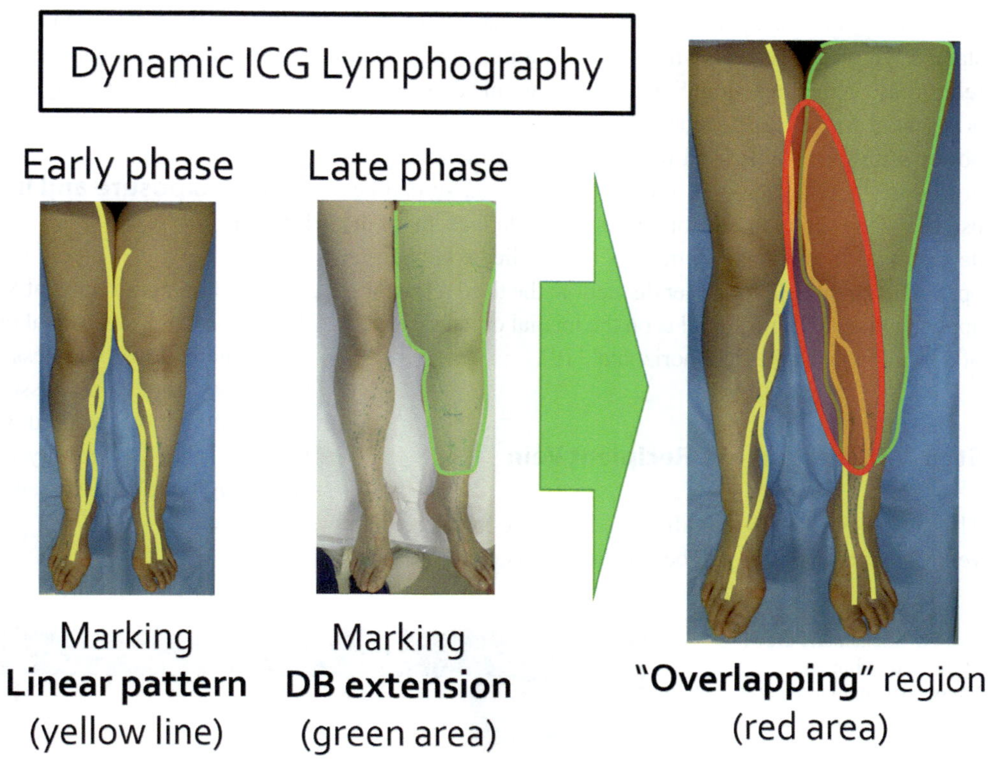

Fig. 9.5 Overlapping region revealed by indocyanine green (ICG) lymphography. DB, dermal backflow

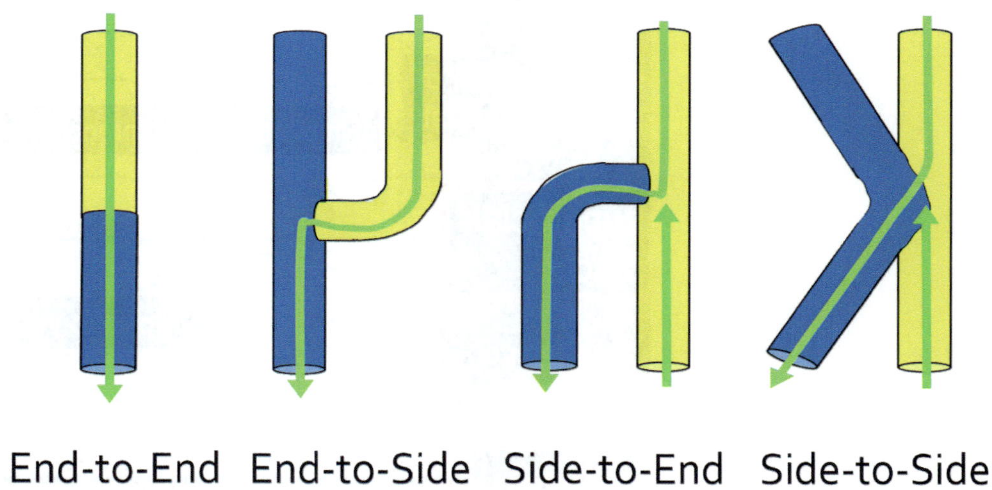

Fig. 9.6 Basic four types of anastomotic configuration for lymphaticovenular anastomosis (LVA)

Step-by-Step Operative Techniques for Lymphaticovenular Anastomosis (LVA) (see supplementary material)

Step 1: Skin Incision and Retraction

The whole procedure, including injection of local anesthesia, is performed under an operative microscope. After infiltration of local anesthetic along the designed skin incision line with 1% lidocaine with 1:100,000 epinephrine, the dermis is incised with a surgical scalpel. We do not use dye injection distal to the field, although some have reported the use of blue dye injection to find the lymphatic vessel; there are many non-stained lymphatic vessels, which can be injured if a surgeon relies only on dye injection. Systematic anatomical dissection is essential for safe and secure LVA. Electrocautery with the power setting at 5–7 is used for most parts of the dissection procedure; a dissector or a fine-tip mosquito is sometimes used for deep vessel dissection. After complete incision of the dermis, two to three skin retractors are applied to obtain an optimal surgical field for easier dissection; the third retractor is applied, when a surgical field is on the medial or lateral aspect of a limb, to make the field horizontal [19].

Step 2: Dissection of a Recipient Vein

The superficial fat layer is dissected to look for a recipient vein. Subdermal veins, just below the dermis, can be used as recipients, but deeper venous branches from the subcutaneous veins such as the saphenous, the cephalic, and the basilic veins are preferred, as they are likely to have intact valves for prevention of venous reflux. Fat lobules should not be destroyed throughout dissection procedures; interlobular dissection is important (Fig. 9.7) [14, 19]. In almost all cases, recipient veins are located superficially to the superficial fascia. A recipient vein should be dissected first before the lymph vessels. A vein is dissected as distal as possible to include as many valves inside as possible. When the vein found is relatively large, it should be dissected proximally and distally to seek a smaller branch suitable for LVA. Once a suitable vein is found and dissected distally enough, the vein is cut as distally as possible with coagulation of the distal stump of the vein (Fig. 9.8).

Step 3. Exposure and Incision of the Superficial Fascia

After obtaining a recipient vein, the next step is anatomical dissection to the superficial fascia (Fig. 9.9); the focus should be on meticulous bloodless interlobular dissection – never try to look for lymph vessels at this stage. The superficial fascia should be exposed widely throughout the surgical field, and then is carefully incised using electrocautery; the collecting lymphatic vessels are found just below the superficial fascia.

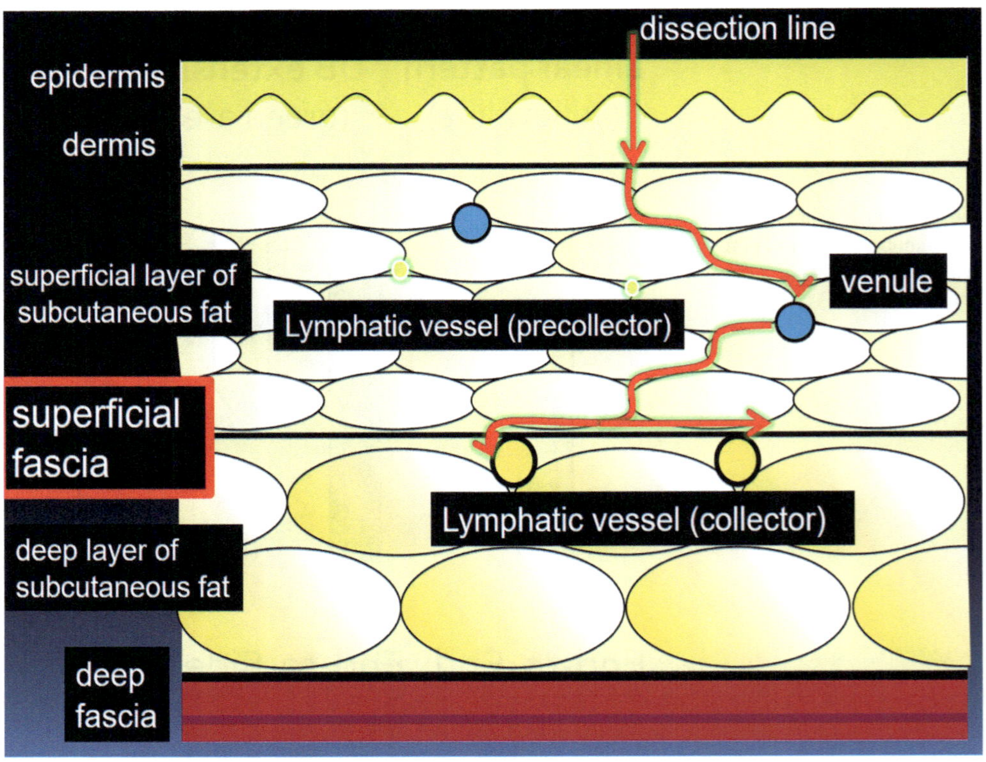

Fig. 9.7 Schematic drawing of dissection line in lymphaticovenular anastomosis (LVA) surgery. Dissection should be done between fat lobules – interlobular dissection

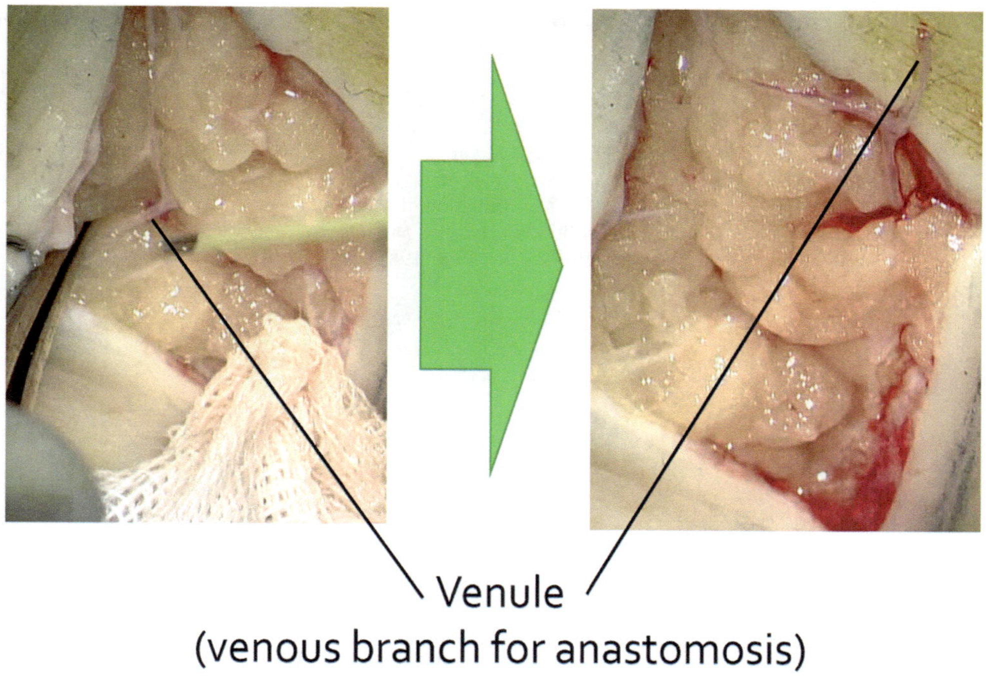

Fig. 9.8 Recipient vein dissection. A vein should be dissected and cut as distally as possible, facilitating deeper layer dissection

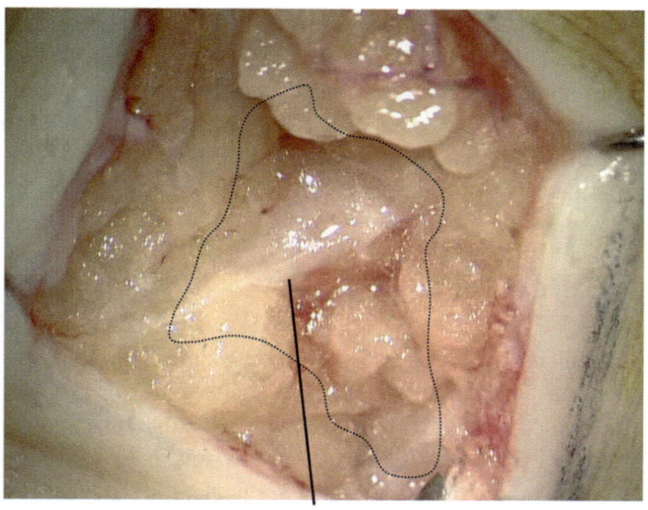

Fig. 9.9 Wide exposure of the superficial fascia

Step 4. Dissection of the Collecting Lymph Vessels

After incision of the superficial fascia is completed, the deep fat layer is dissected between the lobules with a blunt dissector; the tips of a dissector are inserted between fat lobules, and the tips are opened to dissect the deep fat tissue interlobularly. Collecting lymph vessels, if present, lie just below the superficial fascia; dissection therefore should not be performed too deeply [19]. If no lymph vessels have been found after dissection of all interlobular spaces, the skin incision should be elongated to explore other interlobular spaces nearby, or the surgical field should be changed; if there are no lymph vessels there, the surgeon should not dissect deeper. When a lymph vessel is found, a 3-0 nylon thread is placed below the lymph vessel so as not to lose it (Fig. 9.10). The lymph vessel is then dissected as proximally as possible.

Step 5. Preparation of the Vessels for LVA

The adventitia of the vein and lymph vessel are carefully trimmed as in conventional microsurgery. The venous lumen is irrigated with heparinized water to wash out possible micro-clot and to check for venous reflux; a micro-clot can occur during the dissection procedure and should be washed out. When the vein shows reflux, a clamp should be applied to keep the field bloodless during anastomosis. The anastomosis should be completely free from tension, and kinking is not as problematic as in conventional microvascular anastomosis. The vein should not be trimmed to adjust the location of anastomosis site; the vein should be as long as possible to contain as many valves inside; only when there is too much kinking should the lymph vessel be trimmed.

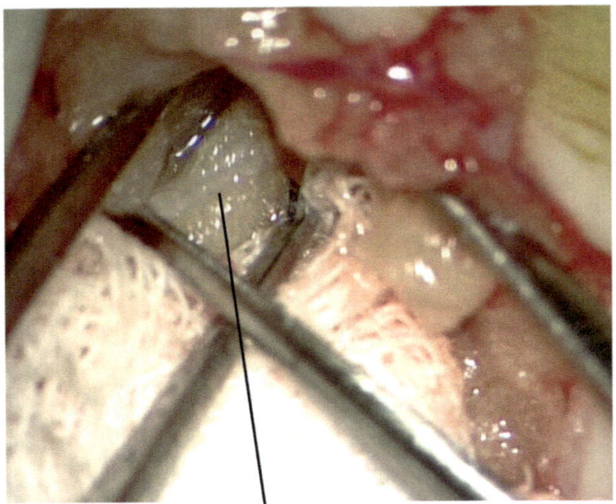

Fig. 9.10 Via interlobular dissection, a lymph vessel is found between the fat lobules just beneath the superficial fascia

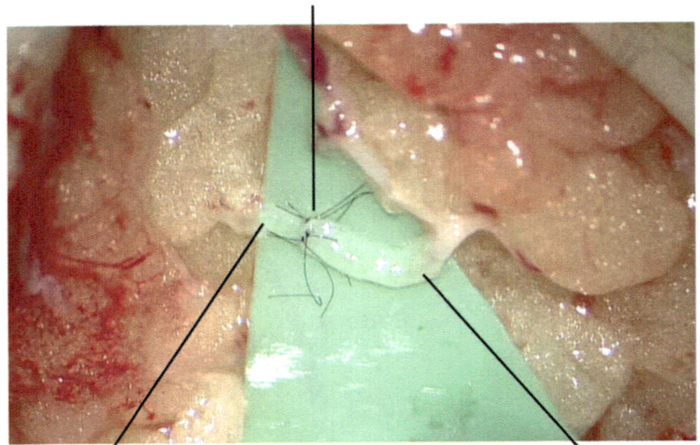

Fig. 9.11 Supermicrosurgical end-to-end (EE) anastomosis in an intima-to-intima coaptation manner

Step 6. "Intima-to-Intima Coaptation" Anastomosis

Irrigation with heparinized water is performed again through the vein stump immediately prior to anastomosis. To prevent anastomotic site thrombosis, no tissue other than the endothelium should be exposed at the anastomosis site. Supermicro-suture is used for anastomosis: 11-0 (65 micron needle) for 0.5–1.0 mm vessels, 12-0 (50 micron needle) for 0.2–0.5 mm vessels, and 12-0s (30 micron needle) for 0.1–0.3 mm vessels [6, 10, 13, 14, 19]. The suture is started on the vessel that is easier for a surgeon, in terms of size and location. If the lumen is hardly identified, a vein-to-lymph stitching sequence may be useful, as the lumen of the vein is usually easier to recognize. An intravascular stent may be also considered to keep the vessel lumen open during anastomosis [4, 19] – a several millimeters-long 3-0 to 7-0 nylon thread, depending on the vessel diameter, is inserted into the lymph vessel. The needle is inserted into and out from the space between the vessel wall and the intravascular stent, significantly facilitating the procedure. For EE anastomosis, the last one or two stitches are left untied to allow removal of the nylon stent from the space between the free vessel ends. Typically, approximately six stiches are applied for an EE anastomosis; four stiches may be enough only when a vessel is smaller than 0.2 mm. Patency is confirmed by the presence of venous expansion with translucent lymph after distal compression with or without intraoperative ICG lymphography confirmation (Fig. 9.11) [4, 6, 15, 16].

Step 7: Protection of the Vessels and Anastomosis Site

After completion of the anastomosis, fat tissues above and below the superficial fascia are undermined to allow easy positioning of the vessels and the anastomotic site underneath it; the vessels should be placed as deep as possible to protect them from sheer stress during wearing of the compression garment postoperatively (Fig. 9.12).

Step 8: Careful Skin Closure

The skin is also closed under an operative microscope. A surgeon has to pay attention especially to the vein, which is usually located in the most superficial layer. Subdermal sutures with 4-0 PDS are placed to close the dermis, taking care not to catch or affect the vessels. Surgical tapes are usually applied after the dermal sutures. If there is a lot of exudate from the field, surface sutures with 6-0 nylon may be applied.

Postoperative Management and Follow-Up

The same compression garment worn preoperatively should be applied immediately after LVA surgery [13, 14, 19]. Without external compression, lymphatic and venous pressures are similar, and lymph flow after LVA can be to-and-fro, which may cause anastomosis site thrombosis. Since the lymphatic system is a closed system in a lymphedematous limb due to lymph flow obstruction, lymphatic pressure becomes higher under external compression. On the other

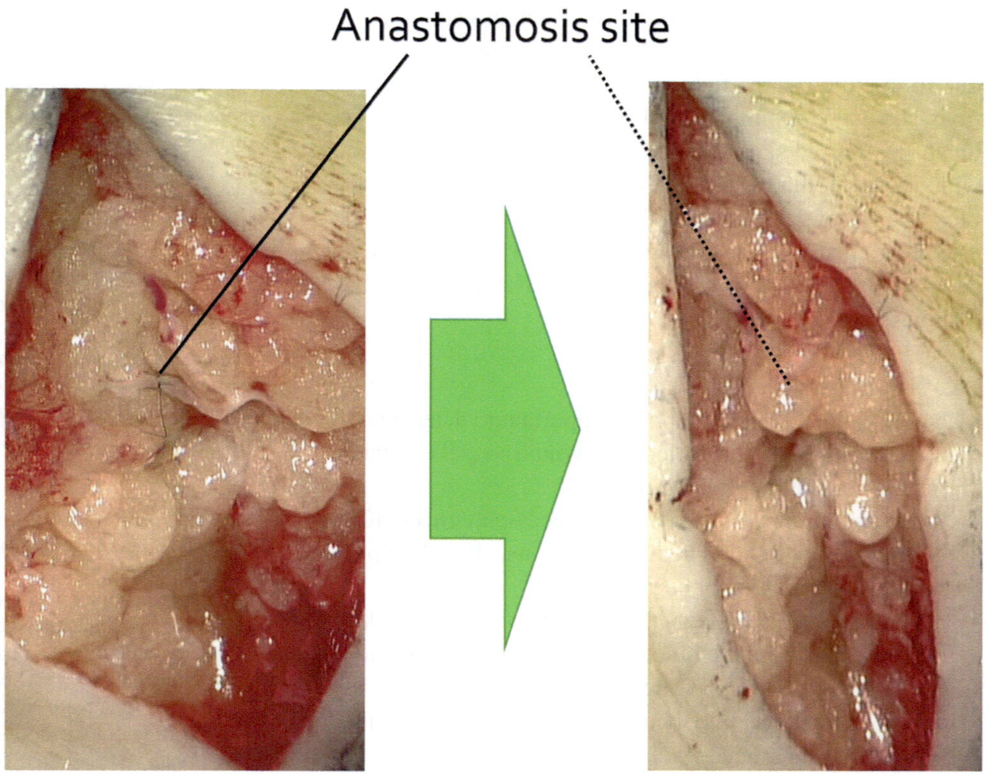

Fig. 9.12 Protection of vessels and anastomosis site by covering them with fat tissue

hand, the venous system is an open system, and venous pressure does not change under external compression; venous blood just moves proximally without pressure change. Therefore, external compression creates a lymph-to-venous pressure gradient and continuous lymph-to-venous flow, preventing anastomotic site thrombosis [19].

Supermicro-sutures are exposed in an anastomosis site and are usually covered with the endothelium within 1–2 weeks [12, 19]. Twenty-four-hour compression is recommended for 2 weeks after LVA; the garment can be removed only when taking a shower or a bath. Two weeks after LVA, the compression garment is used only during the daytime, with no compression used during the nighttime. Wounds are checked the day after surgery and 2 weeks after surgery; when surface sutures are applied, they are removed at 2 weeks postoperatively. Patients are followed every 3 months, evaluating severity of subjective symptoms, occurrence of cellulitis episodes, and circumferential measurements to calculate limb lymphedematous volume [6–10, 28]. Compression garments are renewed every 6 months. ICG lymphography and MR imaging are performed annually to evaluate lymph flow circulation and fat/fluid valance, respectively.

Compression garments are maintained for at least 1 year after LVA. Compression can be gradually reduced, when the following criteria are met: (1) absence of tension-sensation, (2) absence of cellulitis episode, (3) sustained volume reduction, and (4) improvement of lymph circulation on ICG lymphography [13, 19]. Even after complete relief from compression – so-called "cure" status – patients should be followed with annual lymph flow imaging such as ICG lymphography; if ICG lymphography shows re-worsening, compression should be resumed. When the volume is partially reduced but significant volume remains after LVA, repeat LVA may be considered. When LVA is not effective at all, more progressive surgeries such as VLNT should be considered [8, 10, 18, 19].

Complications

Based on the senior author's (T.Y.) experience of over 10,000 lymphatic anastomoses, no serious complications have been observed. However, there are possible risks of postoperative complications, and there are several reports of minor complications after LVA [3, 7, 13, 14, 19]. Surgical site infection and possible subsequent cellulitis can be prevented with conventional preoperative disinfection, intraoperative antibiotics administration (30 min before skin incision), and postoperative skin care [4, 5, 10, 13, 19]. When the skin is fragile due to old age or long-lasting steroid therapy, pressure ulceration caused by the compression garment can occur, and should be avoided by careful skin observation and appropriate garment use [14, 19]. Thermal burns can occur due to the microscope light, and intraoperative skin conditions should be monitored and not allowed to dry out too much [3]. Purple skin color change can be seen after LVA with venous reflux; the color change is due to retrograde blood perfusion into the dermal lymphatic capillaries [5, 7]. The color change usually disappears within 3–4 weeks, and can be prevented and reduced with strict postoperative compression.

Pearls and Pitfalls

- Dynamic ICG lymphography is important to determine if LVA is indicated and to localize lymph vessels suitable for LVA in overlapping regions.
- Intact lymph vessels, shown as Linear pattern on ICG lymphography in non-edematous regions, should be preserved; LVA should not be performed.
- Anatomical layer-by-layer interlobular dissection is key to secure and rapid identification of a recipient vein and a lymph vessel. The superficial fascia is a landmark to dissect lymph vessels; lymph vessels are located just beneath the superficial fascia.
- A recipient vein should be dissected as distally as possible to include many valves for prevention of venous reflux and subsequent anastomosis site thrombosis. A vein should not be trimmed; rather, a lymph vessel should be trimmed when too much kinking is expected.
- Secure intima-to-intima coaptation with 11-0 (65 micron needle) or 12-0 (30 micron needle) suture is essential for successful supermicrosurgical anastomosis.

References

1. Degni M. Surgical management of selected patients with lymphedema of the extremities. J Cardiovasc Surg. 1984;25(6):481–8.
2. Campisi C, Davini D, Bellini C, et al. Lymphatic microsurgery for the treatment of lymphedema. Microsurgery. 2006;26(1):65–9. https://doi.org/10.1002/micr.20214.
3. Yoshida S, Koshima I, Imai H, et al. Microscope-induced thermal burns during lymphaticovenular anastomosis. Ann Plast Surg. 2020;84(5):e24–6.
4. Yamamoto T, Narushima M, Kikuchi K, Yoshimatsu H, Todokoro T, Mihara M, Koshima I. Lambda-shaped anastomosis with intravascular stenting method for safe and effective lymphaticovenular anastomosis. Plast Reconstr Surg. 2011;127(5):1987–92.
5. Yamamoto T, Koshima I, Yoshimatsu H, Narushima M, Mihara M, Iida T. Simultaneous multi-site lymphaticovenular anastomoses for primary lower extremity and genital lymphoedema complicated with severe lymphorrhea. J Plast Reconstr Aesthet Surg. 2011;64(6):812–5.
6. Yamamoto T, Narushima M, Yoshimatsu H, Seki Y, Yamamoto N, Oka A, Hara H, Koshima I. Minimally invasive lymphatic supermicrosurgery (MILS): indocyanine green lymphography-guided simultaneous multi-site lymphaticovenular anastomoses via millimeter skin incisions. Ann Plast Surg. 2014;72(1):67–70.
7. Yamamoto T, Yoshimatsu H, Yamamoto N, Narushima M, Iida T, Koshima I. Side-to-end lymphaticovenular anastomosis through temporary lymphatic expansion. PLoS One. 2013;8(3):e59523.
8. Yamamoto T, Yoshimatsu H, Narushima M, Seki Y, Yamamoto N, Shim TWH, Koshima I. A modified side-to-end lymphaticovenular anastomosis. Microsurgery. 2013;33(2):130–3.
9. Yamamoto T, Yoshimatsu H, Narushima M, Yamamoto N, Shim TWH, Seki Y, Kikuchi K, Karibe J, Azuma S, Koshima I. Sequential anastomosis for lymphatic supermicrosurgery: multiple lymphaticovenular anastomoses on one venule. Ann Plast Surg. 2014;73(1):46–9.
10. Yamamoto T, Yamamoto N, Yamashita M, Furuya M, Hayashi A, Koshima I. Efferent lymphatic vessel anastomosis (ELVA): supermicrosurgical efferent lymphatic vessel-to-venous anastomosis for the prophylactic treatment of subclinical lymphedema. Ann Plast Surg. 2016;76(4):424–7.
11. Yamamoto T, Yamamoto N, Hayashi A, Koshima I. Supermicrosurgical deep lymphatic vessel-to-venous anastomosis for a breast cancer-related arm lymphedema with severe sclerosis of superficial lymphatic vessels. Microsurgery. 2015;37(2):156–9.
12. Ishiura R, Yamamoto T, Siato T, Mito D, Iida T. Comparison of lympho-venous shunt methods in rat model: Supermicrosurgical lymphaticovenular anastomosis versus microsurgical lymphaticovenous implantation. Plast Reconstr Surg. 2017;139(6):1407–13.
13. Yamamoto T, Yamamoto N, Kageyama T, Sakai H, Fuse Y, Tsuihiji K, Tsukuura R. Supermicrosurgery for oncologic reconstructions. Glob Health Med. 2020;2(1):18–23. https://doi.org/10.35772/ghm.2019.01019.
14. Yamamoto T. Onco-reconstructive supermicrosurgery. Eur J Surg Oncol. 2019;45(7):1146–51.
15. Yamamoto T, Yamamoto N, Azuma S, Yoshimatsu H, Seki Y, Narushima M, Koshima I. Near-infrared illumination system-integrated microscope for supermicrosurgical lymphaticovenular anastomosis. Microsurgery. 2014;34(1):23–7.
16. Yamamoto T, Yamamoto N, Numahata T, Yokoyama A, Tashiro K, Yoshimatsu H, Narushima M, Kohima I. Navigation lymphatic supermicrosurgery for the treatment of cancer-related peripheral lymphedema. Vasc Endovasc Surg. 2014;48(2):139–43.
17. Yamamoto T, Yoshimatsu H, Narushima M, Yamamoto N, Hayashi A, Koshima I. Indocyanine green lymphography findings in primary leg lymphedema. Eur J Vasc Endovasc Surg. 2015;49:95–102.
18. Yamamoto T, Yoshimatsu H, Yamamoto N. Complete lymph flow reconstruction: a free vascularized lymph node true perforator flap transfer with efferent lymphaticolymphatic anastomosis. J Plast Reconstr Aesthet Surg. 2016;69(9):1227–33.
19. Yamamoto T, Yamamoto N, Kageyama T, Sakai H, Fuse Y, Tsuihiji K, Tsukuura R. Technical pearls in lymphatic supermicrosurgery. Glob Health Med. 2020;2(1):29–32. https://doi.org/10.35772/ghm.2019.01010.
20. Yamamoto T, Yamamoto N, Yoshimatsu H, Narushima M, Koshima I. Factors associated with lymphosclerosis: an analysis on 962 lymphatic vessels. Plast Reconstr Surg. 2017;140(4):734–41.
21. Yamamoto T, Yamamoto N, Fuse Y, Narushima M, Koshima I. Optimal sites for supermicrosurgical lymphaticovenular anastomosis: an analysis of lymphatic vessel detection rates on 840 surgical fields in lower extremity lymphedema. Plast Reconstr Surg. 2018;142(6):924e–30e.
22. Yamamoto T, Yamamoto N, Yoshimatsu H, Narushima M, Koshima I. Factors associated with lower extremity dysmorphia caused by lower extremity lymphedema. Eur J Vasc Endovasc Surg. 2017;54(1):69–77.
23. Yamamoto T, Narushima M, Koshima I. Lymphatic vessel diameter in female pelvic cancer-related lower extremity lymphedematous limbs. J Surg Oncol. 2018;117(6):1157–63.

24. Yamamoto T, Narushima M, Doi K, Oshima A, Ogata F, Mihara M, Koshima I, Mundinger GS. Characteristic indocyanine green lymphography findings in lower extremity lymphedema: the generation of a novel lymphedema severity staging system using dermal backflow patterns. Plast Reconstr Surg. 2011;127(5):1979–86.
25. Yamamoto T, Yamamoto N, Doi K, Oshima A, Yoshimatsu H, Todokoro T, Ogata F, Mihara M, Narushima M, Iida T, Koshima I. Indocyanine green (ICG)-enhanced lymphography for upper extremity lymphedema: a novel severity staging system using dermal backflow (DB) patterns. Plast Reconstr Surg. 2011;128(4):941–7.
26. Yamamoto T, Matsuda N, Doi K, Oshima A, Yoshimatsu H, Todokoro T, Ogata F, Mihara M, Narushima M, Iida T, Koshima I. The earliest finding of indocyanine green (ICG) lymphography in asymptomatic limbs of lower extremity lymphedema patients secondary to cancer treatment: the modified dermal backflow (DB) stage and concept of subclinical lymphedema. Plast Reconstr Surg. 2011;128(4):314e–21e.
27. Yamamoto T, Yamamoto N, Yoshimatsu H, Hayami S, Narushima M, Koshima I. Indocyanine green lymphography for evaluation of genital lymphedema in secondary lower extremity lymphedema patients. J Vasc Surg Venous Lymphat Disord. 2013;1(4):400–5.
28. Yamamoto T, Matsuda N, Todokoro T, Yoshimatsu H, Narushima M, Mihara M, Uchida G, Koshima I. Lower extremity lymphedema index: a simple method for severity evaluation of lower extremity lymphedema. Ann Plast Surg. 2011;67(6):637–40.
29. Yamamoto T, Narushima M, Yoshimatsu H, Yamamoto N, Oka A, Seki Y, Todokoro T, Iida T, Koshima I. Indocyanine green velocity: lymph transportation capacity deterioration with progression of lymphedema. Ann Plast Surg. 2013;71(5):59–594.
30. Yamamoto T, Narushima M, Yoshimatsu H, Yamamoto N, Kikuchi K, Todokoro T, Iida T, Koshima I. Dynamic indocyanine green lymphography for breast cancer-related arm lymphedema. Ann Plast Surg. 2014;73(6):706–9.

Step-by-Step Instruction: Single Site Multiple Lymphatic-Venous Anastomosis Technique

10

Corrado Cesare Campisi, Lidia Molinari, Pietro Giovanni di Summa, and Corradino Campisi

Introduction

Upper and lower extremity primary and secondary lymphedema remains an often poorly recognized disease that causes significant morbidity in advanced cases, in terms of physical limitations, infection risk, and serious life-threatening conditions [1, 2]. Chronic lymphedema is associated with fibrotic tissue changes and adipose tissue formation ("non-pitting" edema) that is irreversible when untreated or improperly managed [3, 4]. Conservative treatments are time-consuming and expensive, and can be ineffective in halting the progression of the disease [2, 5].

The development, in the past 50 years, of surgical techniques to restore lymphatic flow offers treatments that not only target symptomatic relief but also offer a functional repair of the underlying problem of lymph fluid stasis. Initial procedures involved lymph nodal-venous shunts, but these were associated with a high failure rate due to the thrombogenic effect of the lymph node pulp entering the venous vasculature and/or the re-endothelization of the lymph node surface [6, 7]. Technical modifications have improved the long-term outcomes of lymphatic microsurgery, but the efficacy, in terms of volume reduction and long-term stability, remains highly variable between surgical centers worldwide [8–11].

In this chapter, the author's experience refers to a period between 1973 and 2021, with a clinical registry of 5046 cases, treated by lymphatic microsurgery for extremity lymphedema of both the upper and lower extremities, with primary and secondary etiology, at early and late stages (Fig. 10.1). A key technical modification in the evolution of this experience is that the lymphatic-venous anastomoses are performed at a single site at middle volar surface of the arm or at the inguinal-crural region. Both the superficial and deep lymphatic vessels are anastomosed to collateral branches of the main veins close to the vein valves, to avoid backflow of blood and the consequent closure of the anastomotic site [11]. Planning of this microsurgical approach includes preoperative superficial and deep isotope lymphography or lymphoscintigraphy, combined with calculation of the transport index (TI) [12–14]. The patent blue violet (PBV) lymphochromic test and the fluorescent indocyanine green (ICG) microlymphography test are combined intraoperatively to select both superficial and deep lymph collectors. The single site approach is strategically based on both the anatomical and functional considerations, and also minimizes invasive surgical incisions and thereby potential entry sites for infections.

Typical Indications

- The "single site multiple lymphatic-venous anastomosis" (ss-MLVA) technique is a versatile procedure indicated for the management of upper and lower extremity lymphedema, with primary and secondary etiologies, at early and late stages (Tables 10.1 and 10.2).

Supplementary Information The online version of this chapter (https://doi.org/10.1007/978-3-030-93039-4_10) contains supplementary material, which is available to authorized users.

C. C. Campisi
Plastic, Reconstructive and Aesthetic Surgery, Private Consultant, Genoa, Italy

University of Catania, Genoa & Catania, Italy
e-mail: corrado@campisiclinic.com

L. Molinari
General Surgery, Private Consultant, Genoa, Italy

P. G. di Summa
Department of Plastic, Reconstructive and Hand Surgery, Centre Hospitalier Universitaire Vaudois (CHUV), Lausanne, Switzerland
e-mail: Pietro.di-Summa@chuv.ch

C. Campisi (✉)
General Surgery, Vascular Surgery and Emergency Surgery, Clinical Lymphology, Lymphatic Surgery and Microsurgery, School of Medical Sciences and Pharmaceutics, Department of Surgical Sciences and Integrated Diagnostics – DISC, University of Genoa, Genoa, Italy
e-mail: campisi@unige.it

M. V. Schaverien, J. H. Dayan (eds.), *Multimodal Management of Upper and Lower Extremity Lymphedema*, https://doi.org/10.1007/978-3-030-93039-4_10

- The single site is the middle volar surface of the arm for upper limb lymphedema, and the inguinal-crural region for lower limb lymphedema.
- The ss-MLVA microsurgical approach is planned and guided using preoperative superficial and deep isotope lymphography (lymphoscintigraphy), and by calculation of the TI parameter (Kleinhans's method) – a TI lower than 9 is normal, and TI higher than 9 is pathologic [12–14].
- Both the PBV lymphochromic test, by intradermal, subcutaneous, and subfascial locoregional injection, and fluorescent ICG microlymphography, by intradermal locoregional injection, are used intraoperatively to select both the superficial and deep lymph collectors.
- The stepwise surgical approach includes sampling of the superficial and deep extracellular-interstitial matrix, lymph nodes, superficial and deep afferent and efferent lymph collectors, and fascia, for histopathological-immunohistochemistry evaluation and for diagnostic, staging, and prognostic purposes [15].
- Although indicated for the treatment of established lymphedema, the ss-MLVA microsurgical procedure has an additional role in prophylactic surgery performed at the time of lymphadenectomy [16].

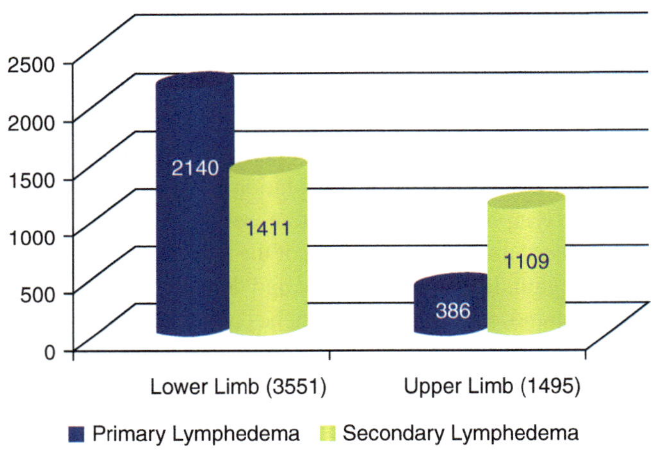

Fig. 10.1 Genoa clinical registry, 1973–2021: 5046 cases treated by lymphatic microsurgery

Anatomy

The vascular architecture of the upper and lower limbs includes a rich network of superficial and deep lymphatic-lymph node pathways that intercommunicate and have a high number of anatomic variants. These arrangements are even more complex in primary lymphedema due to congenital anomalies-malformations, and in secondary lymphedema following lymphadenectomy and/or radiotherapy. For this reason, the most convenient surgical approach to address the altered or damaged locoregional lymph vasculature is target-

Table 10.2 Staging of lymphedema. International Society of Lymphology (ISL) Consensus Document, modified by C. Campisi, 2009

Staging of lymphedema	
Stage I	A. *Latent lymphedema*, without clinical evidence of edema, but with impaired lymph transport capacity (provable by lymphoscintigraphy) and with initial immunohistochemical alterations of lymph nodes, lymph vessels, and extracellular matrix
	B. *Initial lymphedema*, totally or partially decreasing by rest and draining position, with worsening impairment of lymph transport capacity and of immunohistochemical alterations of lymph collectors, nodes, and extracellular matrix
Stage II	A. *Increasing lymphedema*, with "vanishing" lymph transport capacity, relapsing lymphangitis attacks, fibroindurative skin changes, and developing disability.
	B. *"Column-shaped" limb fibrolymphedema*, with lymphostatic skin changes, suppressed lymph transport capacity, and worsening disability
Stage III	A. *Properly called elephantiasis*, with scleroindurative pachydermitis, papillomatous lymphostatic verrucosis, no lymph transport capacity, and life-threatening disability
	B. *Extreme elephantiasis* with total disability
	(ISL Consensus Document, modified by C. Campisi, 2009)

Table 10.1 Lymphedema classification (on etiological basis). C. Campisi, 2001

C.Campisi, 2001

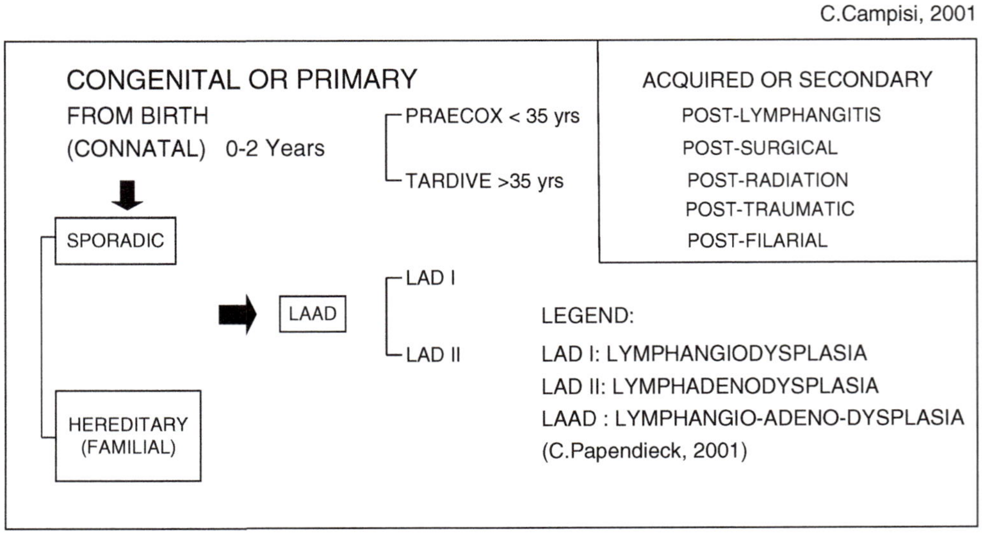

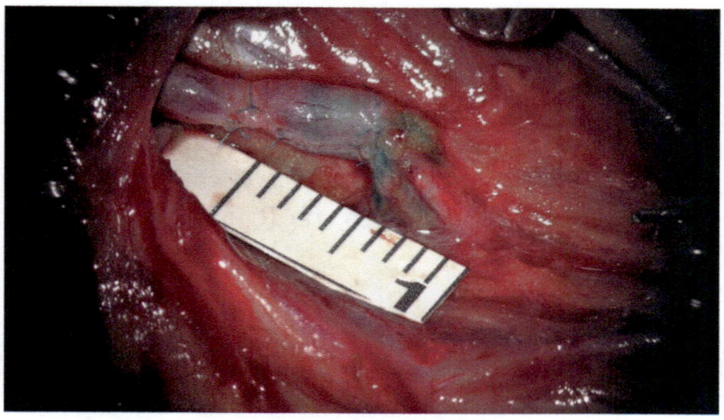

Fig. 10.2 Single site multiple lymphatic-venous anastomosis (ss-MLVA) for the treatment of upper extremity lymphedema. The single surgical site is at the anatomic crossroads of the middle volar surface of the arm, along the bicipital ridge and the corresponding brachial neurovascular bundle

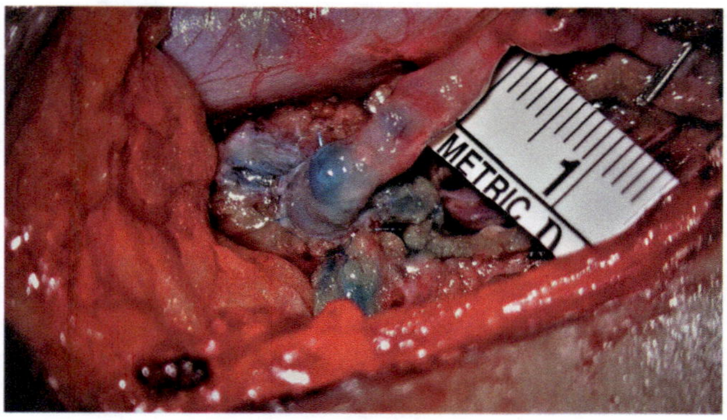

Fig. 10.3 Single site multiple (superficial and deep) lymphatic-venous anastomosis (ss-MLVA) for the treatment of primary lower extremity lymphedema. The single surgical site is at the anatomic crossroads of the left inguinal-crural region; the great saphenous vein and the anastomotic site are shown

ing the anatomic crossroads, which in the arm is located at the middle volar surface along the bicipital ridge and the corresponding brachial neurovascular bundle (Fig. 10.2), and in the lower limb at the inguinal-crural region (Fig. 10.3).

During microsurgical dissection, the superficial and deep lymph vessels are identified using a combination of the PBV and ICG tests, identifying and selecting lymphatic collectors for multiple anastomosis from all three anatomic levels (superficial-subdermal, superficial-epifascial, and subfascial); telescopic end-to-end anastomosis of several lymph vessels with minor vein branches that have competent and well-functioning valve apparatuses allows a greater amount of lymph to flow through the anastomosis, creating a long-lasting positive lymphatic-venous one-way pressure gradient, with constant anatomic and functional patency, both in clinostatism and in orthostatism, thereby avoiding the potential venous-lymphatic backflow gravitational phenomenon with consequent thrombotic occlusion of the anastomosis. There is an additional advantage of the ss-MLVA technique: by creating the anastomosis in close proximity to a valve in the recipient vein, the valvular pumping generates a suction that sucks the lymph through the anastomosis, thus preventing thrombosis by the combination of this "flutter valve micro-pump draining mechanism" in addition to the positive lymphatic-venous one-way pressure gradient generated by the anastomosis of multiple lymph vessels to a single vein.

Patient Selection and Preoperative Investigations

The main indication for lymphatic surgery-microsurgery is in patients that are nonresponsive or only partially responsive to nonoperative conservative treatments [17] [Genoa Protocol: manual and mechanical lymphatic drainage according to the "Combined Physical Therapy (CPT) System," and intermittent negative pressure therapy, in conjunction with an innovative technological physical biocircuit, digitally personalized for each patient, appropriate multilayered bandages, and compressive garments or stockings]. Mechanical lymphatic drainage refers to the use of uniform and sequential-peristaltic pneumatic devices. In addition, manual lymphatic drainage (MLD) is performed by means of a tailored protocol (LPG® Endermologie system). The "Completed Lymphedema Function Therapy" (CLyFT) Protocol is applied in three phases: Phase 1, an intensive/subintensive preoperative phase, maintained for a period of 6–12 months; Phase 2, a surgical phase of approximately 1 week in length; and Phase 3, postoperative rehabilitation and follow-up for a minimum of 5 years (Fig. 10.4).

Due to potential associations of peripheral lymphatic disease with unrecognized pathologies in other locations or other well-known morbidities, each patient affected by upper and lower extremity lymphedema requires a meticulous clinical history, general checkup, and specific locoregional objective physical examination, as well as clinical measurements (including limb water volumetry, circumferences, pitting test, and Stemmer sign). In additional to these clinical parameters, imaging using isotope lymphography or lymphoscintigraphy for the comparative evaluation of the superficial and deep lymphatic pathways is performed with the additional calculation of the TI [12–14], with whole body imaging acquired where indicted. Venous and arterial echo color Doppler is systematically carried out with additional imaging including ultrasound-echography, magnetic resonance lymphography (MRL), and CT, as necessary. In particular, a Duplex scan must be performed in all patients to identify any venous disorder that might be contributing to the edema. In most patients, it is possible to correct venous dysfunction secondary to valve incompetency, at the same time as the microsurgical procedure, such as by performing external valvuloplasty (using 6/0-7/0 nylon sutures).

In a minority of cases, nonsurgically correctable or uncontrolled venous pathology associated with lymphedema can represent a contraindication to performing MLVA. In these selected cases, however, it is possible to reconstruct a new lymphatic pathway by adopting C. Campisi's technique of autologous interpositioned vein grafting between the lymphatics identified above and below the site of obstruction to lymphatic flow [18] (Fig. 10.5). For this procedure, originally named "Multiple Lymphatic-Venous-Lymphatic Anastomosis" or "Lymphatic-Venous-Lymphatic Plasty," the autologous vein graft can be harvested from the same operative site or from the forearm (typically the cephalic

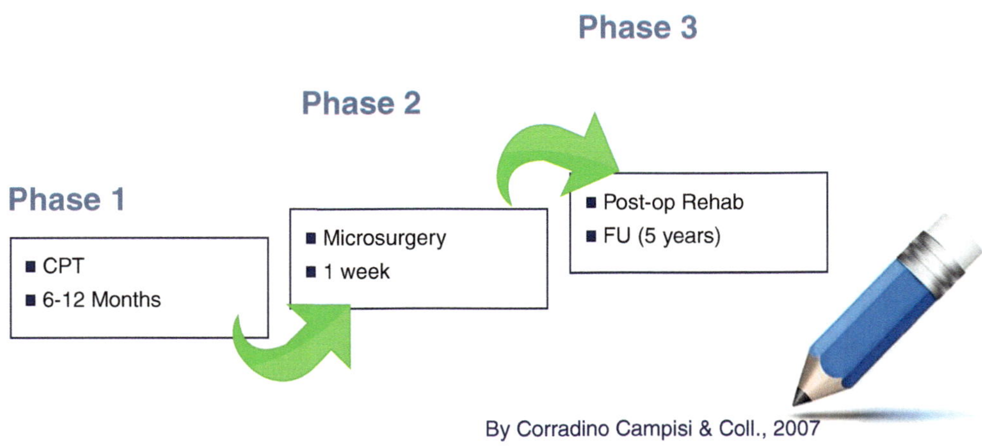

Fig. 10.4 Staging-Guided Complete Lymphedema Functional Treatment (CLyFT). *CPT* Combined Physical Therapy; *FU* Follow-Up

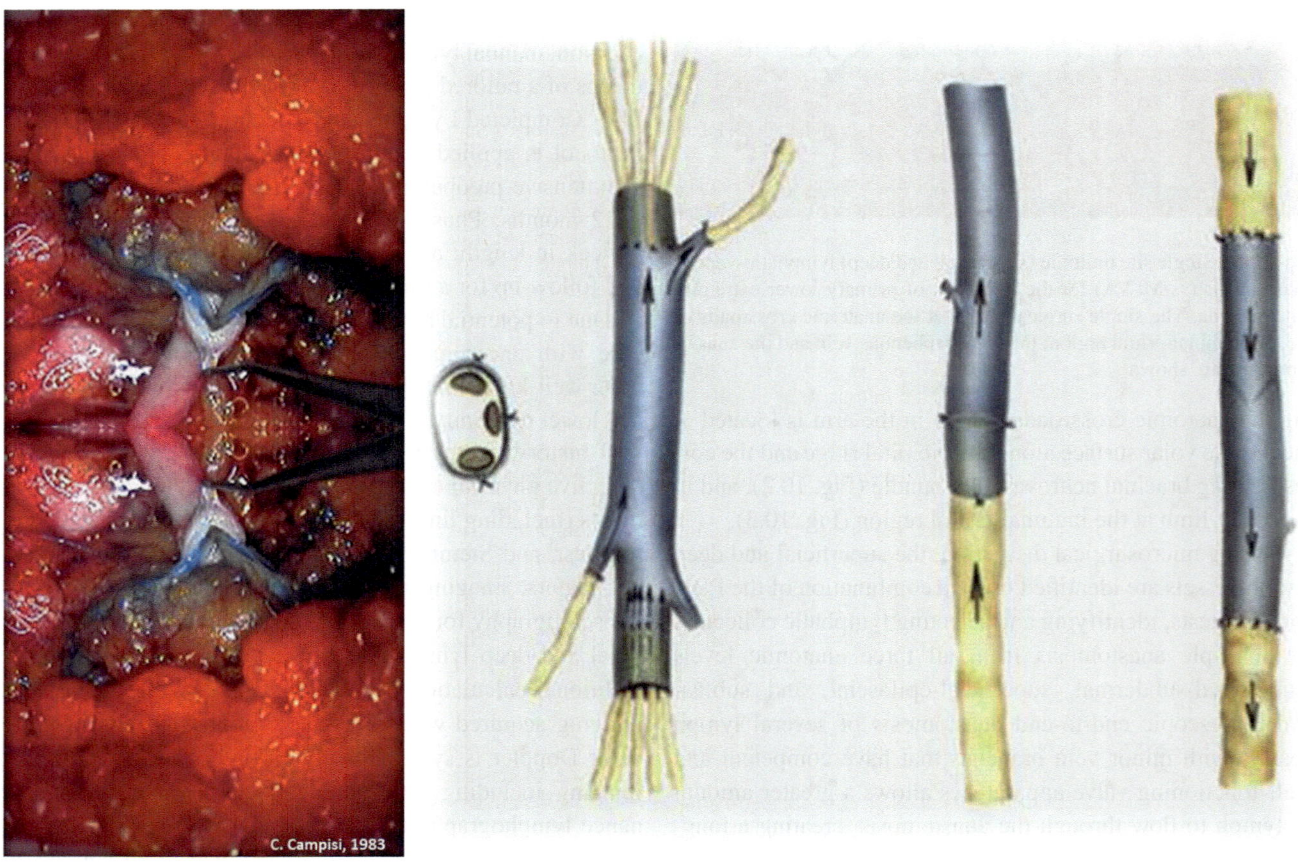

Fig. 10.5 Autologous interpositioned vein grafting. The vein graft is placed between the lymphatics above and below the obstacle to lymph flow, under operating microscope visualization (15×). The original schematic drawing by the author: an alternative microsurgical option for selected cases of phlebo-lymphedema with stable and persistent venous hypertension

vein). The length of the graft can vary from 7 to 15 cm, collecting several lymphatics and anastomosing them (in higher number than at the proximal cut-end) to the distal cut-end of the vein segment, with the valves ensuring that the graft is filled with lymph fluid, thereby addressing the flow in an antigravitational direction by the positive pressure gradient. The technique used at both cut-ends of the vein graft is the same telescopic end-to-end anastomosis technique used and described below for the ss-MLVA procedure.

Relative contraindications to lymphatic microsurgery are few, although specifically include lymphatic-lymph nodal aplasia or agenesis (very uncommon), diffuse metastatic carcinoma, and extremely advanced lymphedema or elephantiasis (Campisi Stage IIIB), or lymphedema unresponsive to conservative therapy in noncompliant patients. The age of the patient is not an absolute consideration in the indications for lymphatic microsurgery. This surgery is usually performed using locoregional subarachnoid anesthesia for lower limb lymphedema, and by plexus block or laryngeal mask for upper limb lymphedema. Therefore, both lymphatic microsurgery and mini-invasive anesthetic techniques are normally available for the majority of the patients, even in those with important general comorbidities, on the condition that those are well-controlled.

It is essential that patients are optimized preoperatively with adherence to maximal medical therapy and conservative measures. In addition, a precise informed consensus must be acquired in detail with the patient during the preoperative period of the clinical assessment, with all information clearly specified, representing a basic written document of fundamental importance not only on the medicolegal point of view but also from clinical, psychological, ethical, and deontological points of view.

Operative Techniques

Principles

The operating theatre, organized for lymphatic microsurgery and particularly for ss-MLVA with the correct equipment, includes the following (Fig. 10.6):

- A single operating microscope.
- A complete surgical and microsurgical armamentarium (two specific side tables).
- Correct equipment for fluorescent ICG microlymphography to monitor all phases of the surgery.
- A specifically skilled technician should be regularly available in the operating theatre, to ensure mechanical working of all technology mentioned above.
- Two widescreen TVs.
- Complementary technology for live broadcast and procedure recording; if possible, including the use of prearranged technology for teleconferencing, Skype or streaming viewing, or online live transmission through the Zoom platform, for surgical education.

Anesthesia

- For upper limb lymphedema, either a brachial plexus block or general anesthesia by laryngeal mask is preferable, unless general endotracheal anesthesia is indicated.
- For lower limb lymphedema, locoregional subarachnoid anesthesia is usually performed.

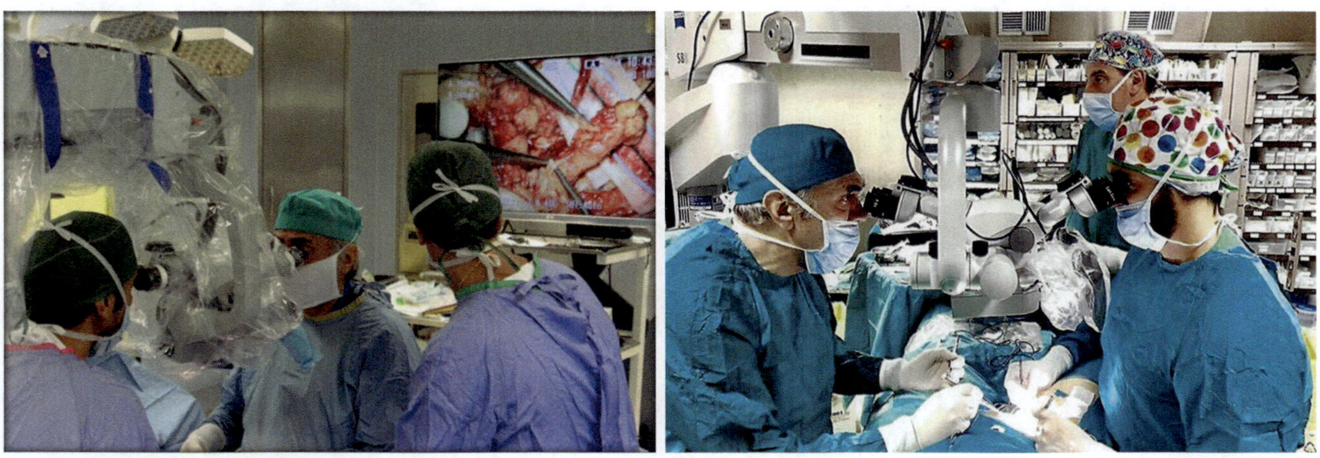

Fig. 10.6 Operating theatre and technological equipment for lymphatic microsurgery

Patient Positioning

- For upper limb lymphedema, the most convenient position is with the arm in abduction, exposing the volar surface.
- For unilateral lower limb lymphedema, the most convenient position is with the extremity in abduction, exposing the inguinal-crural region, and with partial flexion of the leg.
- For bilateral lower limb lymphedema, the most convenient positioning is with the limbs in the "frog-leg" position.

Recipient Site Preparation

Guided by preoperative lymphoscintigraphy, complemented by Duplex ultrasonography to map the locoregional venous tree, recipient site preparation is performed both by injection of 1.5–2.5 ml of BPV dye (intradermal, subcutaneous, and subfascial) and by intradermal injection of 1 ml of ICG solution (25 mg of powder diluted with 5 ml of 5% glucose solution), at the middle third of the volar surface of the arm, or at the middle/superior third of the anteromedial surface of the thigh. Before performing the skin incision, along the bicipital ridge (for the arm), or immediately under the inguinal plica (for the thigh), the surgical area is explored using fluorescent ICG microlymphography to map the superficial (subdermal and subcutaneous) lymphatic pathways.

Loupes and Operating Microscope Surgical Procedure (Figs. 10.7 and 10.8) (see supplementary material)

Preliminary dissection is performed under loupe magnification (3–4x), with gentle dissection of lymphatic structures and contiguous venous vessels. To better identify lymphatic structures, ICG microlymphography (useful in particular for superficial lymph pathways) is repeated "ad hoc" many times during the procedure, with simultaneous additional evaluation using the BPV lymphochromic dye test (useful for deep lymph vessels too). At the same time, micro-sampling for histopathology-immunohistochemistry is performed of the extracellular (interstitial) superficial matrix, perilymphatic and perivenous tissue, and lymphatic-lymph nodal structures, with afferent and efferent superficial and deep collectors, fascia, and extracellular deep matrix. This evaluation is very helpful for the definitive diagnosis, staging, and prognostic evaluation (the available anatomo-histopathologist should be properly skilled in this ambit of pathology).

The next part of the procedure is performed under the operating microscope (generally at 25x magnification). The identified lymphatic vessels are collected in bundles (superficial together with deep lymphatics) and then are anastomosed to the recipient minor venous branch(es) previously dissected. This fine dissection must preserve "vasa vasorum" with "vasa et nervi lymphaticorum" in the peri-adventitial space to avoid any possible injury to the anatomic trophism and regular motility of the lymphangion

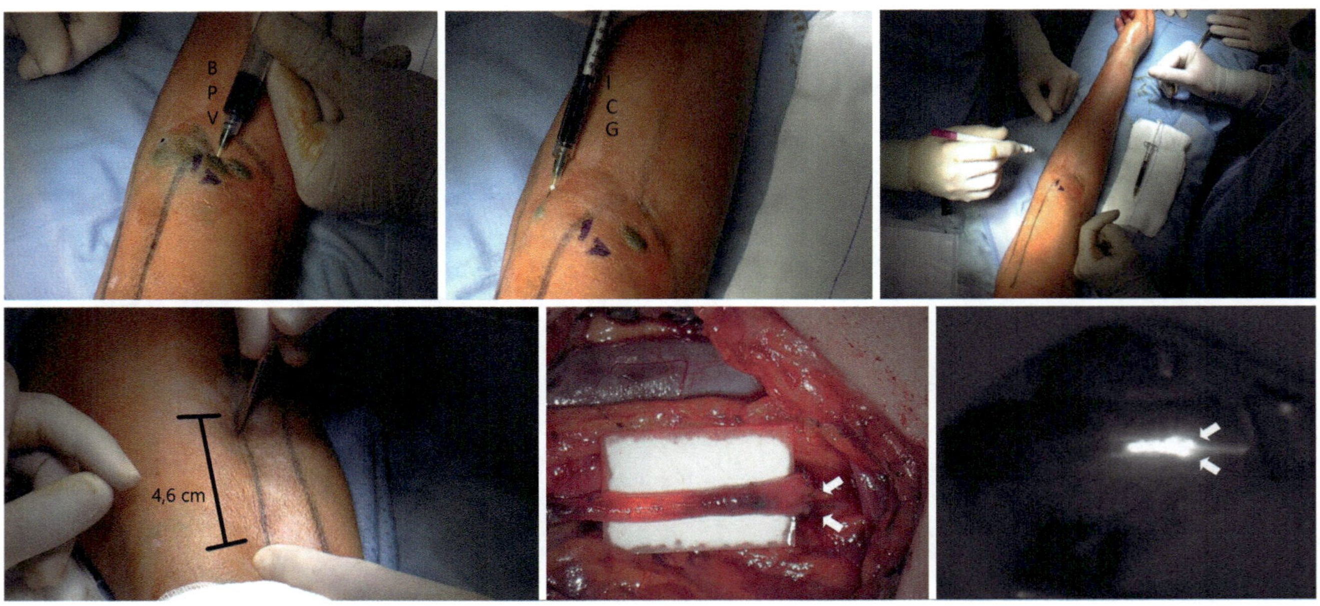

Fig. 10.7 Upper extremity breast cancer-related lymphedema (BCRL): single-site multiple lymphatic-venous anastomosis (ss-MLVA), with very good evidence of patency at the anastomotic site using indocyanine green (ICG) microlymphography (arrows)

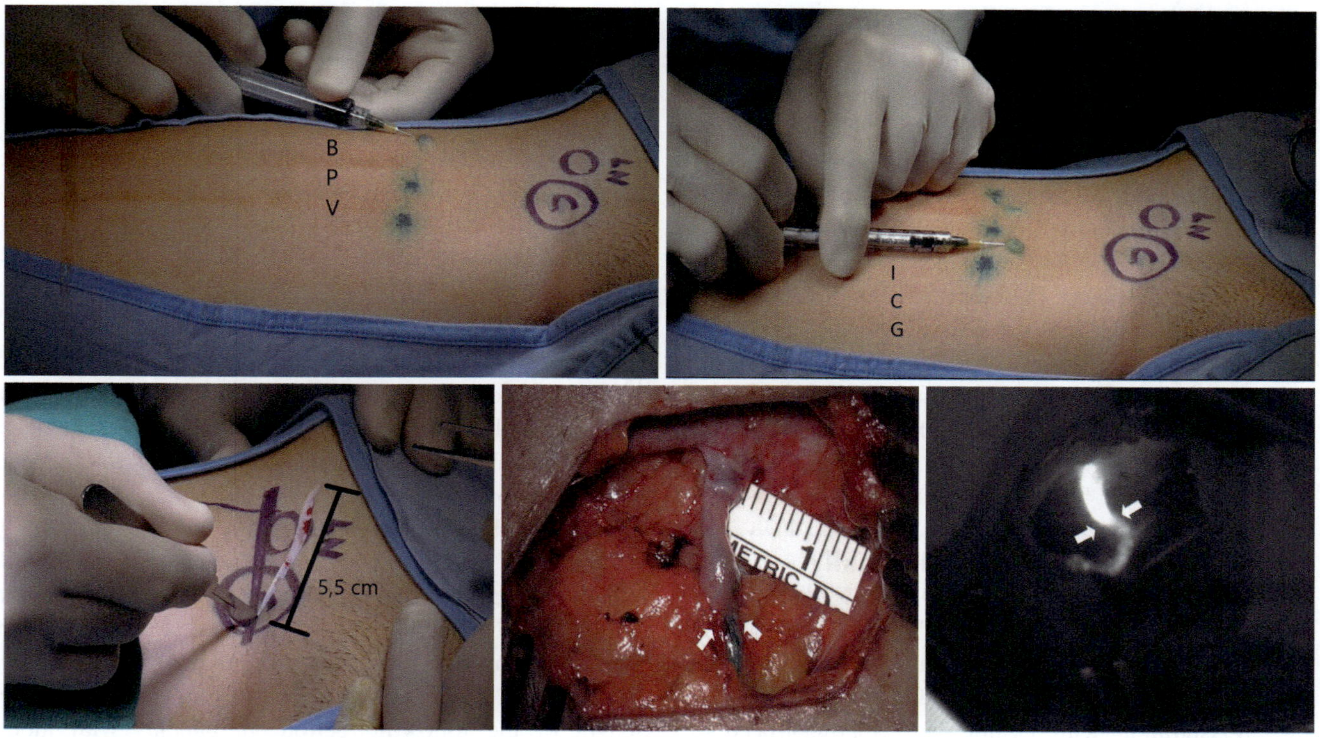

Fig. 10.8 Lower extremity primary lymphedema: single-site multiple lymphatic-venous anastomosis (ss-MLVA), with very good evidence of patency at the anastomotic site using indocyanine green (ICG) microlymphography (arrows)

units in the anastomosed lymphatic vessels [17]. The multiple lympho-venous shunt is performed as an end-to-end telescopic anastomosis, with initial inosculation by only one U-shaped 8/0-9/0-10/0 polypropylene stitch. The completion of the anastomosis is performed by annular peri-adventitial interrupted sutures, anchoring the vein "rima oris" to the peri-adventitial tissue of the anastomosed lymphatic pedicle. At the end, the initial U-shaped stitch is removed. Depending on the number of identified and isolated lymph vessels and the gap that exists between them and recipient vein, more than one MLVA can be performed. In this way, the number of lymph vessels anastomosed can vary from a minimum of 3 to a maximum of 30. The patency of the anastomosis is verified by the BPV/ICG tests, in particular by the progressively increasing flow of fluorescent lymph into the vein visualized using the ICG test.

Following meticulous hemostatic control, gentle washing of the scar bed by physiological solution with gentamicin and ropivacaine, placement of a small tubular drain under low aspiration pressure, and wound closure with absorbable subcutaneous and intradermal sutures, the operation is concluded. A low compressive medical dressing is applied and the limb is then covered by a multilayer functional bandage.

Postoperative Care

- Antibiotic short-term prophylaxis is usually performed, with anti-thromboembolic prophylaxis by daily subcutaneous low molecular weight heparin (LMWH) injections given for 10 days.
- To avoid any possible trauma to the anastomotic site, following the procedure for lower extremity lymphedema, the patient is maintained on 2–3 days of bed rest, with passive and active gentle mobilization: a urinary catheter can be used during these few days. For upper limb lymphedema, the patient can stand up and mobilize a few hours after surgery.
- At 1 week postoperatively, the bandage is removed and replaced by proper elastic garments or stockings.

Preoperative and Postoperative Conservative Treatment

The patient is managed according to the stage-guided CLyFT Protocol developed in Genoa in 2007 (Fig. 10.4). The intensive preoperative Phase 1 of the CLyFT Protocol is targeted to reduce the size of the affected limb(s) as much as possible prior to the surgical approach, followed by a gentle postoperative phase in which the pressures of the lymphatic drainage are gradually increased as healing continues, and finally, by a long-term maintenance phase of daily (often self-managed) manual-mechanical lymphatic drainage, with physical remedial exercises and activity, to strengthen the anastomotic joints over time. Optimal lifestyle, skin care, cosmetic measures, and tailored dietary habits, with scientifically based functional foods, are adhered to [19]. The timing of the treatment protocol depends on the preoperative stage of the disease, but in general, there is 1 or 2 weeks of preoperative CLyFT, followed by surgery, and then 1 or 2 weeks of postoperative CLyFT, before the patient initiates the maintenance phase.

Additional Supplementary Minimally Invasive Procedures

Starting in 2012, the additional sequential minimally invasive technique of selective liposuction (named "Fibro-Lipo-Lymph-Aspiration" with "Lymph Vessel Sparing Procedure": FLLA-LVSP), developed in Genoa by C.C. Campisi, has been applied to late stage lymphedema (Stages IIB–III) previously treated by lymphatic microsurgery with only partial improvement of the disease [20, 21] (Figs. 10.9 and 10.10).

Complications

No significant postoperative complications have occurred in the authors' clinical registry, in the immediate, medium and long-term follow-up period, with the exception of 3% on average of non-compliant patients.

Outcomes (Fig. 10.11)

In the early stages of the disease, there is an absence of (or minimal) fibrosclerotic tissue changes in the lymphatic walls and surrounding tissues, and these microsurgical techniques can be applied to treat peripheral lymphedema with excellent clinical outcomes. Compared with preoperatively, over 90% of patients obtained significant reductions in excess limb volume (ELV), with an average 75% reduction as measured by limb water volumetry and circumferences. These results were stable over an average of 10 years of follow-up. Over 96% of patients with earlier stages of disease (Stage I or IIA) progressively stopped using conservative therapies over the length of the follow-up period. In patients with more advanced lymphedema (Stages IIB and III) treated by previous lymphatic microsurgery with limited improvement and that were subsequently treated by sequential additional FLLA-LVSP (performed from 2012 up to the first half of

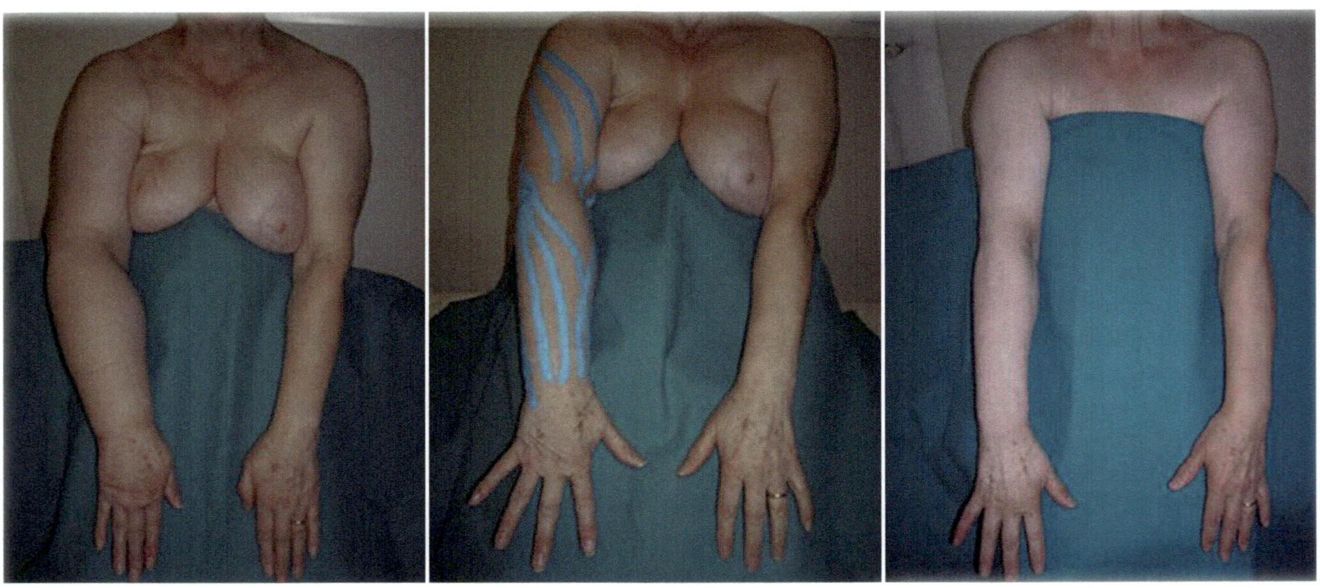

Fig. 10.9 Fibro-Lipo-Lymph-Aspiration with Lymph Vessel Sparing Procedure (FLLA-LVSP), after single-site multiple lymphatic-venous anastomosis (ss-MLVA) for the treatment of advanced breast cancer-related lymphedema (BCRL) of the right upper extremity

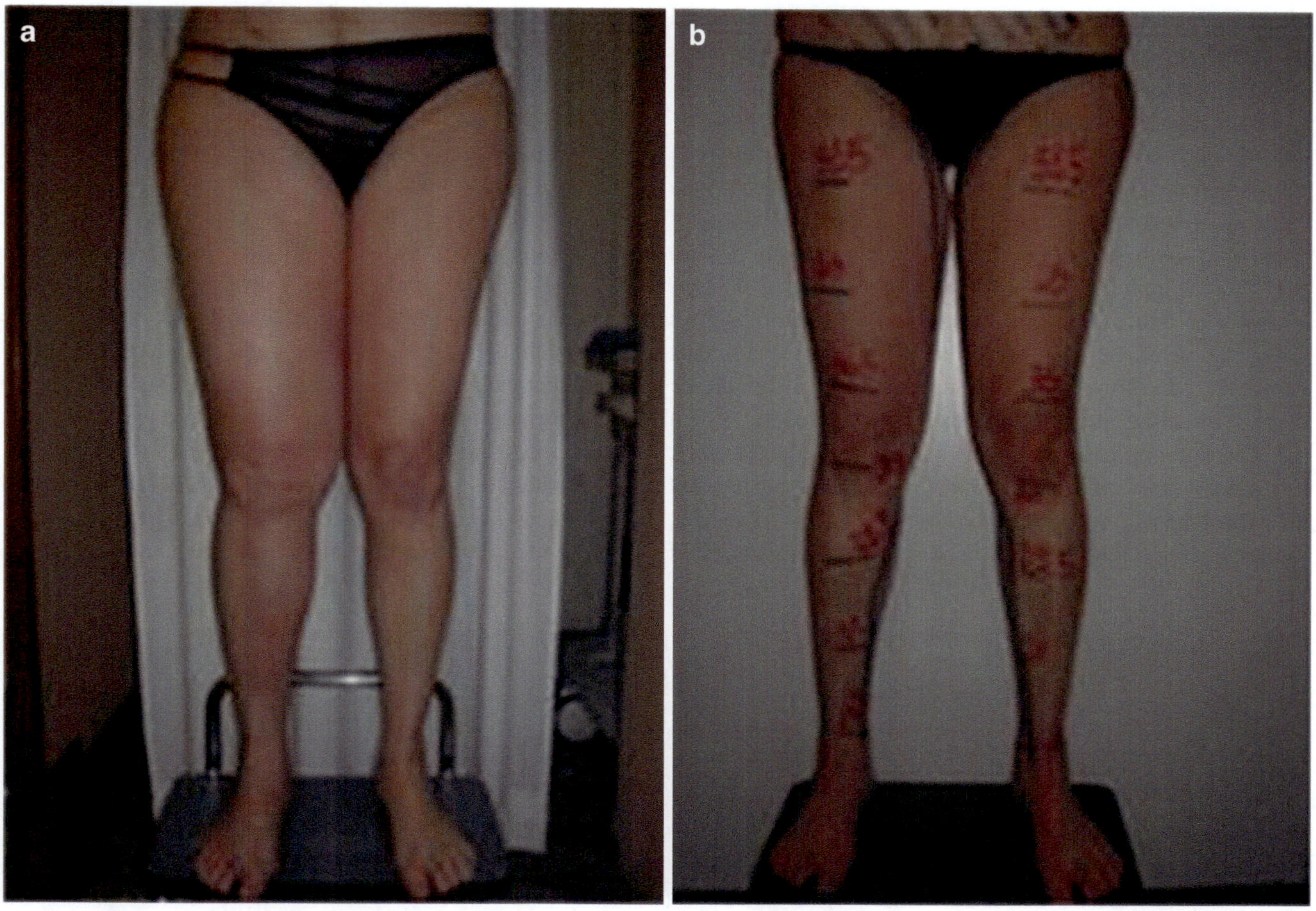

Fig. 10.10 Single-site multiple lymphatic-venous anastomosis (ss-MLVA) and Fibro-Lipo-Lymph-Aspiration with Lymph Vessel Sparing Procedure (FLLA-LVSP) for the treatment of right lower extremity advanced lymphedema related to uterine cervical cancer

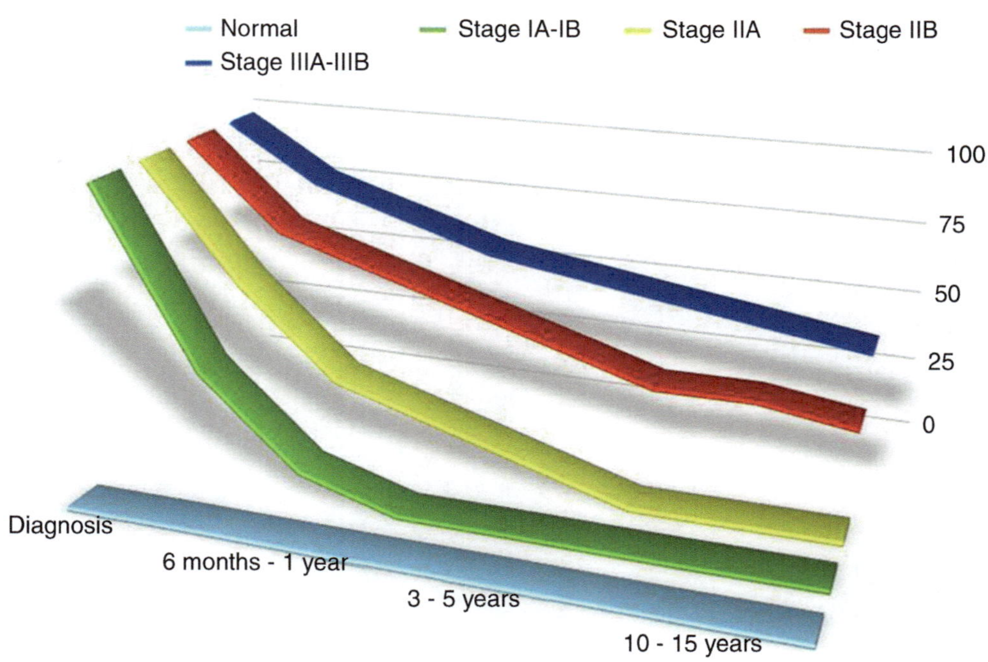

Fig. 10.11 Staging-guided surgical treatment of upper and lower extremity lymphedema: long-term clinical outcomes (by C. Campisi, C.C. Campisi et al.)

2020; 387 patients in total), over 80% significantly decreased the frequency of physical therapies and discontinued compressive garments or stockings.

In all patients, the frequency of cellulitis attacks considerably reduced by over 95%, compared with preoperatively. There were no immediate significant postoperative complications, such as postoperative infections, lymphorrhea, or worsening of their edema. In the past 5 years, fluorescent ICG microlymphography has also been performed postoperatively to confirm anastomotic patency. This method allows visualization of the superficial lymphatic pathways and is valuable to confirm the significant reductions in lymphatic dermal backflow after the microsurgical procedure. When ICG microlymphography is used immediately after surgery, it is possible to verify microsurgical patency and ensure that no thrombosis of the anastomoses has occurred. Lymphoscintigraphy was also used to verify the patency of the microanastomoses in the long term by direct and indirect methods (Figs. 10.12 and 10.13). These included the following: (a) reduced dermal backflow of the tracer and the appearance of preferential lymphatic pathways that were not discernible preoperatively; (b) disappearance of the tracer at the site of the lymphatic-venous anastomoses (MLVA), indicating the passage of the lymph into the venous system, or the visualization of the interpositioned autologous vein graft (MLVLA); and (c) earlier liver uptake of tracer, compared with preoperatively, taken as indirect evidence of the passage of lymph in the vascular system. In the long term, the ongoing reduction in ELV over time, together with follow-up lymphoscintigraphy, provided evidence of the patency of the anastomoses and the absence of thrombosis.

No patient who was compliant with the CLyFT Protocol experienced a worsening of lymphedema. There was anecdotal evidence of significant patient satisfaction with the

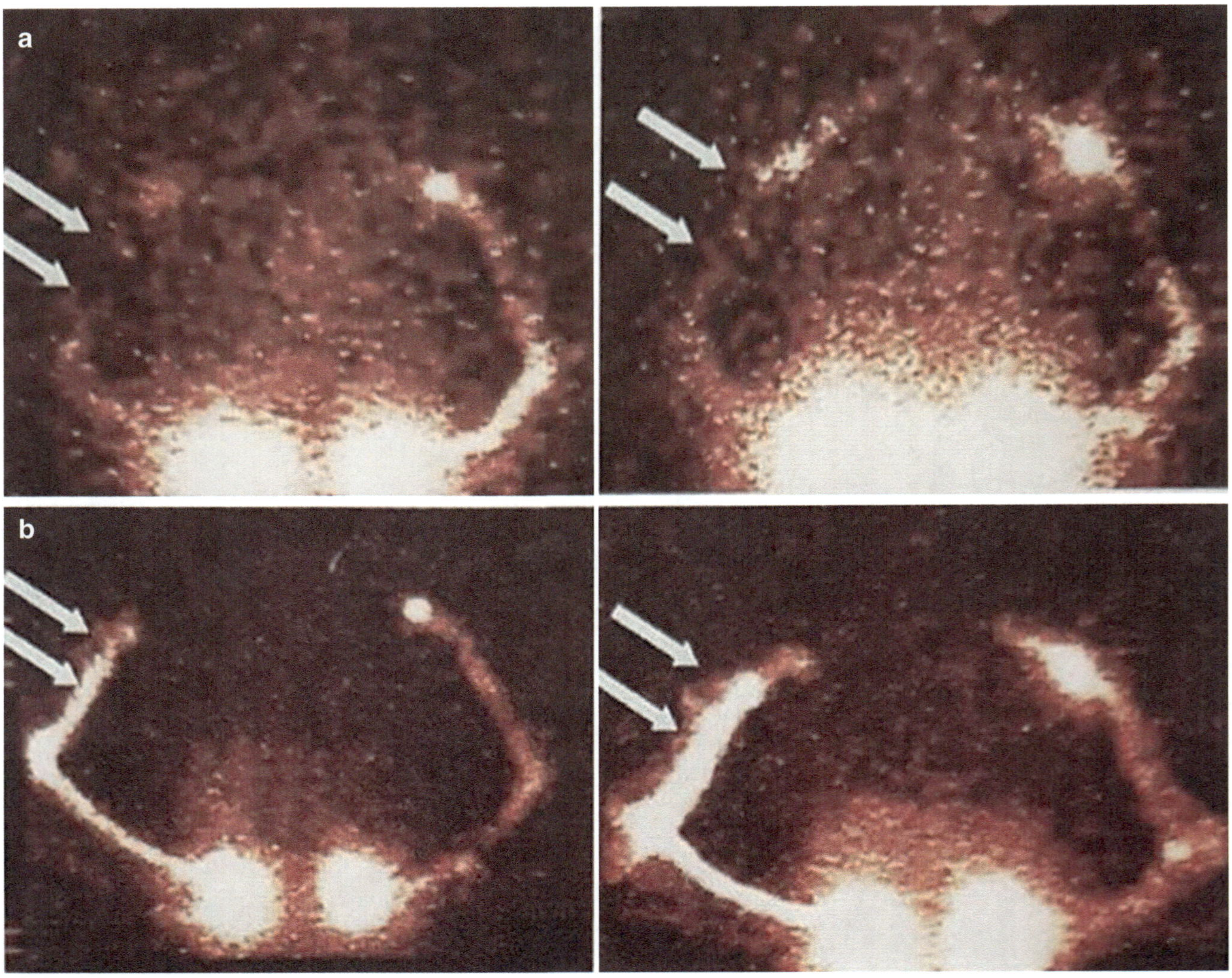

Fig. 10.12 Preoperative lymphoscintigraphy in a patient affected by right arm lymphedema secondary to breast cancer treatment: poor lymphatic transport along the arm can be seen with dermal backflow (arrows) (left). Postoperative lymphoscintigraphy shows the appearance of preferential lymphatic pathways and disappearance of dermal backflow (arrows) (right)

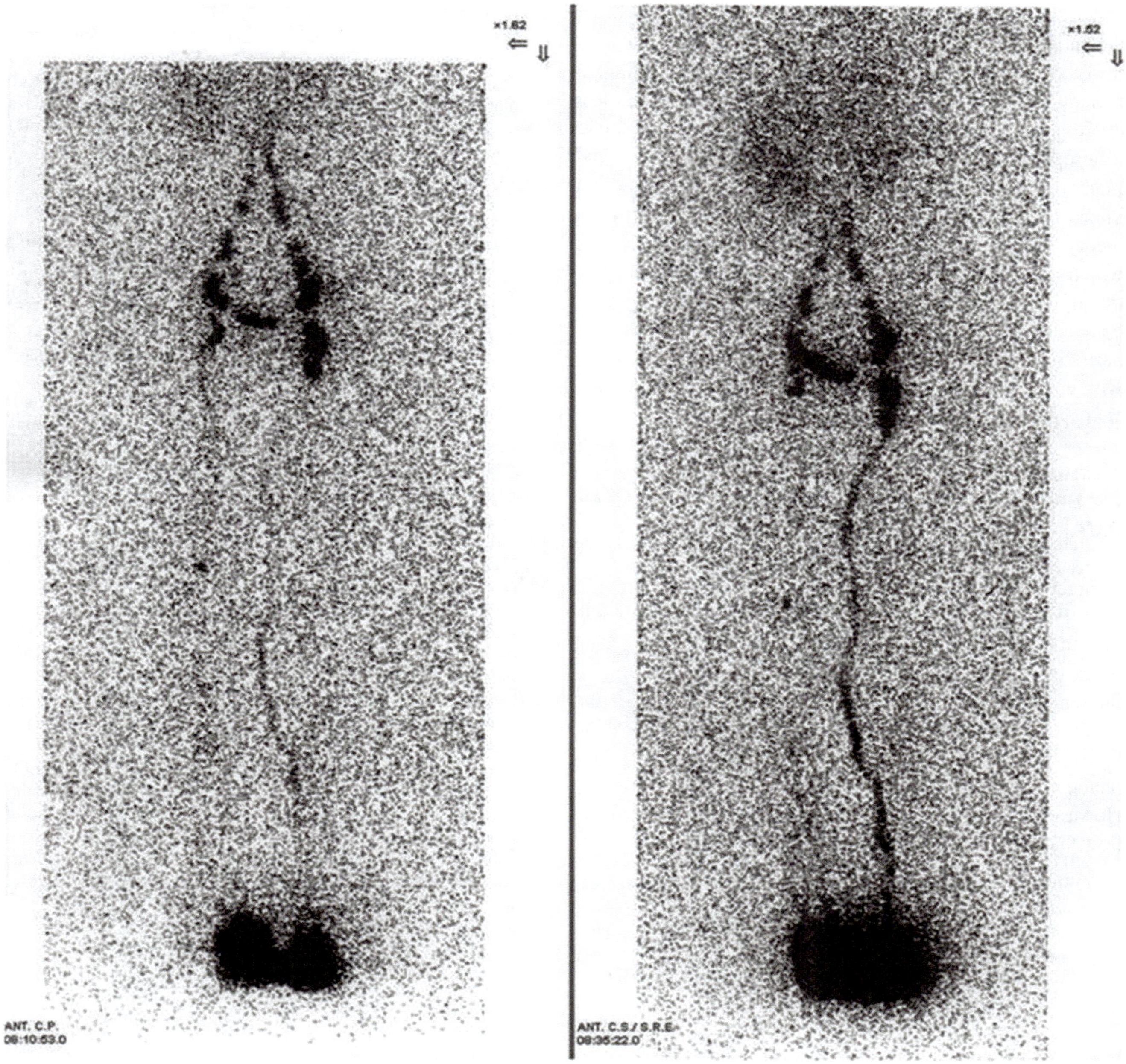

Fig. 10.13 Preoperative lymphoscintigraphy in a patient affected by left lower extremity lymphedema (left). Postoperative lymphoscintigraphy shows the appearance of preferential lymphatic pathways into the inguinal region (right)

achieved clinical outcomes, and this was supported by the fact that the vast majority of patients completed the minimum 5-year follow-up regimen.

Pearls and Pitfalls

- The ss-MVLA technique is a highly versatile procedure available for the management of primary and secondary upper and lower extremity lymphedema. This method can be tailored to the stage-guided requirements of each clinical case, according to the lymphoscintigraphic preoperative evaluation and venous echo-color-Doppler ultrasound findings, allowing both the superficial and deep lymph pathways to be addressed at the same surgical time in a targeted strategic single anatomic site: the middle volar surface of the arm, or the inguinal-crural region of the lower extremity.
- The BPV lymphochromic test and the fluorescent ICG microlymphography test are fundamental intraoperative investigations for surgical planning and strategy.
- To achieve even better long-term clinical results, according to the lymphedema stage, this technique can be subsequently combined with other reconstructive microsurgical procedures, for example, where the lymphedema is associated with significant chronic venous pathology, or with

selective tailored liposuction where there is advanced elephantiasic lymphedema.

- Nonsurgical treatments are very important for surgical preparation and in the follow-up of the patient, performed in accordance with the CLyFT Protocol practiced in Genoa.
- Long-term follow-up during which the maintenance phase of self-managed conservative treatment is adhered to is very important; at a minimum of 5 years after surgical therapy, a 95% long-term patency and effectiveness rate of the MLVA is achieved in compliant patients.

References

1. Morgan PA, Murray S, Moffatt CJ, Honnor A. The challenges of managing complex lymphoedema/chronic oedema in the UK and Canada. Int Wound J. 2012;9(1):54–69.
2. Rutkowsky JM, Davis KE, Scherer PE. Mechanisms of obesity and related pathologies: the macro-and microcirculation of adipose tissue. FEBS J. 2009;276(20):5738–46.
3. Dixon JB. Lymphatic lipid transport: sewer or subway? Trends Endocrinol Metab. 2010;21(8):480–7.
4. Schneider M, Conway EM, Carmeliet P. Lymph makes you fat. Nat Genet. 2005;37(10):1023–4.
5. Lee BB, Laredo J, Neville RF. Current dilemmas and controversy. In: Lee BB, Bergan J, Rockson S, editors. Lymphedema. London: Springer; 2011. p. 381–5.
6. Campisi C, Boccardo F. Lymphedema and microsurgery. Microsurgery. 2002;22(2):74–8.
7. Mehrara BJ, Zampell JC, Suami H, Chang DW. Surgical management of lymphedema: past, present, and future. Lymphat Res Biol. 2011;9(3):159–67.
8. O'Brien BM. Replantation and reconstructive microvascular surgery. Part II. Ann R Coll Surg Engl. 1976;58(3):171–82.
9. Cormier JN, Rourke L, Crosby M, Chang D, Armer J. The surgical treatment of lymphedema: a systematic review of the contemporary literature (2004–2010). Ann Surg Oncol. 2012;19(2):642–51.
10. Penha TR, Ijsbrandy C, Hendrix NAM, et al. Microsurgical techniques for the treatment of breast cancer-related lymphedema: a systematic review. J Reconstr Microsurg. 2013;29(2):99–106.
11. Campisi CC, Ryan M, Boccardo F, Campisi C. A single-site technique of multiple lymphatic-venous anastomoses for the treatment of peripheral lymphedema: long-term clinical outcome. J Reconstr Microsurg. 2016;32(1):42–9.
12. Kleinhans E, Baumeister RGH, et al. Evaluation of transport kinetics in lymphoscintigraphy: follow-up study in patients with transplanted lymphatic vessels. Eur J Nucl Med. 1985;10:349–52.
13. Campisi CC, Villa G, Campisi C, et al. Rationale for the study of deep subfascial lymphatic vessels during lymphoscintigraphy for the diagnosis of peripheral lymphedema. Clin Nucl Med. 2019;44:91–8.
14. Villa G, Campisi CC, Campisi C, et al. Procedural recommendations for lymphoscintigraphy in the diagnosis of peripheral lymphedema: the Genoa protocol. Nucl Med Mol Imaging. 2019;53:47–56.
15. Dellachà A, Boccardo F, Zilli A, Napoli F, Fulcheri E, Campisi C. Unexpected histopathological findings in peripheral lymphedema. Lymphology. 2000;33(Suppl 1):62–4.
16. Campisi CC, Larcher L, et al. Microsurgical primary prevention of lymphatic injuries following breast cancer treatment. Plast Reconstr Surg. 2012;130(5):749e–50e. author reply 750e-751e
17. Földi M, Földi E, editors. Földi's textbook of lymphology. 2nd ed. Munich: Elsevier GmbH, Urban & Fischer Verlag; 2006.
18. Campisi C. Microvenous grafts in reconstructive lymphatic microsurgery: 7 years' clinical results. Vasc Surg. 1991;25(5):345–52.
19. Campisi CC, Ryan M, et al. Inclusion of targeted skin products in the pre-surgical treatment regimen of peripheral lymphedema & lipedema. Lymphology. 2019;52:194–201.
20. Campisi CC, Ryan M, Boccardo F, Campisi C. Fibro-Lipo-lymph-aspiration with a lymph vessel sparing procedure to treat advanced lymphedema after multiple lymphatic-venous anastomoses. The complete treatment protocol. Ann Plast Surg. 2017;78(2):184–90.
21. Campisi CC, Ryan M, Campisi C. Multiple lymphatic-venous anastomoses and multiple lymphatic-venous-lymphatic anastomoses. Fibro-lipo-lymph-aspiration with the lymph vessel-sparing procedure. In: Neligan PC, Masia J, Piller NB, editors. Lymphedema: complete medical and surgical management. Boca Raton: CRC Press Taylor & Francis Group; 2015. p. 447–62.

Reverse Lymphatic Mapping for Vascularized Lymph Node Transplant

11

Joseph H. Dayan

Introduction

The early years following the first clinical description of vascularized lymph node transplant (VLNT) by Becker were met with excitement but also justifiable skepticism and concerns regarding its safety [1]. On one hand, there was a visionary procedure using familiar microsurgical techniques that could potentially treat a disabling and relentlessly progressive disease. On the other hand, the concept of harvesting lymph nodes with a risk of causing iatrogenic lymphedema seemed altogether misguided. I recall arguments for VLNT along the lines of "donor site lymphedema has not been reported," until, of course, reports of iatrogenic lymphedema began to surface [2]. The risk/benefit equation for a procedure with significant uncertainty and significant risk clearly tipped the scale out of favor. Until there would be greater safety and a satisfactory degree of efficacy, the VLNT procedure failed to gain traction for about 20 years since its introduction.

The first major move to tip the scales was increasing the safety of VLNT by differentially mapping lymph nodes that drained the limb from those that drained the trunk. During the formative years of VLNT, the breast surgery world was exploring ways to reduce the risk of lymphedema following axillary lymph node biopsy and dissection. Klimberg had described a technique using blue dye injection into the upper arm and technetium injection for the sentinel lymph node biopsy [3, 4]. This allowed for the identification of lymph nodes providing drainage to the upper limb which could potentially be avoided, and, presumably, lower the risk of lymphedema. Hultborn et al. first described differential mapping of lymph nodes draining the upper limb and breast back in 1971 [5]. Dayan and colleagues built on this concept and applied it to vascularized lymph node harvest for both the groin and axillary donor sites [6]. We initially used blue dye but a major limitation became clear: the critical lymph nodes draining blue dye could not be identified until you were directly in contact with the lymph node, risking injury to the efferent and afferent lymphatics and circulation which could compromise the node. We had modified the technique to use filtered technetium injected into the extremity (hand or foot) and indocyanine green (ICG) dye injected into the trunk. Technetium provided two advantages: (1) critical lymph nodes could be localized prior to the incision and throughout the dissection providing a GPS-like system for maximum safety; and (2) the uptake into any lymph node could be quantified with a 10-second count. This quantification allowed for formal evaluation of the percent of uptake into the harvested lymph nodes compared to the limb sentinel nodes that were left behind. Injection of ICG into the upper limb has since been described, providing a more convenient and cost-effective alternative [7]. The authors still prefer technetium because the uptake can be quantified, unlike ICG, which is either "on" or "off," and allows for earlier identification. Since the author has routinely used VLNT with reverse lymphatic mapping, donor site lymphedema has not been observed in over 200 patients with follow-up ranging from 1 to 10 years. While the data demonstrates a solid safety profile, all patients are informed very clearly of the risk of donor site lymphedema. There is also a risk that there is shared drainage between the sentinel nodes draining the limb and those draining the trunk, in which case one cannot safely complete the lymph node flap harvest. This potential scenario (approximately 5% in our series) should be discussed with the patient prior to surgery and a backup plan should be included in the consent. Most commonly, we will list a second potential donor site. The omentum and supraclavicular lymph nodes are alternative options in this scenario that have virtually eliminated the risk of donor site lymphedema, but are not always feasible depending on the requirements of the defect.

J. H. Dayan (✉)
Division of Plastic and Reconstructive Surgery, Memorial Sloan Kettering Cancer Center, New York, NY, USA
e-mail: dayanj@mskcc.org

M. V. Schaverien, J. H. Dayan (eds.), *Multimodal Management of Upper and Lower Extremity Lymphedema*,
https://doi.org/10.1007/978-3-030-93039-4_11

Following the significant increase in safety with reverse mapping and alternative low risk donor sites, improved efficacy soon followed. As data began to pour out of increasing numbers of lymphatic surgery centers, improved patient selection and technique quickly evolved. The scales have since tipped in favor of VLNT in the appropriately selected patient.

Indications

- Groin or axillary lymph node flap harvest.
- No prior limb swelling or lymphatic compromise.

Procedure Technique

Principles

Reverse lymphatic mapping is used whenever axillary (including lateral thoracic/thoracodorsal nodes) or groin lymph nodes are being harvested for VLNT. Ideally, filtered technetium 99 sulfur colloid is injected into the adjacent limb the morning of surgery as the particle size and uptake are more consistent. However, if not feasible, unfiltered technetium can be used the day prior to surgery which stays in the system much longer. A gamma probe is then used in the operating room to identify and avoid critical nodes. Injection of ICG in the trunk can be used in order to confirm harvested lymph nodes draining the trunk.

A working knowledge of the general location of the sentinel lymph nodes draining the upper and lower limb is critical. In the upper limb, these sentinel nodes consistently lie just posterior to the superolateral border of the pectoralis major muscle [8, 9]. In the lower extremity, the sentinel lymph nodes draining the lower limb always lie below the groin crease along the femoral vessels. The target groin nodes for harvest lie at the confluence of the superficial inferior epigastric vein (SIEV) and superficial circumflex iliac vein (SCIV), above the groin crease. Care should be taken to cross very medial to the SIEV [10].

Algorithm for Reverse Lymphatic Mapping

The axillary (lateral thoracic and/or thoracodorsal nodes) and groin donor sites can be used virtually anywhere with reverse lymphatic mapping. To provide context, we are including our current practice which is always evolving and not meant to be used as a strict algorithm. We use reverse mapping almost exclusively for axillary nodes as they provide more lymph nodes, a more substantial pedicle, and greater soft tissue compared to the groin lymph nodes which we have largely abandoned. Our first choice for VLNT is the omentum for most cases. However, there are circumstances where the omentum is not available, or preferable, such as prior abdominal surgery or a history of ovarian cancer. There are also situations where skin replacement is required, which is a major shortfall of the omentum. In practices where the supraclavicular lymph nodes are routinely used, as was our practice previously, there are situations where this donor site is not ideal – such as right upper extremity lymphedema where the left supraclavicular donor site would be used but also carries a risk of thoracic duct injury or leak.

Reverse Lymphatic Mapping Technique for Axillary Lymph Node Flap Harvest (Fig. 11.1)

- 0.2 millicuries (0.2 ml) of filtered technetium 99 sulfur colloid is injected into the first and third webspaces of the hand adjacent to the donor site the morning of surgery.
- The gamma probe is used to localize the lymph nodes draining the upper limb and this region is marked on the skin.
- Optional: 0.1 ml of indocyanine green dye is injected in four areas approximately 15 cm below the axillary crease across the lateral chest wall; a near-infrared camera is then used to localize the lymphatics and lymph nodes through the skin that drain the trunk.
- A transverse axillary incision is made with subcutaneous flaps elevated exposing the clavipectoral fascia.
- Next, dissection is carried down to the lateral chest wall just posterior to the pectoralis major muscle.
- The distal end of the nodal packet is identified and distal lateral thoracic artery and vein are divided. If the artery is not present, dissection proceeds to the distal thoracodorsal vessels which are then divided.

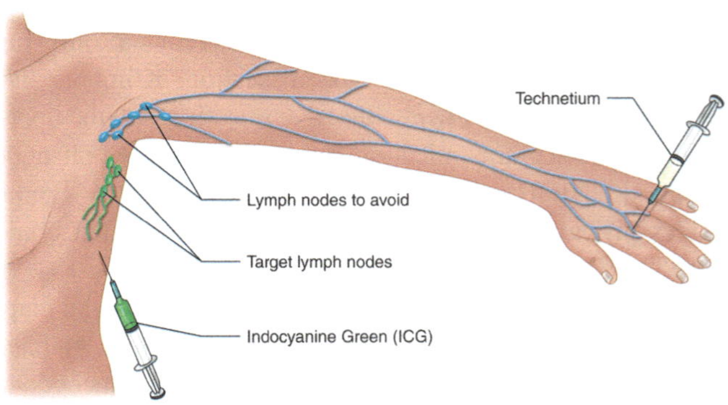

Fig. 11.1 Axillary reverse lymphatic mapping of the upper extremity for lateral thoracic/thoracodorsal vascularized lymph node flap harvest. Filtered technetium is injected into the first and third webspaces of the hand. Indocyanine green (ICG) is injected intradermally into four areas across the lateral chest wall and back to aid inclusion of the target lymph nodes within the flap

- The superior-most region where the nodes remain silent is marked and dissection is carried down straight to the proximal pedicle.
- Typically, the nodes draining the upper limb are anterior. Once these are cleared, one can capture more lymph nodes posteriorly and superiorly.
- The gamma probe is used continuously throughout dissection to ensure critical nodes are not harvested. Dissection never proceeds directly in contact with hot nodes to avoid compromising their lymphatic drainage.
- Once the flap is harvested, a 10-second count of the flap and of the sentinel nodes left behind in the axilla is recorded to quantify the amount of upper limb lymphatic drainage was in the flap. This is typically below 2%.
- The skin is closed in layers over a closed suction drain.

Reverse Lymphatic Mapping for Groin Lymph Node Harvest (Fig. 11.2)

- 0.2 millicuries (0.2 ml) of filtered technetium 99 sulfur colloid is injected into the first and third webspaces of the foot adjacent to the donor site the morning of surgery.
- The gamma probe is used to localize the lymph nodes draining the upper limb and this region is marked on the skin.
- Note that the gamma probe will demonstrate a hot signal above the crease prior to skin incision because it is detecting deeper lymph nodes draining the limb along the iliac chain. Once the superficial groin nodes are elevated, they should be relatively silent on the gamma probe.
- An incision is made above the groin crease along the superficial circumflex iliac pedicle.
- Next, skin flaps are elevated exposing the underlying lymph nodes, or a skin paddle is included if necessary.
- The flap is then elevated from lateral to medial, first off of the sartorius muscle, after which the pedicle is quickly visualized and isolated. If the gamma probe demonstrates hot nodes in the superficial lymph node packet, the procedure is aborted and the skin is closed over a drain.
- If the uptake in the flap is minimal to silent, the flap is then harvested and closure over a closed suction drain is performed.
- A 10-second count is recorded of the flap and the sentinel nodes left in the groin. There is a slightly higher degree of crossover in the groin between the limb and the trunk; this percent uptake in the flap is usually about 5% or less relative to that of the sentinel nodes.
- The historically high risk of seroma is dramatically reduced using absorbable quilting sutures.

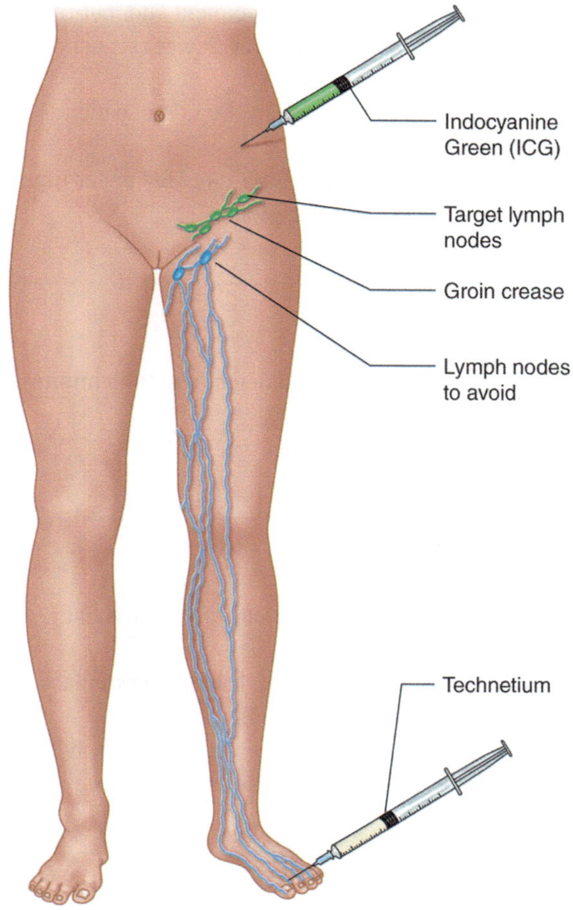

Fig. 11.2 Groin reverse lymphatic mapping of the lower extremity for superficial inguinal (groin) vascularized lymph node flap harvest. Filtered technetium is injected into the first and third webspaces of the foot. Indocyanine green (ICG) is injected intradermally in four areas across the lower abdomen to aid inclusion of the groin lymph nodes in the flap

Postoperative Care

- Drains are removed when less than 20 ml per day.
- Compression shorts are used for 3 weeks for groin harvest.

- Post-op care depends on the recipient site, but in general compression wrapping starts at 2 weeks post-op along with full range of motion.
- For lower extremity recipient sites, the patient is non-weight bearing for 2 weeks.
- DVT prophylaxis is given for 7 days for upper limb, and 30 days for lower limb, recipient sites.

Complications

- Donor site extremity lymphedema (although minimal risk with careful technique).
- Need to abort or switch donor sites (5%).

Pearls and Pitfalls

- Filtered technetium is preferable for consistency, safety, and quantifying uptake.
- Informed consent with an alternative plan in place if during surgery the target nodes are hot.
- Avoid dissecting immediately adjacent to hot lymph nodes to preserve their integrity and function.

References

1. Becker C, Assouad J, Riquet M, Hidden G. Postmastectomy lymphedema: long-term results following microsurgical lymph node transplantation. Ann Surg. 2006;243(3):313–5.
2. Vignes S, Blanchard M, Yannoutsos A, Arrault M. Complications of autologous lymph-node transplantation for limb lymphoedema. Eur J Vasc Endovasc Surg. 2013;45(5):516–20.
3. Tummel E, Ochoa D, Korourian S, Betzold R, Adkins L, McCarthy M, Hung S, Kalkwarf K, Gallagher K, Lee JY, Klimberg VS. Does axillary reverse mapping prevent lymphedema after lymphadenectomy? Ann Surg. 2017;265(5):987–92.
4. Thompson M, Korourian S, Henry-Tillman R, Adkins L, Mumford S, Westbrook KC, Klimberg VS. Axillary reverse mapping (ARM): a new concept to identify and enhance lymphatic preservation. Ann Surg Oncol. 2007;14(6):1890–5.
5. Hultborn A, Hultén L, Roos B, Rosencrantz M, Rosengren B, Ahrén C. Topography of lymph drainage from mammary gland and hand to axillary lymph nodes. Acta Radiol Ther Phys Biol. 1971;10(1):65–72.
6. Dayan JH, Dayan E, Smith ML. Reverse lymphatic mapping: a new technique for maximizing safety in vascularized lymph node transfer. Plast Reconstr Surg. 2015;135(1):277–85.
7. Pons G, Abdelfattah U, Sarria J, Duch J, Masia J. Reverse lymph node mapping using indocyanine green lymphography: a step forward in minimizing donor-site morbidity in vascularized lymph node transfer. Plast Reconstr Surg. 2021;147(2):207e–12e.
8. Coroneos CJ, Woodward WA, Wong FC, Caudle AS, Shaitelman SF, Kuerer HM, Schaverien MV. Anatomy and physiology of the sentinel lymph nodes of the upper extremity: implications for axillary reverse mapping in breast cancer. J Surg Oncol. 2021;123(4):846–53.
9. Nos C, Clough KB, Bonnier P, Lasry S, Le Bouedec G, Flipo B, Classe JM, Missana MC, Doridot V, Giard S, Charitansky H, Charles-Nelson A, Bats AS, Ngo C. Upper outer boundaries of the axillary dissection. Result of the SENTIBRAS protocol: multicentric protocol using axillary reverse mapping in breast cancer patients requiring axillary dissection. Eur J Surg Oncol. 2016;42(12):1827–33.
10. Dayan JH, Dayan E, Kagen A, Cheng MH, Sultan M, Samson W, Smith ML. The use of magnetic resonance angiography in vascularized groin lymph node transfer: an anatomic study. J Reconstr Microsurg. 2014;30(1):41–5.

Key Topic: Vascularized Lymph Node Transplant and Recipient Site Selection

12

Mark V. Schaverien and Joseph H. Dayan

Introduction

The effectiveness of vascularized lymph node transplant (VLNT) for the treatment of advanced lymphedema is supported by several prospective comparative studies and a randomized controlled trial [1–5]. VLNT is indicated in advanced lymphedema where there is significant segmental or confluent dermal backflow with few or no functioning lymphatic vessels on lymphatic imaging to provide new physiological function. The VLN flaps may be harvested from within the regional axillary [6, 7], inguinal [8–11], or cervical lymph node basins [12–16], or from within the intraperitoneal domain including the omental or jejunal mesenteric flaps [17–19], among others [20].

Two main mechanisms of VLNT action have been demonstrated in both experimental and clinical settings [21–25]. The "bridging" mechanism involves lymphangiogenesis with new afferent and efferent lymphatic vessels connecting the transplanted LNs with lymphatic vessels at the recipient site to restore lymphatic fluid drainage; this process is mediated by lymphangiogenic growth factor secretion from the transplanted lymph nodes including vascular endothelial growth factor (VEGF)-C [26, 27]. The "pumping" mechanism involves the development of new lymphatic vessels via neo-lymphangiogenesis to connect the transplanted LNs with lymphatic vessels at the recipient site, allowing new lymphaticovenous drainage within the transplanted lymph nodes driven by perfusion gradients between the arterial inflow and venous outflow [24, 28]. The "bridging" mechanism therefore supports orthotopic proximal placement of the VLNT within an extremity, and the "pumping" mechanism endorses the clinical efficacy of heterotopic distal transfer.

Lymphedema staging scales derived from the severity and distribution of the dermal backflow on contrast-enhanced imaging, in particular indocyanine green (ICG) fluorescent lymphography, are in general agreement that less severe lymphedema is characterized by proximal distribution of dermal backflow within an extremity, contrasting with advanced stage lymphedema that is also distributed distally, finally including the hand or foot once the deep lymphatic system also fails. The decreased contractility of the lymphatic vessel smooth muscle cells that characterizes advanced lymphedema results in this gravity-dependent distribution of lymphedema within the distal extremity, and the distribution of the pitting edema, and in particular the dermal backflow on contrast-enhanced lymphatic imaging, may aid in decision-making between proximal orthotopic and distal heterotopic VLN flap placement. Although studies comparing outcomes of orthotopic [5, 10, 29] and heterotopic [8, 11, 22, 30] VLN flap transfer in both the upper and lower extremities have demonstrated similar results, this is likely the result of confounding – the clinical decision-making regarding proximal versus distal flap placement in these studies may be influenced by the clinical distribution of the lymphedema. Where recipient sites have been compared within the same study, better outcomes have been demonstrated for distal recipient sites for advanced stage lymphedema [8]. Future comparative outcomes studies will better define surgical treatment algorithms, in particular for the more recently introduced VLNT techniques and combination surgical approaches (i.e., combined VLNT and lymphovenous bypass (LVB); dual-level VLNT).

For anatomic and non-anatomic locations, there are particular considerations regarding the choice of specific recipient site locations and recipient vessels, as well as the choice of VLN flaps for these respective locations for the upper and lower extremities (Fig. 12.1). These are detailed below.

M. V. Schaverien (✉)
Department of Plastic Surgery, The University of Texas MD Anderson Cancer Center, Houston, TX, USA
e-mail: mvschaverien@mdanderson.org

J. H. Dayan (✉)
Division of Plastic and Reconstructive Surgery, Memorial Sloan Kettering Cancer Center, New York, NY, USA
e-mail: dayanj@mskcc.org

M. V. Schaverien, J. H. Dayan (eds.), *Multimodal Management of Upper and Lower Extremity Lymphedema*,
https://doi.org/10.1007/978-3-030-93039-4_12

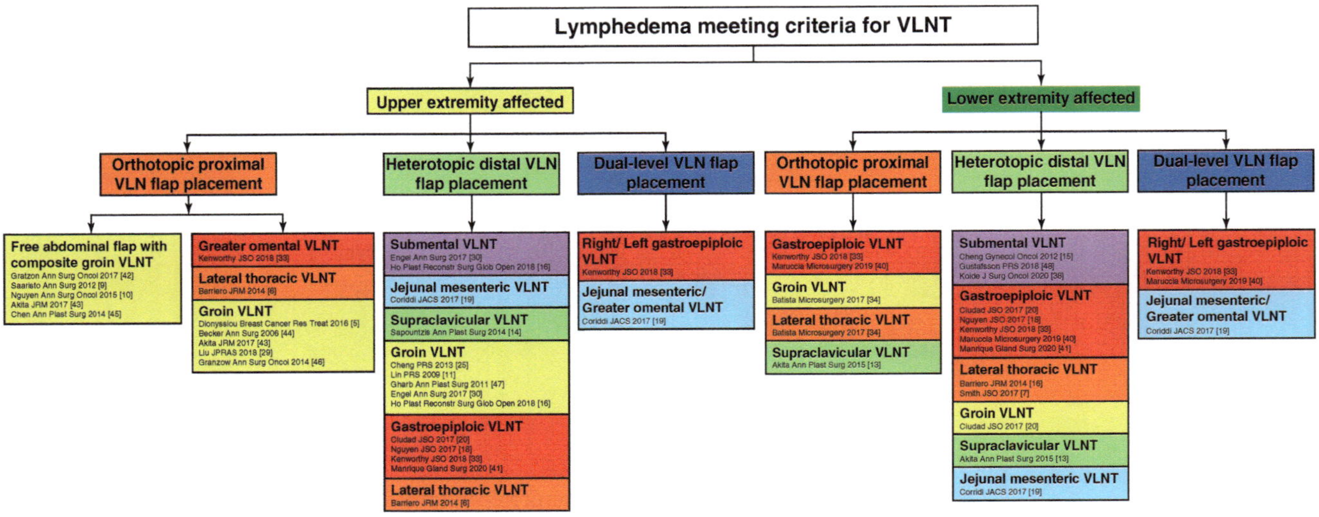

Fig. 12.1 An evidence-based decision aid for the vascularized lymph node flap transplant procedure relative to donor and recipient site locations. The choice of vascularized lymph node flap is individualized based on clinical findings and staging imaging, body habitus, and availability and quality of donor sites. VLN(T) vascularized lymph node (transplant)

Patient Selection for Surgical Intervention

Patients with untreated or uncontrolled cancer (primary, locoregional recurrence, or metastatic disease) are best managed by nonsurgical management, as are those in whom surgery under general anesthetic is contraindicated. Patients with medical comorbidities that increase the risk of complications from surgery should be optimized preoperatively. Surgery is contraindicated in patients with active cellulitis, and therefore, those with recent frequent episodes of cellulitis may benefit from prophylactic antibiotics preoperatively.

Decision-Making for Proximal Anatomic (Orthotopic) Compared with Distal Non-anatomic (Heterotopic) Vascularized Lymph Node Transplant (VLNT) Placement

The decision regarding orthotopic versus heterotopic VLNT is made with respect to symptoms from a focused history, clinical examination findings, and the distribution and severity of dermal backflow on lymphatic imaging. On focused questioning, patients can typically localize their symptoms of heaviness and swelling; in those with a history of cellulitis, the site at which this started can provide additional information. Clinical examination can localize the pitting edema or swelling. Contrast-enhanced imaging, in particular ICG fluorescent lymphography, can demonstrate the distribution of the dermal backflow and the site of greatest intensity of fluorescence with corresponding advanced dermal backflow stage (stardust/diffuse). Lymphoscintigraphy or magnetic resonance lymphography (MRL) may also aid in localizing the dermal backflow distribution and guide recipient site selection.

For the upper extremity, where the upper arm and trunk are most severely affected following prior axillary lymphadenectomy, the VLNT should be placed proximally. Orthotopic VLNT to the axilla allows for scar excision and lysis of scar bands compressing the axillary vein. The resultant scar (typically an extension of the prior axillary lymphadenectomy scar) and flap bulk are well concealed within the axilla, and the dead space is obliterated to prevent scar recurrence. Where the forearm is affected to a lesser degree and obstructed lymphatic vessels are identified on ICG imaging, lymphovenous bypass (LVB) can be performed in the forearm at the time of orthotopic VLNT to the axilla to treat the entire limb, with the elbow region acting as a lymphatic watershed area [31]. Where advanced lymphedema affects the forearm and hand to a similar degree to the upper arm, and axillary lymphadenectomy has been performed previously, dual-level transfer (simultaneous orthotopic proximal VLNT to the axilla and heterotopic distal VLNT to the forearm) is indicated as there are typically few (if any) lymphatic vessels visualized on imaging that are usually sclerotic and therefore unlikely to achieve long-term patency following LVB.

Where the forearm, especially distally, and/or hand, are most greatly affected, then heterotopic transplant placement is indicated as lymphatic fluid transport is severely impaired and distal placement allows for the fluid to be absorbed from the most gravity-dependent position of the limb [8, 15, 22]. In advanced lymphedema where the entire upper extremity is affected, the elbow acts as a watershed area, and therefore, dual-level transfer may improve clinical outcomes by enhancing the lymphatic drainage throughout the affected limb; the intraperitoneal donor site is well suited for this requirement as multiple flaps can be procured from a single donor site to reduce morbidity [19, 32, 33]. Ultimately, decisions regarding VLN flap selection relative to recipient site location are individualized to the patient, taking into account the results of imaging, clinical examination findings, body habitus, and availability and quality of flap donor sites, as well as patient and surgeon preferences.

For the lower extremity, following prior superficial inguinal lymphadenectomy or extirpative resection of the medial thigh, where the thigh/inguinal region is predominantly affected, proximal orthotopic transfer is indicated with concomitant scar release. Where the lower leg and/or foot are affected to a greater degree (typically following pelvic lymphadenectomy), distal heterotopic transfer is indicated, and where obstructed lymphatic vessels are identified on ICG imaging, LVB can be performed in the lower leg synchronously. Distal transfer is also indicated in primary lymphedema as proximal dissection may disrupt functioning lymph nodes/lymphatics. In advanced lymphedema where the entire lower extremity is affected and superficial inguinal lymphadenectomy has been performed previously, the knee acts as a watershed area, and therefore, dual-level transfer (simultaneous orthotopic proximal VLNT to the inguinal region and heterotopic distal VLNT to the lower leg) may improve clinical outcomes by enhancing the lymphatic drainage throughout the affected limb.

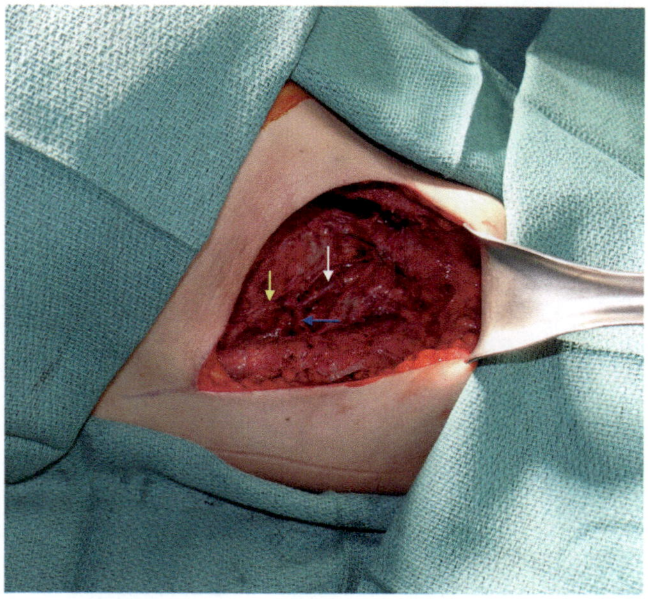

Fig. 12.2 Surgical exposure in the axilla of the subscapular system for proximal orthotopic (anatomic) vascularized lymph node transplant (VLNT). Radical axillary scar release is performed to create space for the lymph node flap and maximize contact surface area, with lysis of any scar bands compressing the axillary vein that may be contributing to venous insufficiency. The thoracodorsal pedicle (*white arrow*) should be preserved where possible, unless the latissimus dorsi flap has already been used for breast reconstruction in which case the thoracodorsal pedicle can be used as the lymph node flap pedicle. The serratus branch (*yellow arrow*) is typically used. Where the axilla is too hostile to safely prepare the recipient vessels due to severe scarring and/or the effects of radiation therapy, or where the subscapular recipient vessels have been previously ligated, the upper medial arm is an alternative donor site using branches of the brachial vessels

Selection of Recipient Site and Vascularized Lymph Node Transplant (VLNT) for Anatomic (Orthotopic) Transfer

In the setting of postmastectomy breast reconstruction, and when lymphedema predominantly affects the upper arm, orthotopic transfer is typically achieved using a deep inferior epigastric artery perforator (DIEP) flap with composite groin VLNT with the internal mammary recipient vessels used to perfuse the DIEP flap, with additional anastomoses between the superficial circumflex iliac vein/ artery (SCIV/SCIA) and branches of the subscapular system. The thoracodorsal pedicle should be avoided to preserve the latissimus dorsi flap as a lifeboat or in the setting of chest wall recurrence, unless the latissimus dorsi flap has already been used for breast reconstruction in which case the thoracodorsal pedicle can be used as the VLN flap pedicle. Radical axillary scar release is performed with lysis of any scar bands compressing the axillary vein that may be contributing to venous insufficiency to create space for the LN flap, and the flap volume obliterates the resultant three-dimensional dead space and maximizes surface area contact for lymphangiogenesis with the recipient bed (Fig. 12.2).

Where the patient has previous had, or does not wish for, breast reconstruction, in setting of breast-conserving surgery, or where lymphadenectomy has been performed for other reasons such as melanoma, the omental lymphatic flap is optimal for orthotopic transfer to the axilla. This may be harvested through a laparoscopic (or robotic) or open approach via a mini-laparotomy incision, depending on the resources available. It may also be performed at the same time as DIEP flap breast reconstruction in selected patients where superficial inguinal (groin) lymph node transfer is contraindicated or not desired by the patient. In patients that have previously undergone DIEP flap breast reconstruction or abdominoplasty, or in a patient desiring abdominoplasty, these incisions may be used for access to either a mini-laparotomy or laparoscopic approach. Another option is the lateral thoracic VLN flap that can be harvested with a variable volume of soft tissue for dead-space obliteration, and the use of the groin VLN flap may also be indicated for orthotopic transfer. Where the axilla is too hostile to safely prepare the recipient vessels due to severe scarring and/or the effects of radiation therapy, or where the subscapular recipient vessels have been previously ligated, the upper medial arm is an alternative donor site using branches of the brachial vessels. A lower volume flap is required, and the flap selection is similar to heterotopic distal transfer. The right gastroepiploic flap is useful as the volume can be tailored to the recipient site requirements. The groin, submental, supraclavicular, and lateral thoracic VLN flaps are also suitable [30].

For the lower extremity, following prior inguinal lymphadenectomy, proximal transfer can be performed either to the

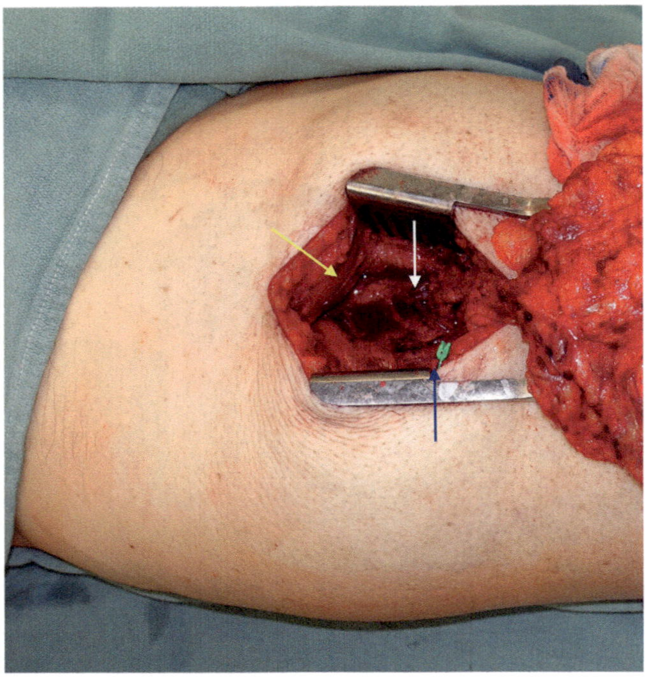

Fig. 12.3 Surgical exposure of the femoral vessel system at the proximal medial thigh for proximal orthotopic (anatomic) vascularized lymph node transplant (VLNT) in the lower extremity, using the medial circumflex femoral vessels, or profunda vessel perforators (*white arrow*). The profunda artery perforators travel through the adductor magnus muscle that is reflected medially (*yellow arrow*). A superficial vein branch of the greater saphenous vein may also be prepared for additional venous anastomosis (*blue arrow*). In this case, right gastroepiploic lymph node flap transfer to the thigh was performed to the second profunda perforator, with the volume well concealed in the proximal thigh

inguinal region using superficial circumflex iliac or superficial inferior epigastric recipient vessels, or occasionally to the deep inferior epigastric vessels [34]; alternatively, including in the setting of prior pelvic lymphadenectomy, transfer to the medial thigh can be performed using the medial circumflex femoral vessels or profunda vessel perforators (Fig. 12.3). Transfer to the anterior thigh can be performed using branches of the lateral circumflex femoral vessels. The greater omental/gastroepiploic is suitable for transfer to the thigh as the volume can be well concealed [33], as is the lateral thoracic VLN flap. The groin and supraclavicular VLN flaps are better indicated for transfer to the inguinal region due to their lower volume [34].

Selection of Recipient Site and Vascularized Lymph Node Transplant (VLNT) for Non-anatomic (Heterotopic) Transfer

Low volume flaps may achieve improved cosmesis in the setting of distal VLNT, reducing the need for revisional surgeries. Where possible, the use of skin grafts should be avoided to reduce the risk of graft-related complications and adverse cosmetic outcomes. Flaps are typically transferred to the proximal volar forearm where the flap bulk can be well concealed (Fig. 12.4). Localized debulking of fibroadipose soft tissues and the typically thickened deep fascia provides a pocket for the LN flap and may allow tension-free primary skin closure. Meticulous excision of perivascular scarring around the recipient veins is necessary to avoid venous outflow obstruction. Low volume flaps including the submental, jejunal mesenteric, and supraclavicular VLN flaps are optimal [14, 19, 30]. Where there is sufficient adipose soft tissue, following localized debulking, bulkier flaps including the groin, lateral thoracic, and right gastroepiploic flaps can be used [6, 8, 17]. The recipient vessels are typically the radial artery, either end-to-side or flow-through depending on the arterial anatomy of the VLN flap chosen, with outflow to the cephalic vein (or another superficial vein) and/or a radial artery vena comitans. The ulnar vessels may also be used in similar fashion although care needs to be taken when mobilizing the vessels in the region of the ulnar nerve, with the use of either the basilic vein (or another superficial vein) or an ulnar artery vena comitans for venous outflow. Where there is pitting edema localized to the dorsoulnar forearm, flap placement at the dorsal distal forearm may be indicated, using the dorsal branch of the radial artery and branches of the cephalic vein [35]. For flap placement in the antecubital fossa, the anterior ulnar recurrent artery can

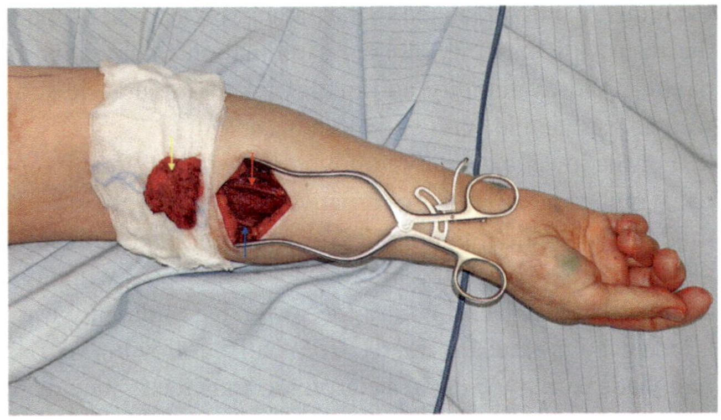

Fig. 12.4 Surgical exposure in the forearm of the radial vessels (*red arrow*) and cephalic vein (*blue arrow*) for heterotopic (non-anatomic) vascularized lymph node transplant (VLNT) to the proximal volar forearm. The recipient vessels are typically the radial artery, either end-to-side or flow-through, depending on the arterial anatomy of the lymph node flap chosen, Venous outflow is via the cephalic vein (or another superficial vein) and/or a radial artery vena comitans. The ulnar vessels may also be used in similar fashion, with the use of either the basilic vein (or another superficial vein) or an ulnar artery vena comitans for outflow. In the proximal volar forearm, the flap bulk can be well concealed; localized debulking of fibroadipose soft tissues (*yellow arrow*) and the typically thickened deep fascia provides a pocket for the lymph node flap and may allow tension-free primary skin closure. Where possible, the use of skin grafts should be avoided to reduce the risk of graft-related complications and adverse cosmetic outcomes

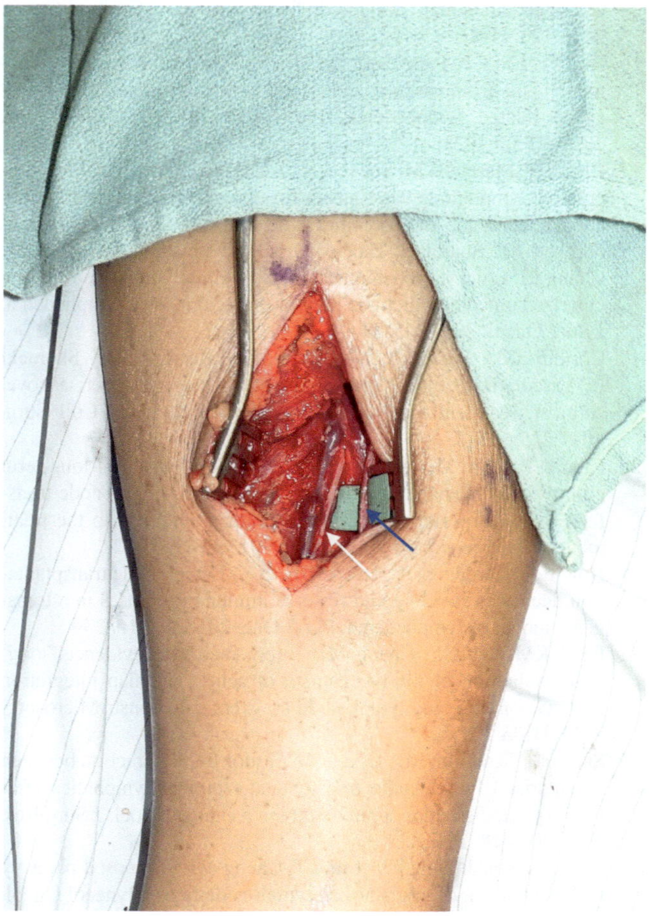

Fig. 12.5 Surgical exposure in the lower leg of the posterior tibial vessels (*white arrow*) and a branch of the greater saphenous vein (*blue arrow*) for heterotopic (non-anatomic) vascularized lymph node transplant (VLNT) to the medial calf area. In this region, distal flap placement can be achieved with acceptable cosmetic results. Anastomosis can either be end-to-side to the posterior tibial artery, or end-to-end to the medial sural vessels. The use of a skin graft should be avoided where possible; where required to avoid compression of the flap, the skin graft can later be excised

be used together with a vena comitans and/or branch of the basilic vein.

For the lower extremity, placement of the flap in the medial calf area achieves distal placement with acceptable cosmetic appearance [7]. This can either be end to side to the posterior tibial artery, or to the medial sural vessels (Fig. 12.5). If there is significant soft tissue excess, then following debulking, the gastroepiploic or lateral thoracic VLN flaps may be indicated [6, 7, 32]. Where lower volume flaps are indicated, options include the submental, groin, supraclavicular, and jejunal mesenteric VLNT [8, 13, 19, 20]. The flap may also be placed anteriorly, end to end to the anterior tibial vessels; however, cosmetic appearance is poor, and the flap may interfere with the choice of footwear.

Selection of Recipient Sites and Vascularized Lymph Node Transplants (VLNT) for Dual-Level Transfer

Where the entire extremity is affected by lymphedema, consideration should be given to simultaneous dual-level orthotopic and heterotopic VLNT. The peritoneal cavity is typically the source for LN flaps in this scenario due to the ability to harvest multiple flaps from a single donor site without increasing morbidity; the omental flap is optimal for orthotopic transfer, and the flap can be split into two, based on the right and left gastroepiploic vessels [32, 33].

For the upper extremity, perhaps the most common approach is to use the omental lymphatic flap based on the left gastroepiploic vessels for orthotopic proximal transfer following prior axillary lymphadenectomy, and the right gastroepiploic VLN flap for distal transfer to the volar forearm. The omental flap can be harvested laparoscopically (or robotically) or via an open approach, in particular through access via prior abdominal DIEP flap incisions. Another approach in those where the right gastroepiploic VLN flap would be too bulky for distal transfer is to use the omental lymphatic flap based on the right gastroepiploic vessels for orthotopic transfer and the jejunal mesenteric LN flap for the volar forearm, harvested via an open mini-laparotomy approach [19]. Alternatively, in patients undergoing DIEP flap breast reconstruction, composite DIEP/groin VLNT can be performed to the axilla, and an open mini-laparotomy or laparoscopic approach can be used for right gastroepiploic VLNT to the volar forearm, or open approach for jejunal mesenteric VLNT harvest, via this surgical exposure.

For the lower extremity, the omental flap is the procedure of choice for dual-level transfer as the flap volume is suitable even for distal transfer: the omental lymphatic flap based on the left gastroepiploic vessels can be used for orthotopic transfer to the medial thigh (following prior inguinal lymphadenectomy), and the right gastroepiploic VLN flap procured for transplantation to the medial lower leg using the posterior tibial or medial sural recipient vessels.

Postoperative Management for the Vascularized Lymph Node Transplant (VLNT) Procedure

The extremity is elevated postoperatively to reduce swelling and aid flap venous drainage. Distal lower extremity flaps typically require a postoperative dangling protocol. For orthotopic transfer to the axilla, the arm is kept away from the side at around 45 degrees to avoid compression or traction to the pedicle; postoperative compression therapy is resumed at 2–4 weeks, especially where LVBs only have been performed synchronously in the forearm. For heterotopic transfer to the forearm and for VLNT to the lower extremity, postoperative compression therapy is reinstituted at 4 weeks postoperatively [5, 7, 9, 33]. Suction-assisted lipectomy to reduce residual soft tissue excess may be performed in staged fashion with limited use of a compression garment postoperatively where indicated [36, 37] (see Chap. 7).

References

1. Chang DW, Masia J, Garza R 3rd, Skoracki R, Neligan PC. Lymphedema: surgical and medical therapy. Plast Reconstr Surg. 2016;138:209–18.
2. Schaverien MV, Coroneos CJ. Surgical treatment of lymphedema. Plast Reconstr Surg. 2019;144(3):738–58.
3. Carl H, Walia G, Bello R, et al. Systematic review of the surgical treatment of extremity lymphedema. J Reconstr Microsurg. 2017;33:412–25.
4. Ozturk CN, Ozturk C, Glasgow M, et al. Free vascularized lymph node transfer for treatment of lymphedema: a systematic evidence based review. J Plast Reconstr Aesthet Surg. 2016;69:1234–47.
5. Dionyssiou D, Demiri E, Tsimponis A, et al. A randomized control study of treating secondary stage II breast cancer-related lymphoedema with free lymph node transfer. Breast Cancer Res Treat. 2016;156:73–9.
6. Barreiro GC, Baptista RR, Kasai KE, et al. Lymph fasciocutaneous lateral thoracic artery flap: anatomical study and clinical use. J Reconstr Microsurg. 2014;30:389–96.
7. Smith ML, Molina BJ, Dayan E, et al. Heterotopic vascularized lymph node transfer to the medial calf without a skin paddle for restoration of lymphatic function: proof of concept. J Surg Oncol. 2017;115:90–5.
8. Cheng MH, Chen SC, Henry SL, et al. Vascularized groin lymph node flap transfer for postmastectomy upper limb lymphedema: flap anatomy, recipient sites, and outcomes. Plast Reconstr Surg. 2013;131:1286.
9. Saaristo AM, Niemi TS, Viitanen TP, Tervala TV, Hartiala P, Suominen EA. Microvascular breast reconstruction and lymph node transfer for postmastectomy lymphedema patients. Ann Surg. 2012;255:468–73.
10. Nguyen AT, Chang EI, Suami H, Chang DW. An algorithmic approach to simultaneous vascularized lymph node transfer with microvascular breast reconstruction. Ann Surg Oncol. 2015;22:2919–24.
11. Lin CH, Ali R, Chen SC, et al. Vascularized groin lymph node transfer using the wrist as a recipient site for management of postmastectomy upper extremity lymphedema. Plast Reconstr Surg. 2009;123:1265–75.
12. Mardonado AA, Chen R, Chang DW. The use of supraclavicular free flap with vascularized lymph node transfer for treatment of lymphedema: a prospective study of 100 consecutive cases. J Surg Oncol. 2017;115:68–71.
13. Akita S, Mitsukawa N, Kuriyama M, et al. Comparison of vascularized supraclavicular lymph node transfer and lymphaticovenular anastomosis for advanced stage lower extremity lymphedema. Ann Plast Surg. 2015;74:573–9.
14. Sapountzis S, Singhal D, Rashid A, et al. Lymph node flap based on the right transverse cervical artery as a donor site for lymph node transfer. Ann Plast Surg. 2014;73:398–401.
15. Cheng MH, Huang JJ, Huang JJ, et al. A novel approach to the treatment of lower extremity lymphedema by transferring a vascularized submental lymph node flap to the ankle. Gynecol Oncol. 2012;126:93–8.
16. Ho OA, Lin CY, Pappalardo M, Cheng MH. Comparisons of submental and groin vascularized lymph node flaps transfer for breast cancer-related lymphedema. Plast Reconstr Surg Glob Open. 2018;6(12):e1923.
17. Ciudad P, Maruccia M, Socas J, et al. The laparoscopic right gastroepiploic lymph node flap transfer for upper and lower limb lymphedema: technique and outcomes. Microsurgery. 2017;37:197–205.
18. Nguyen AT, Suami H, Hanasono MM, Womack VA, Wong FC, Chang EI. Long-term outcomes of the minimally invasive free vascularized omental lymphatic flap for the treatment of lymphedema. J Surg Oncol. 2017;115:84–9.
19. Coriddi M, Wee C, Meyerson J, Eiferman D, Skoracki R. Vascularized jejunal mesenteric lymph node transfer: a novel surgical treatment for extremity lymphedema. J Am Coll Surg. 2017;225:650–7.
20. Ciudad P, Agko M, Perez Coca JJ, et al. Comparison of long-term clinical outcomes among different vascularized lymph node transfers: 6-year experience of a single center's approach to the treatment of lymphedema. J Surg Oncol. 2017;116:671–82.
21. Huang JJ, Gardenier JC, Hespe GE, et al. Lymph node transplantation decreases swelling and restores immune responses in a transgenic model of lymphedema. PLoS One. 2016;11:0168259.
22. Patel KM, Lin CY, Cheng MH. From theory to evidence: long-term evaluation of the mechanism of action and flap integration of distal vascularized lymph node transfers. J Reconstr Microsurg. 2015;31:26–30.
23. Suami H, Scaglioni MF, Dixon KA, Tailor RC. Interaction between vascularized lymph node transfer and recipient lymphatics after lymph node dissection-a pilot study in a canine model. J Surg Res. 2016;204:418–27.
24. Ito R, Zelken J, Yang CY, Lin CY, Cheng MH. Proposed pathway and mechanism of vascularized lymph node flaps. Gynecol Oncol. 2016;141:182–8.
25. Cheng MH, Huang JJ, Wu CW, et al. The mechanism of vascularized lymph node transfer for lymphedema: natural lymphaticovenous drainage. Plast Reconstr Surg. 2014;133:192–8.
26. Viitanen TP, Visuri MT, Hartiala P, et al. Lymphatic vessel function and lymphatic growth factor secretion after microvascular lymph node transfer in lymphedema patients. Plast Reconstr Surg Glob Open. 2013;1:1–9.
27. Aschen SZ, Farias-Eisner G, Cuzzone DA, et al. Lymph node transplantation results in spontaneous lymphatic reconnection and restoration of lymphatic flow. Plast Reconstr Surg. 2014;133:301–10.
28. Yan A, Avraham T, Zampell JC, Aschen SZ, Mehrara BJ. Mechanisms of lymphatic regeneration after tissue transfer. PLoS One. 2011;6:17201.
29. Liu HL, Pang SY, Lee CC, Wong MM, Chung HP, Chan YW. Orthotopic transfer of vascularized groin lymph node flap in the treatment of breast cancer-related lymphedema: clinical results, lymphoscintigraphy findings, and proposed mechanism. J Plast Reconstr Aesthet Surg. 2018;71:1033–40.
30. Engel H, Lin CY, Huang JJ, Cheng MH. Outcomes of lymphedema microsurgery for breast cancer-related lymphedema with or without microvascular breast reconstruction. Ann Surg. 2018;268(6):1076–83.
31. Beederman M, Garza RM, Agarwal S, Chang DW. Outcomes for physiologic microsurgical treatment of secondary lymphedema involving the extremity. Ann Surg. 2020.
32. Ciudad P, Manrique OJ, Date S, et al. Double gastroepiploic vascularized lymph node transfers to middle and distal limb for the treatment of lymphedema. Microsurgery. 2017;37:771–9.
33. Kenworthy EO, Nelson JA, Verma R, Mbabuike J, Mehrara BJ, Dayan JH. Double vascularized omentum lymphatic trans-

plant (VOLT) for the treatment of lymphedema. J Surg Oncol. 2018;117:1413–9.
34. Batista BN, Germain M, Faria JC, Becker C. Lymph node flap transfer for patients with secondary lower limb lymphedema. Microsurgery. 2017;37:29–33.
35. Aljaaly HA, Fries CA, Cheng MH. Dorsal wrist placement for vascularized submental lymph node transfer significantly improves breast cancer-related lymphedema. Plast Reconstr Surg Glob Open. 2019;7(2):e2149.
36. Agko M, Ciudad P, Chen HC. Staged surgical treatment of extremity lymphedema with dual gastroepiploic vascularized lymph node transfers followed by suction-assisted lipectomy-A prospective study. J Surg Oncol. 2018;117:1148–56.
37. Nicoli F, Constantinides J, Ciudad P, et al. Free lymph node flap transfer and laser-assisted liposuction: a combined technique for the treatment of moderate upper limb lymphedema. Lasers Med Sci. 2015;30:1377–85.

Step-by-Step Instruction: Superficial Inguinal (Groin) Vascularized Lymph Node Transplant Procedure

13

Ketan M. Patel

Introduction

The concept of using the tissue containing lymphatic ducts in the arm as a flap was first introduced in the literature by Gillies et al. as an attempt to treat lower limb lymphedema, reported as early as 1935 [1]. Almost four decades later, Shesol et al. successfully demonstrated the restoration of lymphatic function with the transfer of the pedicled groin lymph node flap to the popliteal region using a rat model in 1979 [2]. This was followed by observations by Clodius et al. who reported the first clinical use of the groin lymph node flap in human subjects. The first vascularized groin lymph node (VGLN) flap was partially successful in two patients in 1982 [3]. This landmark clinical study led the way for further investigation in animal models regarding the viability of vascularized lymph node transfer (VLNT) [4, 5].

Chen et al. successfully performed VLNT as a treatment for obstructive lymphedema in a canine model in 1990 [5]. The superficial inguinal lymph node containing tissue from a normal hind limb was moved to the popliteal region of the lymphedematous leg as a free vascularized flap. At this time, Becker et al. also proposed that a functional VLNT can drain lymphatic fluid in patients with postmastectomy upper limb lymphedema [4]. It was later described by Cheng et al. that transferring the VLNT flap with a skin paddle to a distal lymphedematous site demonstrated promising and improved results for providing a new pathway for lymphatic drainage, as well as for providing a tension free closure of the donor site and an external mode for monitoring the vascular integrity of the flap [6, 7].

The mechanism of action of VLNT is based on two chief physiologic hypotheses [7–10]. The first proposes that improved lymphatic drainage is simply due to the transposition of non-diseased lymph tissue, which decreases interstitial pressure within the affected area allowing for more efficient drainage. The premise of lymphangiogenesis has also been proposed, which describes the growth of new lymphatic channels in the affected limb as an outcome of improved function secondary to healthy lymphatic tissue in the flap [11]. The former has been demonstrated in both animal and human studies using fluorescence to detect lymphatic uptake [7, 8].

The VGLN flap can be independently transferred to the axilla, elbow, or wrist to improve upper extremity lymphatic drainage, with promising results demonstrating success or improvement in greater than 80% of secondary lymphedema patients [6, 12]. The VGLN flap may also be transferred simultaneously, either as an independent free flap at the time of deep inferior epigastric artery perforator (DIEP) flap breast reconstruction or by a modified DIEP flap that includes lymph nodes and fascia [13]. It may also be transferred to the contralateral lower extremity. The groin flap has a great number of lymph nodes, rich lymphaticovenous connections for drainage, and a hidden donor site scar in the groin crease [14, 15]. Although it may confer the disadvantage of possible iatrogenic lymphedema of the operated lower extremity, careful dissection and reverse lymphatic mapping can avoid this complication [16]. Given these auspicious properties, the VGLN flap has been described as the preferred choice in International Society of Lymphology (ISL) Stage II–III breast cancer-related lymphedema and is the overall most commonly used donor site in the treatment of both primary and secondary lymphedema [17].

Supplementary Information The online version of this chapter (https://doi.org/10.1007/978-3-030-93039-4_13) contains supplementary material, which is available to authorized users.

K. M. Patel (✉)
Center for Advanced Lymphedema Treatment & Surgery, Division of Plastic and Reconstructive Surgery, Department of Surgery, Keck School of Medicine, University of Southern California, Los Angeles, CA, USA
e-mail: Ketan.Patel@med.usc.edu

M. V. Schaverien, J. H. Dayan (eds.), *Multimodal Management of Upper and Lower Extremity Lymphedema*,
https://doi.org/10.1007/978-3-030-93039-4_13

Typical Indications

- Although early lymphedema can be managed by lymphovenous bypass (LVB) alone, in long-standing lymphedema the lymphatic vessels become sclerosed and nonviable, and LVB fails to provide continued long-term results – in these patients VLNT is indicated to provide new physiologic function [14].
- VLNT may be indicated at the time of LVB in surgical candidates to improve long-term results in these patients [18].
- The VGLN flap can be transferred for upper limb lymphedema simultaneously with the lower abdominal flap transfer in the setting of delayed breast reconstruction with concomitant upper limb lymphedema [13].
- Preferable in patients who value minimal visibility of their scars, as the donor site is the most discreet of all VLNT donor site choices.
- Indicated in those patients for whom the wrist or axilla is the most appropriate recipient site for management of postmastectomy upper extremity lymphedema, especially in the early stages of disease [19].
- It is also indicated for treatment of established lymphedema of the upper extremity in the setting of postmastectomy lymphedema [20].
- Indicated in lower extremity lymphedema where a contralateral flap is transferred to the lower leg.
- Abundant surrounding soft tissue makes the VGLN flap suitable for cases where a moderate to large skin paddle is necessary for recipient site closure [21].

Anatomy

Within the groin region, the superficial inguinal lymph nodes are located in the femoral triangle of Scarpa, inferior to the inguinal ligament, medial to the sartorius muscle, and lateral to the adductor longus (Fig. 13.1). Based on the anatomical study by Assouad et al., the superficial groin nodes primarily drain the lymphatic fluid from the lower abdomen, which is also drained by the deeper inguinal nodes [22]. It is therefore this series of lymph nodes that can be sacrificed and transferred as a vascularized flap without significant donor site morbidity (Fig. 13.1).

A cadaveric study by Zeltzer et al. illustrated that there are 6.5 viable and sizeable (>0.5 mm) superficial nodes on average that may be harvested between the inguinal ligament and groin crease, with a mean size of 7.8 mm [23]. These are distributed in two groups – a superior row based on the superficial circumflex iliac artery (SCIA) and a secondary medial column based on the medial artery of the common femoral artery. Dayan et al. further investigated the groin lymph nodes and characterized an average of 8.2 lymph nodes found 3 cm below the inguinal ligament and above the groin crease, cen-

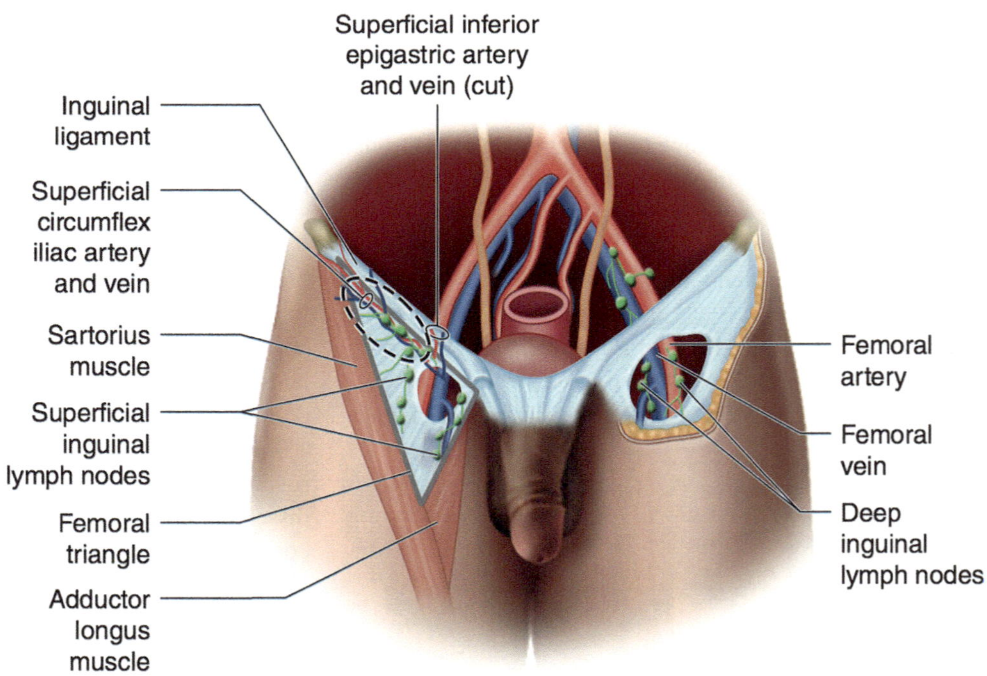

Fig. 13.1 Anatomy of the inguinal region. The superficial groin inguinal lymph nodes are located within the femoral triangle marked by the borders of the inguinal ligament, sartorius muscle, and adductor longus muscles (gray triangle), deep to Scarpa's fascia (patient's right side). The deep inguinal nodes are located deep to the deep fascia along the femoral vessels – care must be taken not to disrupt these nodes during dissection (patient's left side). [Illustrated provided courtesy of Springer]

tered one-third of the distance lateral to the pubic tubercle along the inguinal ligament [24]. Most lymph nodes were found in three primary locations – the junction of the superficial inferior epigastric vein (SIEV) and superficial circumflex iliac vein (SCIV) (67%), medial to the SCIV (19%), and inferior to the SCIV (14%). Overall, these studies support a refined technique of harvest inferior to the inguinal ligament, deep to Scarpa's fascia, and superficial to the deep fascia.

Patient Selection

The VGLN flap is appropriate for patients with ISL Stage I–III lymphedema, even in cases of elephantiasis. It is indicated in patients with lymphedema with pain and palsy, lymphedema with recurrent or chronic infections, in cases where there is a desire to reconstruct the breast simultaneously, or in cases of lymphedema where there is marked fibrosis and scarring of the axilla. In cases of excess fibrosis, it has been suggested that scar release with fat grafting can enhance patient quality of life [25].

Indications for VGLN flap transfer for upper limb lymphedema include total proximal occlusion on lymphoscintigraphy or magnetic resonance lymphangiography (MRL), failure of complex decongestive or debulking treatment, or recurrent cellulitis for greater than 6 months [26]. The only absolute contraindications for VGLN flap transfer are local cancer recurrence or the presence of distal metastasis [6, 7]. Brachial plexus neuritis is a relative contraindication, but decompression of the axilla with flap transfer can still greatly enhance quality of life in these patients.

Operative Technique

Principles

In the setting of VGLN flap transfer for the treatment of upper extremity lymphedema, the total number of available and reliable vascularized superficial lymph nodes in the groin is a prognostic factor. Duplex ultrasonography or computed tomographic angiography (CTA) can be used to detect significant nodes that are greater than 0.5 mm in diameter (Fig. 13.2) [27]. Magnetic resonance imaging (MRI) can also be used to completely survey the inguinal region for lymph nodes in greater detail. Reverse lymphatic mapping may also be used preoperatively to minimize the chance of harvesting important deeper draining lymph nodes of the operated extremity [16]. The donor site is then selected according to these preoperative studies. The flap may be designed with or without a skin paddle.

Recipient Site

The three most common recipient sites that have been reported in the literature for successful VGLN flaps include transfer to the axilla, elbow, and wrist. The most common

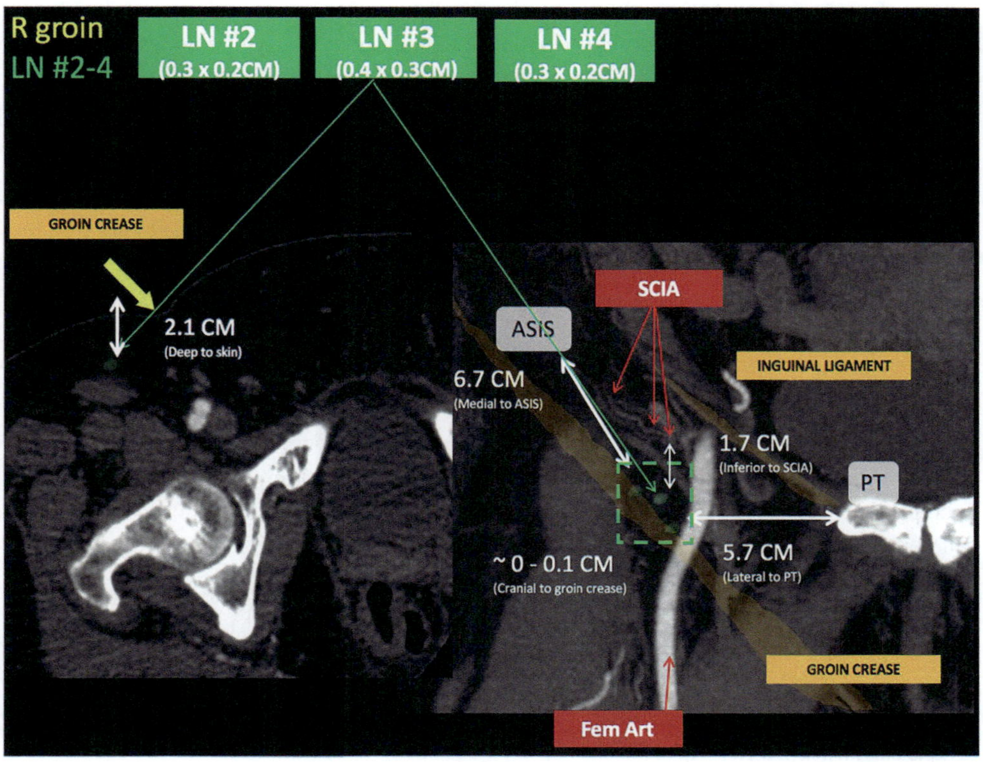

Fig. 13.2 Preplanning computed tomographic angiography (CTA) identifies the number of harvestable nodes and vascular anatomy. LN, lymph node; ASIS, anterior superior iliac spine; SCIA, superficial circumflex iliac artery; PT, pubic tubercle; Fem Art, femoral artery

indication is for transfer to the axilla, and this may be performed via the preexisting axillary lymphadenectomy scar. Radical scar release is also performed at this time, including any scar contracture around the subclavian vein. Branches of the subscapular artery and vein are prepared with lysis of perivascular scar tissue, preserving the thoracodorsal pedicle if possible, for conservation of a future latissimus dorsi flap if necessary. Two veins are prepared for recipient anastomosis, with time and care taken to identify anatomical continuity with the subscapular system and to select veins without significant venous backflow. In most cases, one recipient artery and two veins (preferably one from the superficial system and one from the vena comitans) are prepared for anastomosis to the vascularized flap. In the forearm, either the radial or ulnar artery is used.

For lower extremity lymphedema, the flap is harvested contralateral to the affected extremity and transferred to the lower leg where the posterior tibial artery is typically favored as the recipient vessel. Preoperative vascular imaging of the lower extremity, preferably using CTA, can be helpful in patients with primary lymphedema where there may be anatomical variabilities in the presence, caliber, flow, and course of the posterior tibial artery.

Flap Harvest: Skin Paddle (see supplementary material)

- A technetium lymphoscintogram is performed to identify main drainage pathways the night before surgery or the day of surgery. Appropriate identification of pathways of drainage of the lower extremity is crucial prior to undergoing surgery. Aliquots (0.01 cc) of indocyanine green (ICG) are injected into the lower abdomen in four to six spots. The ICG dye is then massaged into the tissues in order to be captured by the superficial lymphatic system, and ultimately carried to the superficial inguinal lymph nodes.
- A near-infrared camera is used to confirm that ICG dye has been absorbed by these lymph nodes prior to first incision.
- A pencil style narrow beam Doppler can be used to detect the perforators of the SCIA.
- The inguinal ligament from the anterior superior iliac spine to the pubic tubercle is marked in the supine position. The groin crease is also marked, with the target lymph nodes existing deep to Scarpa's fascia in between these two landmarks.
- An ellipse of skin is then marked in between the two landmarks previously marked, with the medial edge overlying the femoral pulse, as the branches of the SCIA system exist directly off the femoral artery (Fig. 13.3).
- The superior incision is made first, followed by lateral and medial incisions, and the SCIA and SCIV are clipped and dissection is made to the level of the deep fascia. The incisions are carried out laterally and superiorly and the dissection proceeds medially (Fig. 13.4).
- Dissection proceeds along the Scarpal plane toward to the fascial defect over the femoral vessels where the perforators from the SCIA system emerge.
- During the medial dissection, the near-infrared camera and gamma probe are used again to identify and harvest the superficial nodes.
- Medial dissection is carefully performed to isolate the main trunk of the SCIA, and care is taken to avoid dissecting more superficial structures, as this can devitalize the lymph nodes and flap.
- Extra care is taken upon dissection of the venous structures - the lymph nodes primarily drain from the SIEV

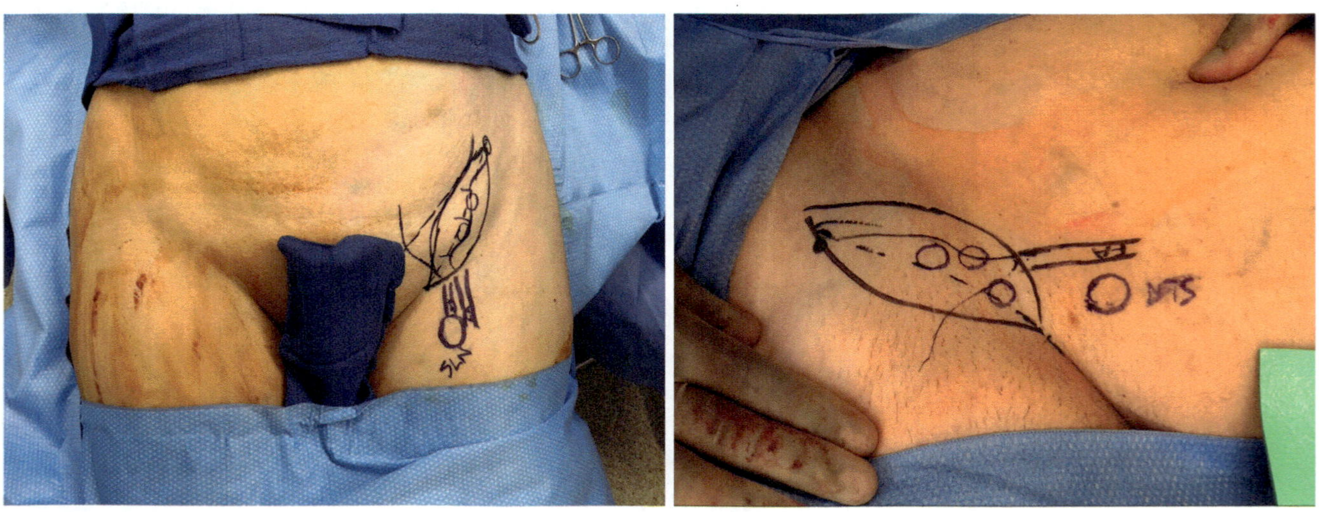

Fig. 13.3 An ellipse of the skin (left) is marked between the inguinal ligament marking and the groin crease, with the medial edge overlying the femoral pulse (right). SLN, sentinel lymph node

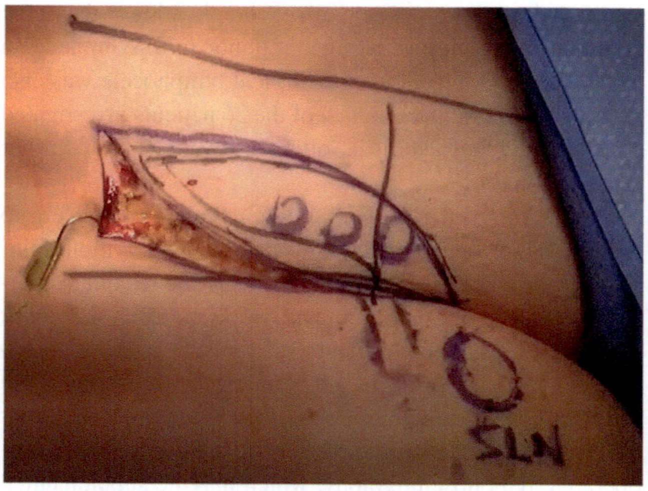

Fig. 13.4 The superior incision is made first, followed by lateral and medial incisions marked in this figure. SLN, sentinel lymph node

and SCIV systems, while more lateral nodes tend to drain from SCIV system; therefore, it is important to dissect this structure (Fig. 13.4).

- More proximal dissection reveals varying branching patterns: it is important to be aware that in one setting, the SCIV and SIEV have common origin off the saphenous vein; in another setting, these two veins have separate origins, and there needs to be careful decision-making in terms of where to harvest the vein. The common origin tends to be greater than 3 mm in caliber, and therefore the matching recipient vein needs to be taken into consideration when choosing this.
- Overdissection around the convergence of the saphenous vein to the femoral vein can disrupt axial lymphatics from the lower extremity; therefore, a cautious approach to this area is recommended.
- Typically, a lymph node exists at this saphenous bulb region - this node tends to drain the lower extremity and will elicit radioactivity with a gamma probe.
- Dual venous drainage is commonly preferred; the vena comitans to the SCIA is very small, but does match distal extremity recipient sites very well. The superficial veins are significantly larger, and therefore superficial veins in the recipient area or larger veins are preferred for size match.
- The great saphenous vein is preserved if possible since it does not primarily drain the superficial inguinal nodes.
- After the pedicle is identified and dissected, a soft tissue paddle is harvested appropriate in size to the receipt site and raised in a parallel orientation to the inguinal ligament (Fig. 13.5).
- The majority of superior row lymph nodes may be included in the flap since they are usually located at the junction of the SCIV and SIEV.

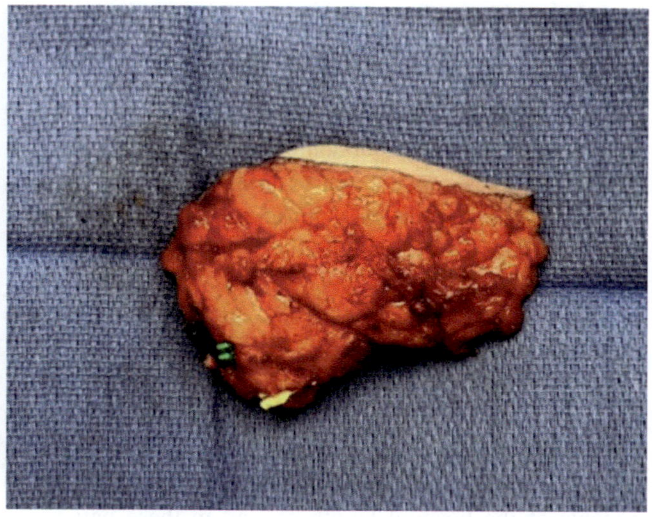

Fig. 13.5 Soft tissue skin paddle (top) is dissected in a parallel orientation to the inguinal ligament which includes the vascularized lymph node flap

- Care is made to use bipolar cautery and vascular clips in flap dissection if possible, in order to minimize injury to the vascular pedicle or any other significant surrounding lymphatic channels and nodes.

The author preferentially harvests the VGLN flap with a skin paddle in all patients as described above, which may then be discarded later if not needed, can be deepithelialized, or can be used to monitor the flap postoperatively. The harvest of additional soft tissue and overlying skin with the VGLNs can be performed by several different techniques. The flap may be supported by including perfusing vessels from the SCIA system, the SIEA system, or the medial-most branch of the femoral artery system. It is important to consider the desired orientation of the skin paddle when choosing which system to use, as each one will impact the final direction of the flap. The most commonly used are the SCIA and SIEA systems, which allow the skin and subcutaneous tissue to be harvested from the lower abdomen at the level of the inguinal ligament, with the SCIA system preferentially used by the author. The use of the femoral arterial system or other techniques places the skin island in a lower configuration, far inferior to the inguinal ligament. In the dissection of vessels from the SCIA and SIEA systems, the final result is a transverse-oriented skin island of the lower abdomen. This standard dissection allows for inclusion of additional subcutaneous tissue with the harvested superficial lymph nodes. As is true in harvesting of the VGLN flap without a skin paddle, continued dissection proximally along the SCIV and SIEV to their junction allows for inclusion of more superior row lymph nodes in the skin paddle. In the setting of axial recipient sites, the senior author prefers to use a deepithelialized skin paddle and uses that as an anchor to the proximal arm, as the skin and subdermal plexus have a rich and reliable blood supply.

The VGLN flap may also be modified to be combined with any of the available abdominal flaps in the reconstruction of the breast, such as the transverse rectus abdominis musculocutaneous (TRAM), muscle-sparing (ms-)TRAM, DIEP, or SIEA flaps [28].

Postoperative Care

The postoperative course following VGLN transfer is very similar to that of other microsurgical procedures involving vascularized flap transfer. One of the most important determinants of the hospital length of stay in these patients is based on the inclusion of a monitoring skin paddle. Not only does the addition of a skin paddle allow for tension-free closure of the recipient site (more often the wrist or elbow), but it also allows for much more accurate monitoring of flap perfusion. This provides for more predictable evaluations of flap success based on the assurance of lymph node viability given the presence of a well-perfused skin flap. When an axillary recipient site is chosen, however, the VGLN transfer is often buried, without use of a skin flap for a more cosmetic appearance. In this case, postoperative vascular compromise may often go undetected; however, hospital stay is usually shorter.

Postoperative re-exploration of the VGLN flap occurs more often than in other microvascular flap procedures. This is likely due to the often comorbid venous pathology in the affected limb of patients that require operative treatment of lymphedema. Complications may also be secondary to significant lymphatic fluid shifts and rapid absorption by the transferred flap causing immediate and non-native microcirculatory changes. Prompt and early recognition of perfusion compromise followed by immediate re-exploration and surgical management may ultimately prevent flap failure.

Complications

Donor site morbidity is of the utmost concern in VGLN flap harvest, given the high incidence of iatrogenic lower limb lymphedema that has been reported in the literature. A study by Viitanen et al. reported the results of donor site morbidity in 13 patients who underwent VGLN harvest for upper limb lymphedema [29]. Although patients did not have significant changes to lower limb circumference, there were some patients that demonstrated pathologic changes to postoperative lymphoscintigraphy and lymphatic transport indices in the donor limb. In addition, a recent study by Vignes et al. found that 38% of their patients undergoing VGLN flap transfer developed postoperative complications, the most common of which was iatrogenic donor limb lymphedema [30]. The development of postsurgical lymphocele was also reported as a complication in 4 of the 26 patients investigated by the study; however, this often resolved without further intervention.

If swelling of the ipsilateral donor limb is of concern to the patient postoperatively, ultrasound Doppler, lymphoscintigraphy, or MRI can be used to evaluate the residual superficial and deep draining inguinal lymph nodes at the donor site [15]. It is therefore critical to avoid harvesting any sentinel lymph nodes from the groin that may be draining the lower extremity, and to avoid harvesting any of the deeper inguinal nodes. The authors highly recommended using preoperative lymphoscintigraphy, which may be supplemented by intraoperative gamma probe guidance to detect sites of radionuclide tracer accumulation to minimize the risk of harvesting of sentinel nodes draining the lower extremity.

References

1. Gillies H, Fraser F. Treatment of Lymphoedema by plastic operation:(a preliminary report). Br Med J. 1935;1(3863):96.
2. Shesol BF, Nakashima R, Alavi A, Hamilton RW. Successful lymph node transplantation in rats, with restoration of lymphatic function. Plast Reconstr Surg. 1979;63(6):817–23.
3. Clodius L, Smith P, Bruna J, Serafin D. The lymphatics of the groin flap. Ann Plast Surg. 1982;9(6):447–58.
4. Becker C, Hidden G. Transfert de lambeaux lymphatiques libres. Microchirurgie et étude anatomique. J Mal Vascul. 1988;13:199–22.
5. Chen H-C, O'Brien BM, Rogers I, Pribaz J, Eaton C. Lymph node transfer for the treatment of obstructive lymphoedema in the canine model. Br J Plast Surg. 1990;43(5):578–86.
6. Cheng M-H, Chen S-C, Henry SL, Tan BK, Lin MC-Y, Huang J-J. Vascularized groin lymph node flap transfer for postmastectomy upper limb lymphedema: flap anatomy, recipient sites, and outcomes. Plast Reconstr Surg. 2013;131(6):1286–98.
7. Cheng M-H, Huang J-J, Wu C-W, et al. The mechanism of vascularized lymph node transfer for lymphedema: natural lymphaticovenous drainage. Plast Reconstr Surg. 2014;133(2):192e–8e.
8. Ito R, Zelken J, Yang C-Y, Lin C-Y, Cheng M-H. Proposed pathway and mechanism of vascularized lymph node flaps. Gynecol Oncol. 2016;141(1):182–8.
9. Patel KM, Lin C-Y, Cheng M-H. From theory to evidence: long-term evaluation of the mechanism of action and flap integration of distal vascularized lymph node transfers. J Reconstr Microsurg. 2015;31(01):026–30.
10. Yan A, Avraham T, Zampell JC, Aschen SZ, Mehrara BJ. Mechanisms of lymphatic regeneration after tissue transfer. PLoS One. 2011;6(2):e17201.
11. Aschen SZ, Farias-Eisner G, Cuzzone DA, et al. Lymph node transplantation results in spontaneous lymphatic reconnection and restoration of lymphatic flow. Plast Reconstr Surg. 2014;133(2):301.
12. Lin C-H, Ali R, Chen S-C, et al. Vascularized groin lymph node transfer using the wrist as a recipient site for management of postmastectomy upper extremity lymphedema. Plast Reconstr Surg. 2009;123(4):1265–75.
13. Akita S, Tokumoto H, Yamaji Y, et al. Contribution of simultaneous breast reconstruction by deep inferior epigastric artery perforator flap to the efficacy of vascularized lymph node transfer in patients

with breast cancer-related lymphedema. J Reconstr Microsurg. 2017;33(08):571–8.
14. Schaverien MV, Badash I, Patel KM, Selber JC, Cheng M-H. Vascularized lymph node transfer for lymphedema. Paper presented at: Seminars in plastic surgery 2018.
15. Liu H-L, Pang S-Y, Lee C-C. Donor limb assessment after vascularized groin lymph node transfer for the treatment of breast cancer-related lymphedema: clinical and lymphoscintigraphy findings. J Plast Reconstr Aesthet Surg. 2019;72(2):216–24.
16. Dayan JH, Dayan E, Smith ML. Reverse lymphatic mapping: a new technique for maximizing safety in vascularized lymph node transfer. Plast Reconstr Surg. 2015;135(1):277–85.
17. Committee E. The diagnosis and treatment of peripheral lymphedema: 2016 consensus document of the International Society of Lymphology. Lymphology. 2016;49(4):170–84.
18. Chang DW, Masia J, Garza R III, Skoracki R, Neligan PC. Lymphedema: surgical and medical therapy. Plast Reconstr Surg. 2016;138(3S):209S–18S.
19. Scaglioni MF, Suami H. Lymphatic anatomy of the inguinal region in aid of vascularized lymph node flap harvesting. J Plast Reconstr Aesthet Surg. 2015;68(3):419–27.
20. Poortmans PJTL. Postmastectomy radiation in breast cancer with one to three involved lymph nodes: ending the debate. Lancet. 2014;383(9935):2104–6.
21. Chang EI, Chu CK, Hanson SE, Selber JC, Hanasono MM, Schaverien MV. Comprehensive overview of available donor sites for vascularized lymph node transfer. Plastic Reconstruct Surg Global Open. 2020;8(3):e2675.
22. Assouad J, Becker C, Hidden G, Riquet M. The cutaneo-lymph node flap of the superficial circumflex artery. Surg Radiol Anat. 2002;24(2):87–90.
23. Zeltzer AA, Anzarut A, Braeckmans D, et al. The vascularized groin lymph node flap (VGLN): anatomical study and flap planning using multi-detector CT scanner. The golden triangle for flap harvesting. J Surg Oncol. 2017;116(3):378–83.
24. Dayan JH, Dayan E, Kagen A, et al. The use of magnetic resonance angiography in vascularized groin lymph node transfer: an anatomic study. J Reconstr Microsurg. 2014;30(01):041–6.
25. Maruccia M, Elia R, Ciudad P, et al. Postmastectomy upper limb lymphedema: combined vascularized lymph node transfer and scar release with fat graft expedites surgical and patients' related outcomes. A retrospective comparative study. J Plast Reconstr Aesthet Surg. 2019;72(6):892–901.
26. Fumiere E, Leduc O, Fourcade S, et al. MR imaging, proton MR spectroscopy, ultrasonographic, histologic findings in patients with chronic lymphedema. Lymphology. 2007;40(4):157–62.
27. Patel KM, Chu S-Y, Huang J-J, Wu C-W, Lin C-Y, Cheng M-H. Preplanning vascularized lymph node transfer with duplex ultrasonography: an evaluation of 3 donor sites. Plast Reconstr Surg Glob Open. 2014;2(8).
28. Nguyen AT, Chang EI, Suami H, Chang DW. An algorithmic approach to simultaneous vascularized lymph node transfer with microvascular breast reconstruction. Ann Surg Oncol. 2015;22(9):2919–24.
29. Viitanen TP, Mäki MT, Seppänen MP, Suominen EA, Saaristo AM. Donor-site lymphatic function after microvascular lymph node transfer. Plast Reconstr Surg. 2012;130(6):1246–53.
30. Vignes S, Blanchard M, Yannoutsos A, Arrault M. Complications of autologous lymph-node transplantation for limb lymphoedema. Eur J Vasc Endovasc Surg. 2013;45(5):516–20.

14 Step-by-Step Instruction: Combined Microvascular Breast Reconstruction and Groin Vascularized Lymph Node Transplant Procedure

Jaume Masia, Gemma Pons, and Cristhian Pomata

Introduction

In 2012, Saaristo et al. published the first description of simultaneous breast and lymphatic reconstruction with an autologous composite flap [1]. The technique involved the transfer of tissue from the lower abdomen together with vascularized lymph nodes (VLN) from the groin. Several groups have since published their experience using this combined procedure, including variants in flap design and optimization of flap vascularization [2–6].

Although several potential donor sites have been described for autologous breast reconstruction and VLN transplant (VLNT), harvesting both components from the lower abdominal wall allows the transfer "en bloc" of a single composite flap. In addition, this approach not only eliminates the need for additional scars but also improves the shape of the abdomen. The main advantage of this combined approach is that it provides an aesthetic, definitive, total breast anatomy restoration (TBAR) while treating or preventing upper limb lymphedema in a single operation [7].

Indications

- *Delayed breast reconstruction and treatment of breast cancer-related lymphedema (BCRL)*
  - Patients with a previous mastectomy and axillary lymph node dissection (ALND) who seek delayed breast reconstruction, and present with:
    - (a) Clinical manifestations of upper extremity lymphedema
    - (b) Subclinical upper extremity lymphedema detected by indocyanine green (ICG) lymphography assessment (linear pattern with areas of dermal backflow)
- *Immediate breast reconstruction and prevention of breast cancer-related lymphedema (BCRL)*
  - Patients undergoing mastectomy with ALND

Anatomy

The blood supply of the inferior abdominal tissue comes from perforators of the deep inferior epigastric artery/vein (DIEA/V). The DIEA originates from the medial aspect of the external iliac artery, approximately 1 cm above the inguinal ligament. It ascends from the lateral aspect of the rectus abdominis muscle, between the transversalis fascia and the peritoneum. It then penetrates the posterior aspect of the rectus abdominis muscle, after which it branches out in different patterns with an average of 5(±2) perforators supplying the skin. Finally, the DIEA forms anastomoses with the superior epigastric vessels above the umbilicus (Fig. 14.1) [8, 9].

The inguinal region is supplied by the superficial circumflex iliac artery/vein (SCIA/V) or the superficial inferior epigastric artery/vein (SIEA/V) and unnamed branches from the common femoral artery (Fig. 14.1) [10]. The inguinal lymph nodes responsible for abdominal lymphatic drainage are located along the lower edge of the inguinal ligament (until 3 cm below) [11]. To maintain the functionality of these lymph nodes, they must be harvested with a wide strip of surrounding adipofascial tissue containing the tridimensional architecture of the lymphatic system – the VLN flap is generally based on the SCIA.

When the VLN flap is being harvested, neither the lymphatic vessels nor the vascular pedicle should be skeletonized as devascularization of the lymph nodes must be

J. Masia (✉) · G. Pons (✉)
Plastic and Reconstructive Surgery, Hospital de la Santa Creu i Sant Pau and Clinica Planas, Barcelona, Spain
e-mail: jmasia@santpau.cat; gponsp@santpau.cat

C. Pomata (✉)
Plastic and Reconstructive Surgery, Clinica Planas, Barcelona, Spain
e-mail: cpomata@clinicaplanas.com

M. V. Schaverien, J. H. Dayan (eds.), *Multimodal Management of Upper and Lower Extremity Lymphedema*,
https://doi.org/10.1007/978-3-030-93039-4_14

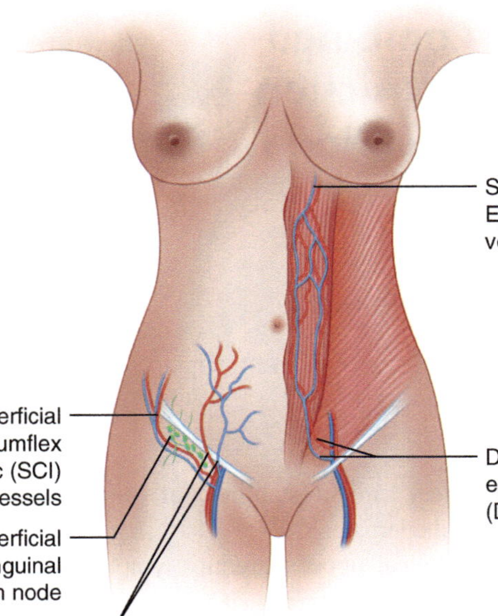

Fig. 14.1 Vascular anatomy of the lower abdomen and inguinal region

avoided. Special attention is required to ensure that the deep inguinal lymphatic system responsible for lower extremity lymphatic drainage is not damaged. If dissection is excessive, the risk of lower extremity lymphedema at the donor site is significant [12]. Reverse lymphatic mapping of the lower extremity with ICG lymphography is therefore mandatory to identify and preserve the deep inguinal lymph nodes during dissection [13].

The composite flap is typically designed with the VLNT contralateral to the DIE vessels in order to facilitate the composite flap inset in the axilla and thorax (Fig. 14.2). However, if the amount of tissue from a single hemiabdomen is sufficient for breast reconstruction, the VLNT can be elevated from the ipsilateral inguinal region.

Regarding the recipient vessels, the internal mammary vessels are usually the first option for the DIEP flap pedicle, and the thoracodorsal vessels are the first-line choice as recipient vessels for the VLNT pedicle. When the thoracodorsal vessels are not suitable due to extensive scarring, the circumflex scapular, the serratus branch, or the lateral thoracic vessels can be used as recipient vessels.

Patient Selection and Preoperative Assessment

When a patient with a previous mastectomy and ALND returns to the office seeking delayed breast reconstruction, clinical evaluation of the ipsilateral upper extremity is mandatory. If the patient already demonstrates clinical manifestations of upper limb lymphedema, ICG lymphography and lymphoscintigraphy assessment should be performed to evaluate the structure and functionality of the superficial and deep lymphatic system. If the patient does not have clinical manifestations of upper extremity lymphedema, assessment with ICG lymphography is recommended to detect or exclude subclinical lymphedema. Once the decision has been made to perform a combined microvascular breast reconstruction with VLNT (see indications), a preoperative computed tomography angiogram (CTA) is obtained to assess the vascular anatomy of the abdominal wall in which the combined flap will be based and to determine the number and location of superficial and deep lymph nodes in the groin regions [14, 15].

When a candidate for delayed TBAR demonstrates proximal degeneration of the lymphatic channels with distal functioning lymphatic channels, distal lymphovenous anastomosis (LVA) is recommended. In order to plan the LVA surgery, magnetic resonance lymphangiography (MRL) may be necessary to provide more precise information about the lymphatic system [16, 17]. When planning immediate TBAR after the ablative surgery, the targeted lymphatic axillary restoration (TLAR) approach should also be considered for prevention of breast cancer-related lymphedema (BCRL). The TLAR approach involves multiple axillary lymphatic-venous anastomoses performed immediately following ALND.

Absolute contraindications for this combined reconstruction include poor overall medical condition, unresectable chest wall disease, uncontrolled metastatic disease, and previous abdominal surgeries that make the abdomen unsuitable as a donor site. Relative contraindications include previous abdominal liposuction, multiple abdominal scars, active cellulitis, and lymphangitis in the affected upper extremity. Smoking is not a contraindication for free flaps, but patients are requested to cease smoking at least 1 month before surgery and warned of the high risk of associated complications.

Presurgical Markings

Chest

- A vertical line is marked from the suprasternal notch to the xiphoid process.
- Curvilinear lines are marked at the level of the two inframammary folds, correcting the positions when necessary.
- The second or third intercostal space is marked, indicating the location of the recipient vessels.
  – If a simultaneous symmetrization procedure is planned for the healthy breast (mastopexy or reduction mammoplasty), a Wise (inverted T) pattern is designed (Fig. 14.3).

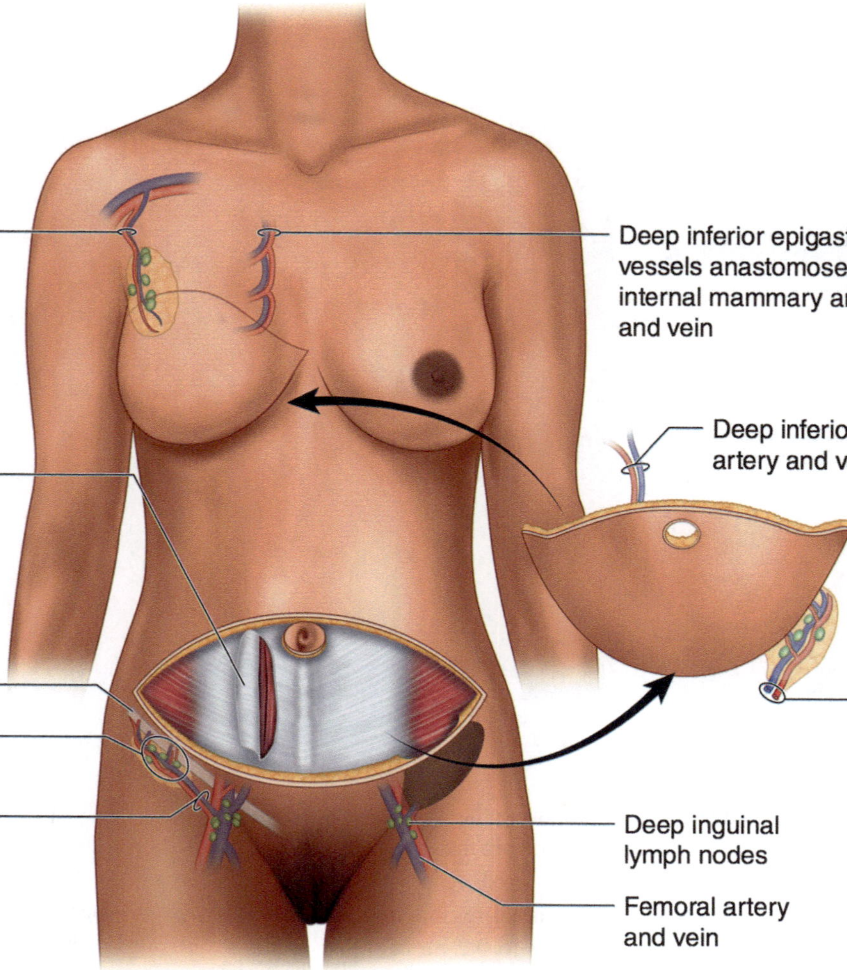

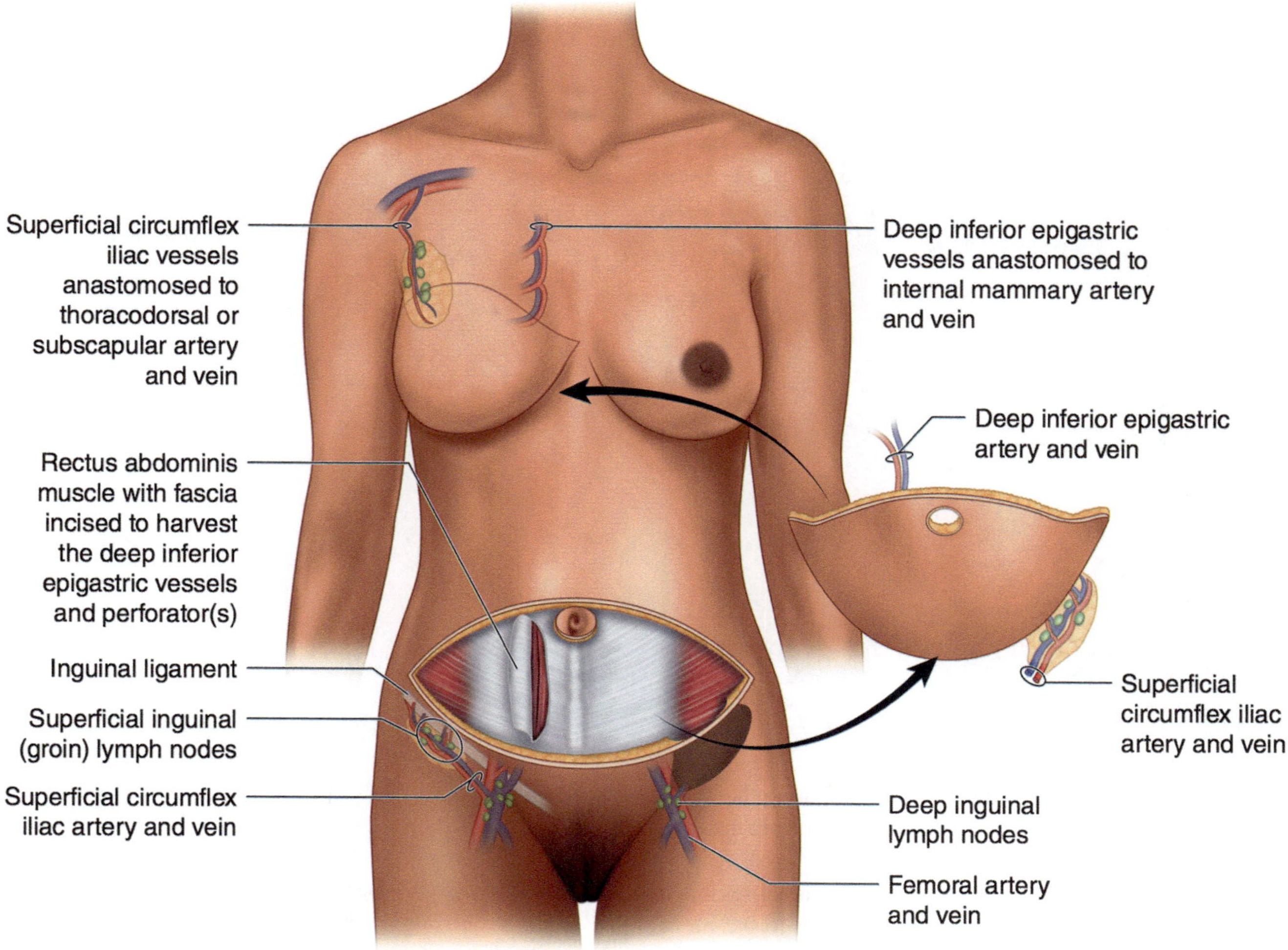

Fig. 14.2 Delayed breast reconstruction using a composite deep inferior epigastric artery perforator flap with contralateral superficial inguinal (groin) vascularized lymph node transplant. (Illustration provided courtesy of Springer)

Abdomen

- In the standing position, a suprapubic line is marked.
- In the supine position, a periumbilical 1 cm grid system is drawn (Cartesian plane) with the umbilicus as "point zero" for the x- and y-axes.
- Based on the coordinates informed by the CTA, DIEA perforator locations are marked on the patient's abdomen, and the position is confirmed by Doppler ultrasound. The dominant perforator is selected and marked according to its location, trajectory, and size from the CTA information. In the same way, the bilateral SIEA and SCIA are located in the inguinal regions using Doppler ultrasound, from medial to lateral and from lateral to medial, respectively.
- The inguinal lymph nodes located between the SIE and SCI vessels are marked based on the coordinates informed by the CTA. The lower limit of the abdominal skin flap is marked by a curvilinear line connecting the right and left anterior superior iliac spines (ASIS), crossing 1–2 cm below the previously marked suprapubic line. The fusiform design is completed when the upper limit of the abdominal skin flap is marked by a curvilinear line connecting the right and left ASIS crossing the umbilicus (Fig. 14.3).
  - When simultaneous distal upper extremity LVA is planned, presurgical ICG lymphography is performed to mark the superficial lymphatic system. Based on the coordinates informed by MRL, the most suitable functioning lymphatic vessels are then also located and marked. The locations where both studies meet represent the best locations for LVA.

Operative Techniques

The patient is placed in the supine position with the arm in the abducted position. A two-team approach can start the sur-

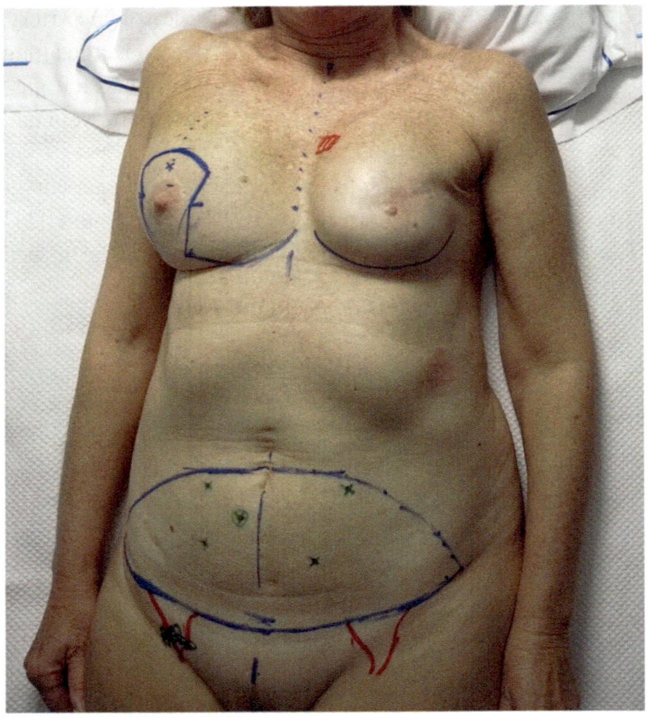

Fig. 14.3 Presurgical markings

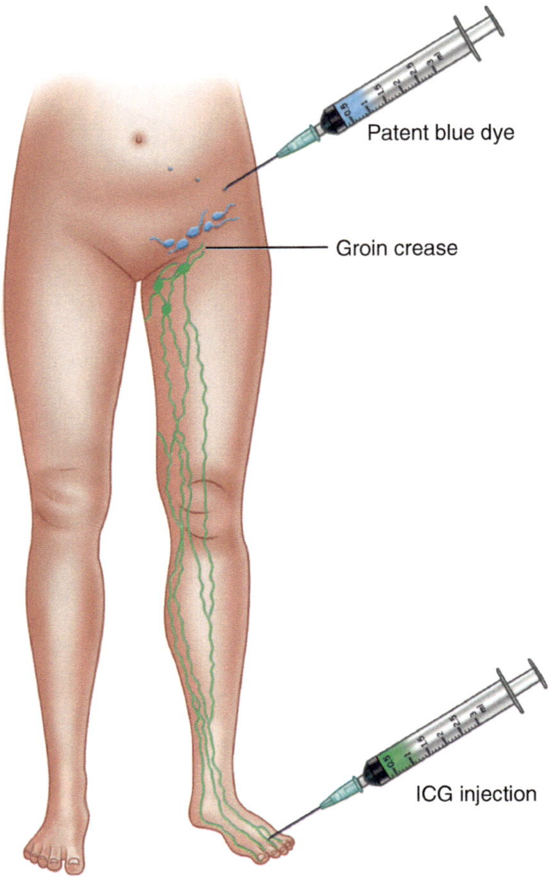

Fig. 14.4 Reverse groin lymph node mapping with indocyanine green (ICG) and injection of patent blue dye in the lower abdomen above the inguinal region

gery simultaneously. One team will start preparing the recipient vessels in the thoracic area, while the other team harvests the abdominal flaps. Before the surgery is started, reverse lymph node mapping of the pre-selected inguinal region is performed using subcutaneous injection of 0.1 to 0.2 ml of ICG at the second and fourth interdigital web spaces of the foot. Subsequently, 0.2 to 0.4 ml of 2.5% patent blue dye is injected intradermally in two or three spots above the inguinal region (Fig. 14.4) [13].

Flap Harvest Technique

- The umbilicus is incised circumferentially down to the abdominal wall.
- The superior edge of the lower abdominal flap is incised, from side-to-side, reaching up to the fascia.
- The upper abdominal flap is turned over superiorly so that the skin edges can be stapled by pulling the upper abdominal skin/fat in static cephalad retraction (Fig. 14.5).
- The inferior edge of the lower abdominal flap is carefully incised, from side-to-side, keeping in a very superficial subdermal plane so as to avoid damaging the superficial vessels.
- At the suprapubic level, the inferior edge of the flap is incised down to the fascia to check the thickness of the flap. In this segment, there is no risk of injuring any superficial vessels.
- From the suprapubic incision, the dissection proceeds laterally on both sides until the SIE vessels are located.
- On the side where the VLNT will be harvested, careful dissection is carried out, from lateral to medial, along the lower edge of the flap until the SCI vessels are identified.
- Once the SIE and SCI vessels have been located, the abdominal flap is raised, from lateral to medial, in a suprafascial plane, up to the lateral edge of the ipsilateral rectus abdominis.
- The VLN tissue to be harvested is centered over the superficial system. Blunt dissection is performed in a subdermal plane toward the inguinal region. The wide adipofascial tissue base between the superficial system is tapered on approaching the origin of the superficial vessels. Care should be taken to avoid damaging the afferent lymphatic channels stained blue.
- Intraoperative ICG lymphography is performed to identify the fluorescence of the deep lymph nodes draining the lower limb to ensure they are not included in the flap (Fig. 14.6).

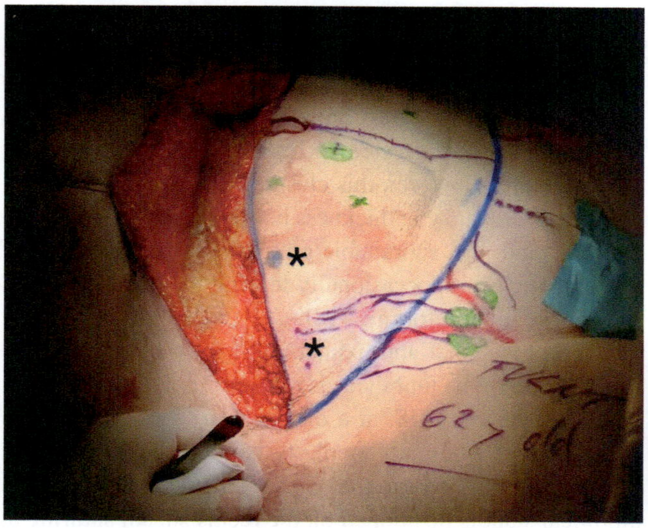

Fig. 14.5 Incision of the superior edge of the flap. Blue patent dye injections spots (asterisks)

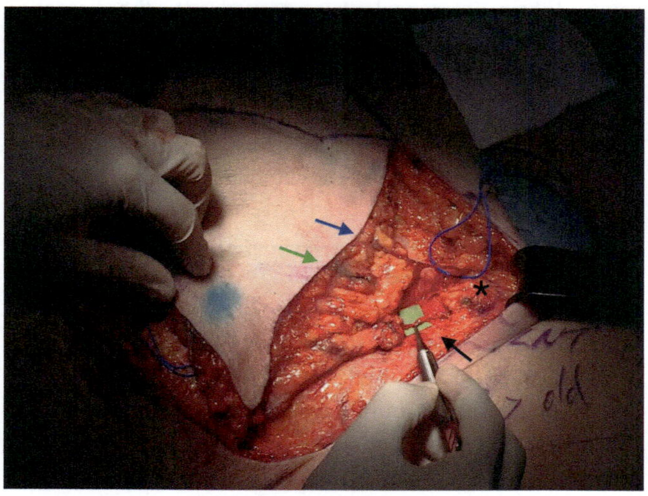

Fig. 14.6 The groin vascularized lymph node flap. The superficial inferior epigastric vein (blue arrow), afferent lymphatic vessel (green arrow), and superficial circumflex iliac artery (black arrow) are demonstrated, and the deep lymph nodes are marked after intraoperative indocyanine green (ICG) lymphography (asterisk)

- The abdominal flap is dissected on the side where the dominant DIE perforator was selected preoperatively. It is performed in a suprafascial plane, from lateral to medial and from superior to inferior, until the perforator is identified.
- An incision is made at the point where the perforator pierces the anterior rectus fascia and is followed through its intramuscular or paramuscular trajectory (Fig. 14.7).
- The upper continuation of the DIE vessels is ligated and divided.
- The SIE and SCI vessels of the VLN flap are then ligated and transected.
- Dissection of the DIE vessels continues inferiorly, in a retromuscular plane, until the pedicle length and diameter of the vessels are adequate.
- Intraoperative ICG angiography is performed to assess DIEP flap perfusion and boundaries.
- The DIE vessels are ligated and transected near their origin at the external iliac vessels, and the composite abdominal flap is transferred "en bloc" to the chest (Figs. 14.7 and 14.8).

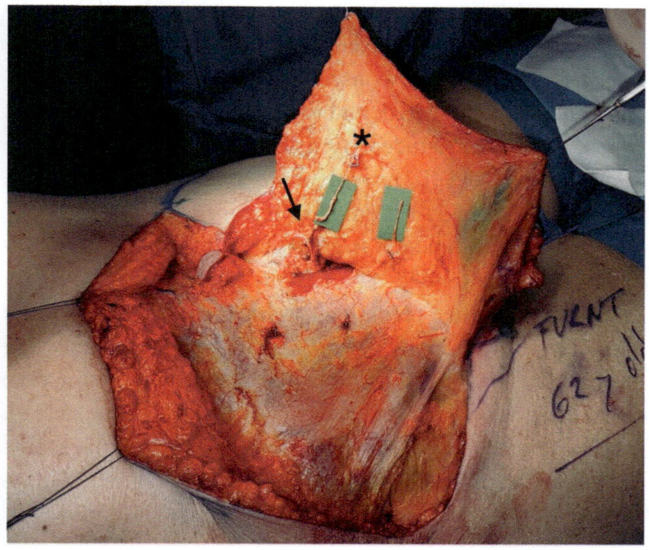

Fig. 14.7 Deep inferior epigastric artery perforator (arrow) and nerve (asterisk)

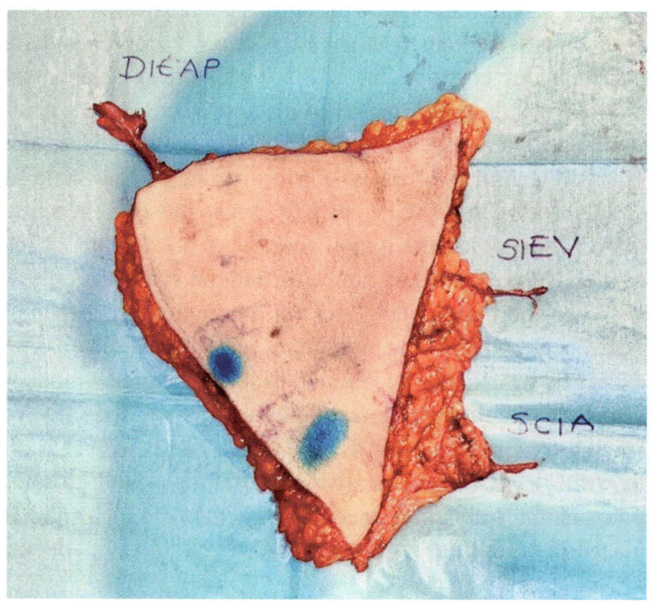

Fig. 14.8 Composite flap: lower right hemiabdomen with ipsilateral superficial inguinal (groin) lymph node flap. DIEAP, deep inferior epigastric pedicle; SIEV, superficial inferior epigastric vein; SCIA, superficial circumflex iliac artery

Recipient Site Preparation

In patients with a previous total mastectomy, the skin of the chest wall is elevated through the prior transverse scar. A wide space is created for the flap inset by dissecting the skin up to the clavicle superiorly and the inframammary fold inferiorly. In patients who have undergone a previous breast reconstruction with a retropectoral prosthetic device, the pectoralis muscle is released from the skin flap and tacked back down on the chest wall. To prepare the internal mammary vessels, a transverse incision is made parallel to the fibers of the pectoralis muscle at the second or third intercostal space, exposing two consecutive rib cartilages. The intercostal muscle is resected, and the internal mammary vessels can be found surrounded by a thin layer of fat under the intercostal muscle. To provide more space for anastomosis, the rib cartilage may be removed in some cases.

Next, the axillary area is approached to dissect the thoracodorsal vessels or the regional alternative vessels. A very important step when preparing this recipient site is to remove all scar tissue, especially along the axillary vessels. Releasing all the adhesions in the axilla can also considerably improve the axillary venous flow. When a TLAR approach is planned, axillary reverse mapping using ICG and patent blue dye is carried out in the corresponding upper extremity in order to identify the afferent lymphatic vessels in the axilla during ALND.

Revascularization and Flap Inset

The composite flap is transferred to the chest wall with the abdominal DIEP flap located in the mammary region and the lymph nodes covering the axillary plexus. The flap must therefore be properly rotated to place it in the correct position. The DIE vessels are anastomosed end-to-end to the internal mammary vessels. Performing a second arterial (SCIA) and venous (SCIV or SIEV) anastomosis in the axilla is mandatory to ensure lymph node survival. If a distal LVA or a TLAR is planned, it can be carried out synchronously.

When the flap is being shaped, the potentially ischemic areas identified by ICG angiography should be resected. The excess tissue can also be resected to shape the breast mound. The flap can then be de-epithelialized as needed, always leaving a monitoring skin island, which can be resected on the fifth or sixth postoperative day. Before wound closure, two suction drains are placed in the chest area and one is placed in the axilla.

Donor Site Closure

The anterior rectus sheath is repaired using a two-layer suture technique. The muscle can be repaired when necessary. The upper abdomen is selectively undermined in the suprafascial plane, within the medial thirds of the rectus abdominis muscle, up to the xiphoid appendix. Plication of the rectus abdominis muscle diastasis is performed when needed using two-layer suture, from the xiphoid appendix to the pubic symphysis. To eliminate dead space at the VLN flap donor site, the created space is closed with a running barbed suture. However, this closure can sometimes exacerbate the discrepancy in thickness between the upper abdominal flap and the suprapubic/groin tissue at the time of abdominal closure, occasionally leaving the patient with an inguinal contour deformity [18].

With provisional approximation of the abdominal flaps, the insertion of the umbilicus is marked 2 cm above the joining points of the ASIS, at a distance of 8–11 cm from the resulting scar. The umbilicoplasty is performed along with fat trimming to shape the periumbilical concavity. The umbilical stalk is positioned on the rectus sheath suturing at 12, 3, and 9 o'clock points. Before tying, these same sutures are used to anchor the umbilicoplasty dermis, helping to pull down the periumbilical abdominal flap accentuating the concavity. Fibrin tissue sealant is sprayed onto the dissection bed, and two suction drains are placed transversely in the lower abdomen. Meticulous wound closure is performed in three layers (Scarpa's fascia, the deep dermal layer, and the epidermal layer) with the patient in a semi-Fowler's position and with slight flexion of the lower extremities.

Postoperative Care

Patients are monitored postoperatively for 5 days following the standard protocol used for other microsurgical procedures. Perioperative antibiotics are indicated to reduce the risk of infection at the donor and recipient sites, and particularly to avoid cellulitis or lymphangitis of the affected upper limb. Muscle activation of the arm is initiated in the first postoperative day by having the patient perform isometric exercises with a rubber handball. Suction drains from the chest, axilla, and abdominal wounds are removed when drainage is less than 30 mL/day.

For most patients with lymphedema, passive antigravitational gymnastics and lymphatic drainage with the Godoy technique is started on the second postoperative day [19]. Manual lymphatic drainage (MLD) should be directed toward the transplanted lymph nodes so as to stimulate neo-lymphangiogenesis. Compression garments are useful in the immediate postoperative period and can be worn for the first 6 months. Patients are generally discharged on postoperative day 6 or 7. Normal physical activities and sports can resume at 6 weeks postoperatively.

Complications

Recipient site complications include venous congestion, hematoma, seroma, wound infection or dehiscence, mastectomy skin flap necrosis, fat necrosis, and partial or total flap loss. Donor site complications include groin seroma, abdominal wall hematoma, wound infection or dehiscence, umbilical stalk necrosis, abdominal bulge or hernia, and secondary lymphedema of the lower extremity.

Pearls and Pitfalls

- Preoperative CTA is a highly effective assessment to precisely locate the superficial lymph nodes in the groin region.
- Reverse lymphatic mapping is crucial to avoid donor site lymphedema. Intraoperative navigation with ICG lymphography helps to identify the deep lymph nodes draining the lower extremity, ensuring that they are not included in the VLN flap.
- When dissecting the VLN flap, it is important to incorporate a considerable amount of surrounding adipose tissue, taking care not to skeletonize the pedicle and ensuring the viability of the afferent lymphatic channels that will maintain the functionality of the VLN flap.
- Releasing the scar compressing the axillary vein is essential because it improves venous drainage from the affected upper extremity and ameliorates the range of shoulder motion and arm mobility.

References

1. Saaristo AM, Niemi TS, Viitanen TP, Tervala TV, Hartiala P, Suominen EA. Microvascular breast reconstruction and lymph node transfer for postmastectomy lymphedema patients. Ann Surg. 2012;255:468–73.
2. Dancey A, Nassimizadeh A, Nassimizadeh M, Warner RM, Waters R. A chimeric vascularised groin lymph node flap and DIEP flap for the management of lymphoedema secondary to breast cancer. J Plast Reconstr Aesthetic Surg. 2013;66:735–7.
3. Chen R, Mu L, Zhang H, Xin M, Luan J, Mu D, et al. Simultaneous breast reconstruction and treatment of breast cancer-related upper arm lymphedema with lymphatic lower abdominal flap. Ann Plast Surg. 2014;73:S12–7.
4. Nguyen AT, Chang EI, Suami H, Chang DW. An algorithmic approach to simultaneous vascularized lymph node transfer with microvascular breast reconstruction. Ann Surg Oncol. 2015;22:2919–24.
5. De Brucker B, Zeltzer A, Seidenstuecker K, Hendrickx B, Adriaenssens N, Hamdi M. Breast cancer-related lymphedema: quality of life after lymph node transfer. Plast Reconstr Surg. 2016;137:1673–80.
6. Montag E, Okada AY, Arruda EGP, Fonseca AS, Bromley M, Munhoz AM, et al. Influence of vascularized lymph node transfer (VLNT) flap positioning on the response to breast cancer-related lymphedema treatment. Rev Col Bras Cir. 2019;46:e2156.
7. Masià J, Pons G, Rodríguez-Bauzà E. Barcelona lymphedema algorithm for surgical treatment in breast cancer-related lymphedema. J Reconstr Microsurg. 2016;32:329–35.
8. Boyd JB, Taylor GI, Corlett R. The vascular territories of the superior epigastric and the deep inferior epigastric systems. Plast Reconstr Surg. 1984;73:1–16.
9. Kikuchi N, Murakami G, Kashiwa H, Homma K, Sato TJ, Ogino T. Morphometrical study of the arterial perforators of the deep inferior epigastric perforator flap. Surg Radiol Anat. 2001;23:375–81.
10. Scaglioni MF, Suami H. Lymphatic anatomy of the inguinal region in aid of vascularized lymph node flap harvesting. J Plast Reconstr Aesthetic Surg. 2015;68:419–27.
11. Dayan JH, Dayan E, Kagen A, Cheng M-H, Sultan M, Samson W, et al. The use of magnetic resonance angiography in vascularized groin lymph node transfer: an anatomic study. J Reconstr Microsurg. 2014;30:41–5.
12. Pons G, Masia J, Loschi P, Nardulli ML, Duch J. A case of donor-site lymphoedema after lymph node-superficial circumflex iliac artery perforator flap transfer. J Plast Reconstr Aesthetic Surg. 2014;67:119–23.
13. Pons G, Abdelfattah U, Sarria J, Duch J, Masia J. Reverse lymph node mapping using indocyanine green lymphography: a step forward in minimizing donor-site morbidity in vascularized lymph node transfer. Plast Reconstr Surg. 2021;147:207e.
14. Masia J, Clavero JA, Larrañaga J, Vives L, Pons G. Preoperative planning of the abdominal perforator flap with multidetector row computed tomography: 3 years of experience. Plast Reconstr Surg. 2008;122:80e–1e.
15. Bontumasi N, Jacobson JA, Caoili E, Brandon C, Kim SM, Jamadar D. Inguinal lymph nodes: size, number, and other characteristics in asymptomatic patients by CT. Surg Radiol Anat. 2014;36:1051–5.
16. Neligan PC, Kung TA, Maki JH. MR lymphangiography in the treatment of lymphedema. J Surg Oncol. 2017;115:18–22.
17. Pons G, Clavero JA, Alomar X, Rodríguez-Bauza E, Tom LK, Masia J. Preoperative planning of lymphaticovenous anastomosis: the use of magnetic resonance lymphangiography as a complement to indocyanine green lymphography. J Plast Reconstr Aesthetic Surg. 2019;72:884–91.
18. Maldonado AA, Garza RM, Artz J, Song DH, Chang DW. Abdominal flap for closing the donor site after groin lymph node transfer. J Surg Oncol. 2017;115:390–1.
19. de Godoy JMP, de Godoy ACP, de FGG M. Evolution of Godoy & Godoy manual lymph drainage. Technique with linear movements. Clin Pract. 2017;7:1006.

Step-by-Step Instruction: Submental Vascularized Lymph Node Transplant Procedure

15

Ming-Huei Cheng and Olivia Ho

Background

The vascularized submental lymph node (VSLN) flap is based on the submental-facial artery as its arterial supply and represents a valuable option when choosing a VLN source [1–3]. The submental artery is a consistent branch of the facial artery. The common facial vein serves as the major venous outflow of the flap. Occasionally, the facial artery's comitant vein can be encountered and incorporated as a secondary venous outflow of the flap. In this flap, VLNs include the level I lymph nodes in the submental (IA) and submandibular (IB) regions [4] (Fig. 15.1).

Patient Selection

Patients with extremity lymphedema with Cheng's Lymphedema Grade II–IV, a symptom duration longer than 5 years; total obstruction stages T-4, T-5, or T-6 on the Taiwan Lymphoscintigraphy Staging (TLS) system; or partial obstruction stages P-2-P3 without patent lymphatic vessels on indocyanine green (ICG) lymphography are indicated for a VSLN flap transfer [4, 5]. Those with extremity lymphedema with Cheng's Lymphedema Grade I to early Grade II; a shorter duration of symptoms of less than 5 years; partial obstruction on the TLS system P-1, P-2, or P-3; and patent lymphatic ducts identified by ICG lymphography were selected for lymphovenous anastomosis (LVA) [4, 5].

M.-H. Cheng (✉)
Department of Plastic and Reconstructive Surgery, Mayo Clinic, Jacksonville, FL, USA

Section of Plastic Surgery, The University of Michigan, Ann Arbor, Michigan, USA

O. Ho
Department of Plastic and Reconstructive Surgery, Chang Gung Memorial Hospital, College of Medicine, Chang Gung University, Taoyuan, Taiwan

Patients with a prior history of radiation to the neck and submental region should be carefully evaluated for possible injury of the VSLN flap anatomy [6–10]. Patients with facial nerve palsy, significant pre-platysmal fat, or excess ptotic skin should be carefully evaluated and counseled on the possibilities of asymmetries and contour irregularities postoperatively. It should also be discussed with these patients that balancing contralateral neck procedures may be required. Preoperative imaging with duplex ultrasonography or magnetic resonance imaging (MRI) may be helpful in evaluation of the lymph node basin and vascular anatomy [8–10].

Flap Markings

Patients are usually marked in the supine position. The facial artery is palpated and identified, usually 2 cm anterior to the mandibular angle. The axis of the submental artery can then be determined by the relationship of the facial-submental artery and the inferior border of the mandible. The submental artery is a reliable branch of the facial artery and is usually located at approximately 0.5 cm inferior to the lower edge of the mandible [11]. An elliptical skin paddle is designed oriented along the axis of the submental artery (Fig. 15.2) [12–15]. This will incorporate the perforating vessels to the skin. Furthermore, careful design of the skin paddle will also capture the cutaneous perforators to the skin paddle, most significant number of lymph nodes within the flap, harness the mechanism of action, and optimize clinical outcomes [16–34]. The skin paddle will allow for postoperative flap monitoring and assist with recipient site closure without tension.

It is essential to limit the superior half of this ellipse to approximately 1 cm inferior to the lower border of the mandible to avoid visibility of the scar during donor site closure. The inferior half of this ellipse is planned based on the neck skin laxity to allow for donor site closure. The standard skin paddle measures approximately 10 × 5 cm to 6 × 2.5 cm,

M. V. Schaverien, J. H. Dayan (eds.), *Multimodal Management of Upper and Lower Extremity Lymphedema*,
https://doi.org/10.1007/978-3-030-93039-4_15

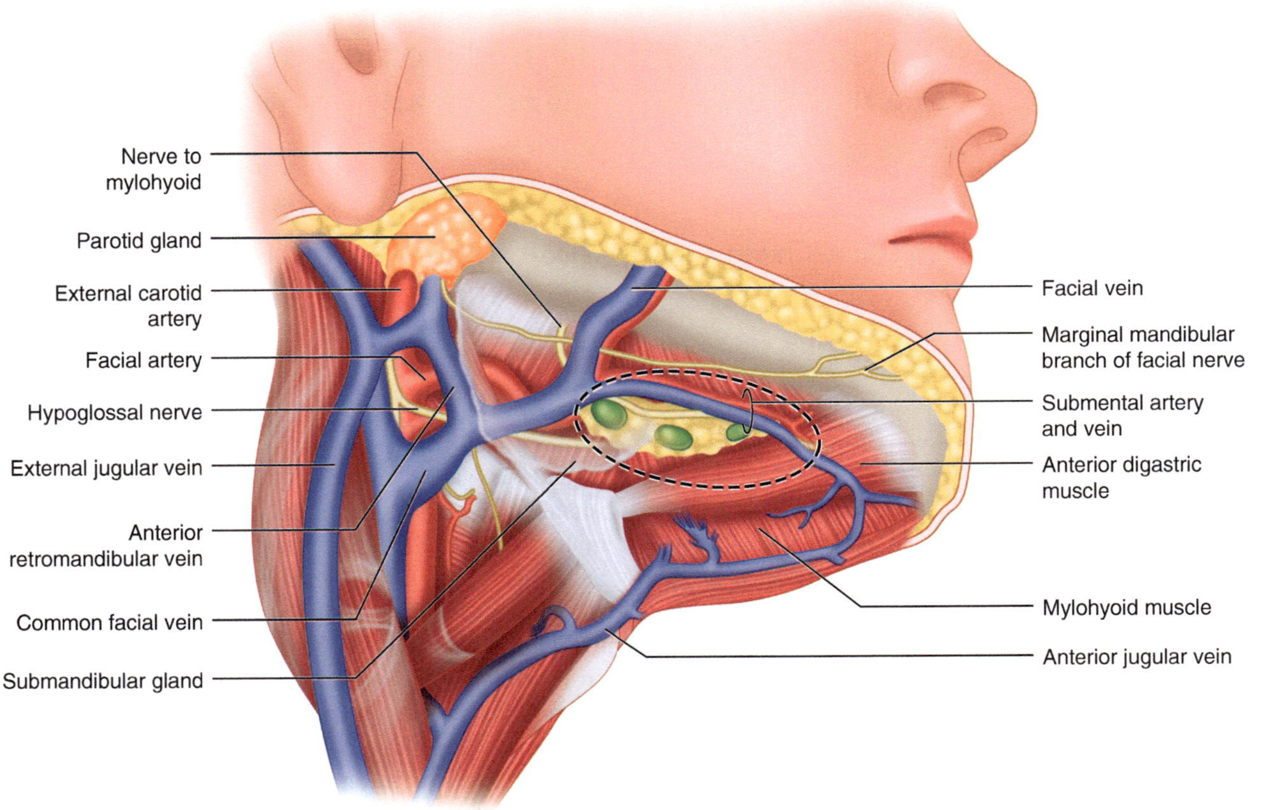

Fig. 15.1 Anatomy of the vascularized submental lymph node flap. (Illustration provided courtesy of Springer)

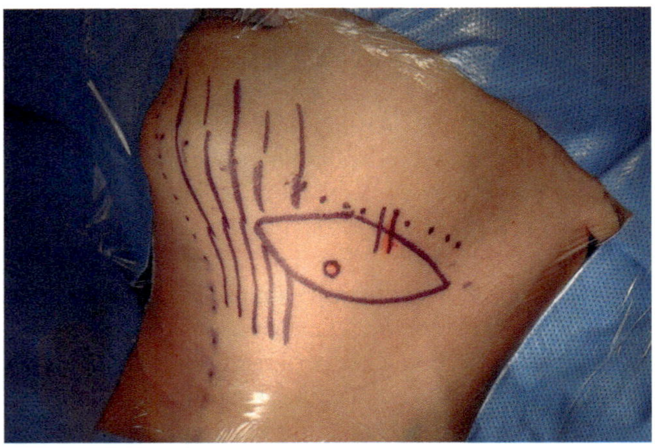

Fig. 15.2 A 70-year-old female was a victim of right upper extremity lymphedema for 2 years post axillary and supraclavicular lymph node dissection due to metastasis of ovarian cancer. A left vascularized submental lymph node flap 6 × 2.5 cm was designed below the lower margin of the mandible with one skin perforator mapped. Medial platysma 5 cm in width was preserved

depending on the skin perforator, with a 5 cm width of medial platysma preservation (Fig. 15.2). The donor site can be easily primary closed with an inconspicuous scar. Generally, the medial most extent of the ellipse should not pass the neck midline.

Flap Dissection

A shoulder roll is placed on the ipsilateral side. Draping of the donor site should allow for movement of the patient's neck during surgery. Clear adhesive dressings are recommended at the sterile drapes border to maintain sterility while providing mobility freedom during the case. Draping of the neck, lower face, corner of the mouth, and the lateral aspects of the lips should be visualized through the clear adhesive dressing. When the marginal mandibular nerve is stimulated and tested with a nerve stimulator intraoperatively, the motion of the lips and face can be easily visualized. Assessment of the facial mimetic muscles should be allowed, especially during dissection around the facial nerve. The neck is extended and rotated to the contralateral side away from the side of the flap harvest. The upper aspect of the ellipse is incised first using a No. 15 blade. Using a Colorado tip monopolar cautery on a lower setting, dissection is carried down to the platysma muscle level. The platysma muscle is carefully dissected through to the subplatysmal plane. Instrumental dissection is performed to visualize the marginal mandibular nerve and the facial vessels, which can be found approximately 2.0 to 2.5 cm anterior to the mandibular angle at the level of the inferior mandibular border under microscope.

Approximately 0.5 cm inferior to this point, the submental artery can be found originating as an anterior branch from the facial artery. On average, the emergence of the submental artery is in close relationship to the submandibular gland. Variations in this anatomy have been noted where in most cases the facial artery is found between the inferior border of the mandible and the submandibular gland [11]. The submental artery frequently travels above the submandibular gland (76%) or travels through the lobes of the gland itself (24%). The artery then travels on the superficial surface of the mylohyoid muscle, supplying perforators through the platysma muscle to nourish the overlying skin. The distal submental artery most commonly travels deep to the digastric muscle (70%), although it may lie superficial to it. The submental vein drains into the anterior facial vein, which most commonly follows the facial artery (31%), although their courses may diverge [1].

One to three branches of the marginal mandibular branch of the facial nerve, which supplies the depressor anguli oris (DAO) and depressor labii inferioris (DLI) muscles, are identified and are usually found near and vertical to the facial artery at the inferior border of the mandible. The marginal mandibular nerve emerges from the lower portion of the parotid gland and courses adjacent to the mandibular angle approximately 0–1.5 cm inferior to the mandibular border; however, it can be displaced 1–2 cm inferiorly when the neck is extended. Branches to the mentalis and DLI usually are located inferior to the mandibular lower border (Fig. 15.3) [12–14]. The larger branch to the DAO is commonly located anterior to the facial artery and above the mandibular border and courses deeply to innervate this muscle. During dissection of the marginal mandibular nerve branches, manipulation should always be gentle and performed under a microscope to prevent unintentional injury or neuropraxia. White vessel loops can be utilized to mark the nerve branches and act as a gentle retractor to avoid injury (Fig. 15.3). Using a nerve stimulator, the small branches of the marginal mandibular nerves can be identified during dissection and their function verified after isolation of the nerves. The corner of the mouth should be easily visualized during testing with the nerve stimulator using the draping technique described above.

The distal ends of the facial artery and vein are then dissected and divided (Fig. 15.4). Once the facial artery and the marginal mandibular nerve branches are isolated, flap elevation is performed from the medial to the lateral direction. The medial part of the platysma, 5 cm in width, is preserved to decrease the morbidity of the weakness of the lower lip (so-called pseudoparalysis of the marginal mandibular nerve) (Fig. 15.5). In this direction, the anterior belly of the digastric muscle is encountered distally and preserved. The distal submental artery is commonly located deep to, or sometimes superficial to, the digastric muscle and included within the flap. The distal portion of the submental artery is isolated and ligated. The inferior half of the elliptical skin paddle markings can be incised. Using a combination of tenotomy scissors and monopolar cautery with a Colorado tip on a low setting, dissection is made subcutaneously to the platysma muscle, preserving the medial platysma 5 cm in width.

During dissection through the subcutaneous adipose layer, care is taken to look for accessory veins that can be used as a secondary outflow vein. As the flap is elevated from the distal aspect, usually, one lymph node may be encoun-

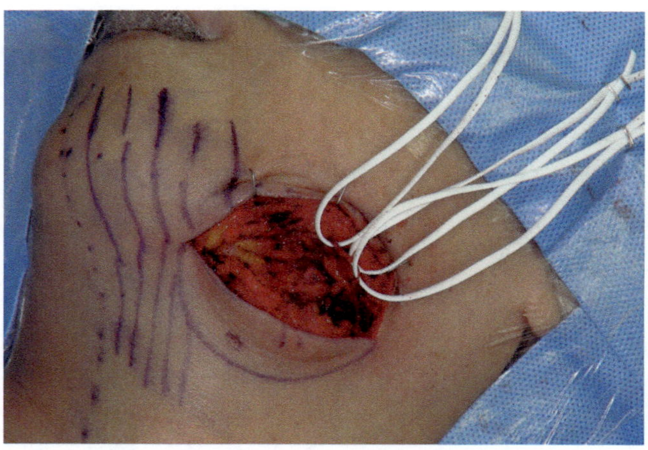

Fig. 15.3 The upper margin of the flap was incised and retracted. Three marginal mandibular nerves were identified and protected with white loops

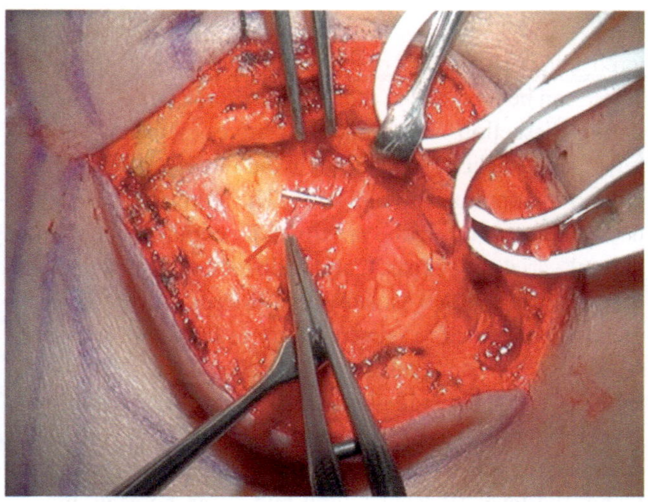

Fig. 15.4 The distal facial artery (red arrow) and vein were dissected and divided

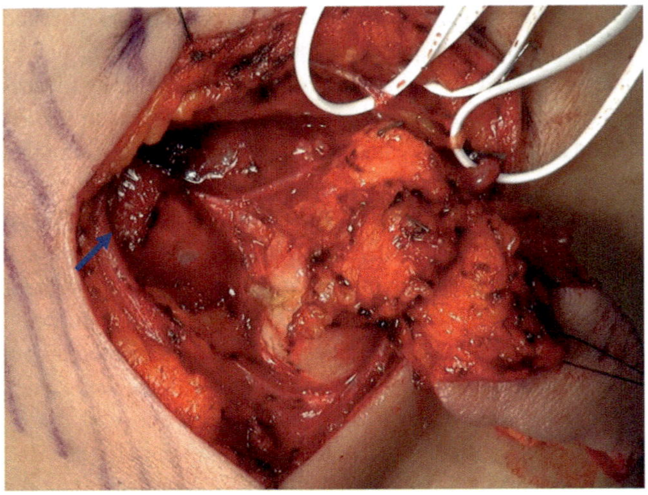

Fig. 15.5 The medial part of the platysma, 5 cm in width, was preserved to decrease the morbidity of the weakness of the lower lip (blue arrow)

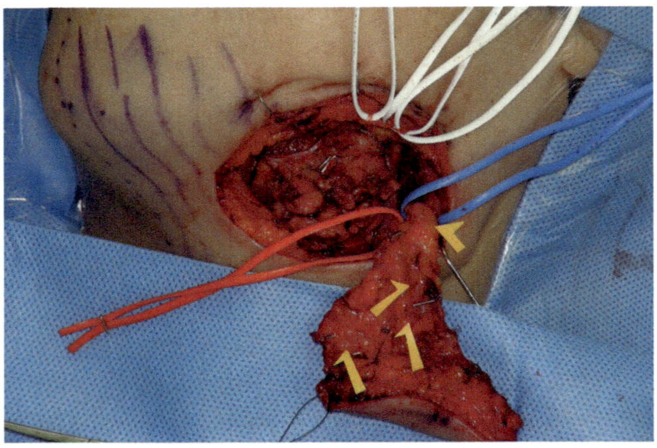

Fig. 15.6 Several sizable level IB level lymph nodes (yellow arrows) can be seen around the proximal facial vessels and were dissected out of the submandibular gland

tered at the distal aspect of the flap, the level IA lymph nodes. These can be included in the flap and protected from damage during dissection. The submental artery is then identified, traveling superficial to the mylohyoid muscle, and this plane is used to continue flap elevation. The submandibular gland is encountered during the proximal dissection. This is where arterial variability exists. Careful dissection around the submandibular gland to isolate large arterial branches to the gland is performed to prevent injury to the facial-submental artery axis. In some cases, this artery will travel within the lobes of the submandibular gland, which takes 30 minutes longer to dissect to the facial artery proximally to obtain the adequate length of the pedicle. Near the submandibular gland, the level IB level lymph nodes can be seen and are carefully incorporated into the flap without devascularization (Fig. 15.6). The remaining dissection around the periphery and the base of the flap is performed. As part of the flap, the harvested sizable lymph nodes, ranging from 3–6, can be visualized on the deep layer of the flap.

Donor Site Closure

The closure of the donor site should receive just as much care to optimize the aesthetic result. Before closure is performed, the shoulder roll should be removed. A small suction drain is placed and secured. The platysma muscle layer is not closed since a segmental resection is performed at the lateral portion. The skin layer is closed with two layers to perform exact approximation to avoid dog ear skin redundancy at the extents of the incision and avoid undue tension, resulting in a widened scar. Surgical strip tapes can be applied to further disperse the tension at the incision.

Insetting of the Flap at the Recipient Site

General postoperative swelling can often occur in the lymphedematous limb, especially when combined with the VLN flap absorbing lymphedema fluid. We recommend using delayed primary retention sutures for the periphery of the flap in the distal recipient site (Fig. 15.7) [35]. These interrupted loose shoelace-type sutures can be loosened if necessary at the bedside in the initial postoperative period. Typically, 5–7 days postoperatively, when the swelling has decreased, these can be tied down and secured.

Postoperative Care

Slight elevation of the extremity can be performed with pillows in the initial postoperative period. Compression of the flap or recipient site is not recommended immediate postop-

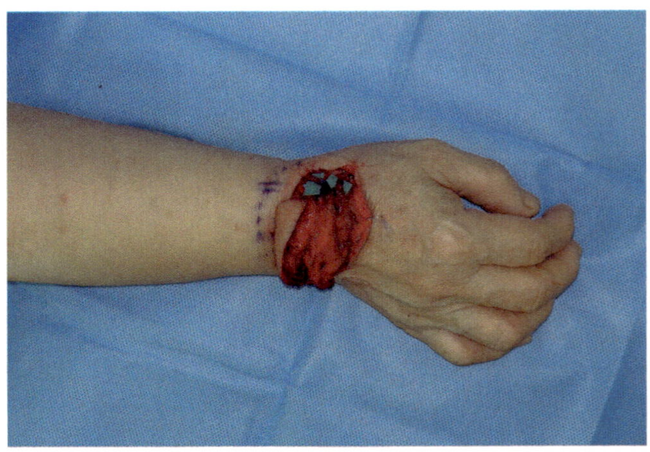

Fig. 15.7 The vascularized submental lymph node flap was transferred to the wrist distal recipient site with anastomoses of the pedicle to the radial artery dorsal branch and cephalic vein (green backgrounds)

eratively. It is suggested that all patients have the VSLN transfer flap inset using the delayed primary retention suture method [35]. This technique can be utilized in both upper and lower extremity recipient sites and any other VLN flaps. The delayed primary retention suture technique allows the tension of the closure to be adjusted to be looser or tighter at the bedside, especially during the critical first few days postoperatively. Loosening the sutures allows for flap and limb swelling while preventing excess pressure at the anastomoses. The flexibility of adjusting the wound tension allows tightening and loosening as needed during the first 5–7 days after surgery. After the swelling has subsided and stabilized, these sutures can be formally secured and tied down at the bedside.

Key Points

- One of the biggest concerns of VLN flap harvest for transfer is the possibility of causing iatrogenic lymphedema at the donor site. The VSLN transfer has not been reported or observed to be associated with lymphedema of the head and face.
- Identification and protection of the marginal mandibular branches of the facial nerve are of utmost importance as an otherwise successful lymphedema-related surgical result will be overshadowed by the morbidity of injury to this critical structure [2]. Morbidity associated with marginal mandibular nerve injury includes weakness or inability to move the ipsilateral lower lip in a downward and lateral direction, which is usually preventable by delicate dissection under microscope with a nerve stimulator.
- The VSLN flap has the advantages of greater number of lymph nodes, reliable skin paddle for flap observation, and larger pedicle facial vein for lymphatic drainage for greater functional improvement of extremity lymphedema.

References

1. Cheng MH, Lin CY, Patel KM. A prospective clinical assessment of anatomic variability of the submental vascularized lymph node flap. J Surg Oncol. 2017;115(1):43–7.
2. Chang TN, Lee CH, Lin JA, Cheng MH. Morbidity of marginal mandibular nerve post vascularized submental lymph node flap transplantation. J Surg Oncol. 2020;122(8):1747–54.
3. Poccia I, Lin CY, Cheng MH. Platysma-sparing vascularized submental lymph node flap transfer for extremity lymphedema. J Surg Oncol J Surg Oncol. 2017;115(1):48–53.
4. Cheng, Ming-Huei, Chang David W, Patel, Ketan M. Principles and practice of lymphedema surgery. Elsevier 2016. Print.
5. Pappalardo M, Cheng MH. Lymphoscintigraphy for the diagnosis of extremity lymphedema: current controversies regarding protocol, interpretation, and clinical application. J Surg Oncol. 2020;121(1):37–47.
6. Dayan JH, Dayan E, Kagen A, Cheng MH, Sultan M, Samson W, Smith ML. The use of magnetic resonance angiography in vascularized groin lymph node transfer: an anatomic study. J Reconstr Microsurg. 2014;30(1):41–5.
7. Dayan JH, Dayan E, Smith ML. Reverse lymphatic mapping: a new technique for maximizing safety in vascularized lymph node transfer. Plast Reconstr Surg. 2015;135:277–85.
8. Patel KM, Chu SY, Huang JJ, Wu CW, Lin CY, Cheng MH. Preplanning vascularized lymph node transfer with duplex ultrasonography: an evaluation of 3 donor sites. Plast Reconstr Surg Glob Open. 2014;2(8):e193.
9. Wu MC, Hsu MY, Shie RF, Cheng MH, Chu FI, Lin CY, Fan YP, Chu SY. Non-contrast-enhanced magnetic resonance angiography of facial arteries for pre-operative evaluation of vascularized submental lymph node flaps. BMC Med Imaging. 2019;19(1):68. https://doi.org/10.1186/s12880-019-0368-7.
10. Asuncion MO, Chu SY, Huang YL, Lin CY, Cheng MH. Accurate prediction of submental lymph nodes using magnetic resonance imaging for lymphedema surgery. Plast Reconstr Surg Glob Open. 2018;6(3):e1691.
11. Tzou CJ, Meng S, Ines T, Reissig L, Pichler U, Steinbacher J, Pona I, Roka-Palkovits J, Rath T, Weninger WJ, Cheng MH. Surgical anatomy of the vascularized submental lymph node flap: anatomic study of correlation of submental artery perforators and quantity of submental lymph node. J Surg Oncol. 2016;115:54.
12. Nason RW, Binahmed A, Torchia MG, et al. Clinical observations of the anatomy and function of the marginal mandibular nerve. Int J Oral Maxillofac Surg. 2007;36:712–5.
13. Dingman R, Grabb W. Surgical anatomy of the mandibular ramus of the facial nerve based on the dissection of 100 facial halves. Plast Reconstr Surg. 1962;29:266–72.
14. Nelson D, Gingrass R. Anatomy of the mandibular branches of the facial nerve. Plast Reconstr Surg. 1979;64:479–82.
15. Cheng MH, Huang JJ, Nguyen DH, Saint-Cyr M, Zenn MR, Tan BK, Lee CL. A novel approach to the treatment of lower extremity lymphedema by transferring a vascularized submental lymph node flap to the ankle. Gynecol Oncol. 2012;126(1):93–8.
16. Cheng MH, Huang JJ, Wu CW, Yang CY, Lin CY, Henry SL, Kolios L. The mechanism of vascularized lymph node transfer for lymphedema: natural lymphaticovenous drainage. Plast Reconstr Surg. 2014;133(2):192e–8e.
17. Patel KM, Lin CY, Cheng MH. From theory to evidence: long-term evaluation of the mechanism of action and flap integration of distal vascularized lymph node transfers. J Reconstr Microsurg. 2015;31(1):26–30.
18. Ito R, Zelken J, Yang CY, Lin CY, Cheng MH. Proposed pathway and mechanism of vascularized lymph node flaps. Gynecol Oncol. 2016;141(1):182–8.
19. Nguyen DH, Chou PY, Hsieh YH, Momeni A, Fang YH, Patel KM, Yang CY, Cheng MH. Quantity of lymph nodes correlates with improvement in lymphatic drainage in treatment of hind limb lymphedema with lymph node flap transfer in rats. Microsurgery. 2016;36(3):239–45.
20. Koide S, Lin CY, Chen C, Cheng MH. Long-term outcome of lower extremity lymphedema treated with vascularized lymph node flap transfer with or without venous complications. J Surg Oncol. 2020;121(1):129–37.
21. Yang CY, Ho OA, Cheng MH, Hsiao HY. Critical ischemia time, perfusion, and drainage function of vascularized lymph nodes. Plast Reconstr Surg. 2018;142(3):688–97.
22. Tinhofer IE, Yang CY, Chen C, Cheng MH. Impacts of arterial ischemia or venous occlusion on vascularized groin lymph nodes in a rat model. J Surg Oncol. 2020;121(1):153.
23. Aljaaly HA, Fries CA, Cheng MH. Dorsal wrist placement for vascularized submental lymph node transfer significantly improves breast cancer-related lymphedema. Plast Reconstr Surg Glob Open. 2019;7(2):e2149–62.

24. Ho OA, Chu SY, Huang YL, Chen WH, Lin CY, Cheng MH. Effectiveness of vascularized lymph node transfer for extremity lymphedema using volumetric and circumferential differences. Plast Reconstr Surg Glob Open. 2019;7(2):e2003.
25. Cheng MH, Loh CYY, Lin CY. Outcomes of vascularized lymph node transfer and Lymphovenous anastomosis for treatment of primary lymphedema. Plast Reconstr Surg Glob Open. 2018;6(12):e2056.
26. Ho OA, Lin CY, Pappalardo M, Cheng MH. Comparisons of submental and groin vascularized lymph node flaps transfer for breast cancer-related lymphedema. Plast Reconstr Surg Glob Open. 2018;6(12):e1923.
27. Gould DJ, Mehrara BJ, Neligan P, Cheng MH, Patel KM. Lymph node transplantation for the treatment of lymphedema. J Surg Oncol. 2018;118(5):736–42.
28. Gustafsson J, Chu SY, Chan WH, Cheng MH. Correlation between quantity of transferred lymph nodes and outcome in vascularized submental lymph node flap transfer for lower limb lymphedema. Plast Reconstr Surg. 2018;142(4):1056–63.
29. Pappalardo M, Patel K, Cheng MH. Vascularized lymph node transfer for treatment of extremity lymphedema: an overview of current controversies regarding donor sites, recipient sites and outcomes. J Surg Oncol. 2018;117(7):1420–31.
30. Ito R, Wu CT, Lin MC, Cheng MH. Successful treatment of early-stage lower extremity lymphedema with side-to-end lymphovenous anastomosis with indocyanine green lymphography assisted. Microsurgery. 2016;36(4):310–5.
31. Schaverien MV, Badash I, Patel KM, Selber JC, Cheng MH. Vascularized lymph node transfer for lymphedema. Semin Plast Surg. 2018;32(1):28–35.
32. Patel KM, Lin CY, Cheng MH. A prospective evaluation of lymphedema-specific quality-of-life outcomes following vascularized lymph node transfer. Ann Surg Oncol. 2015;22(7):2424–30.
33. Engel H, Lin CY, Huang JJ, Cheng MH. Outcomes of lymphedema microsurgery for breast cancer-related lymphedema with or without microvascular breast reconstruction. Ann Surg. 2018;268(6):1076–83.
34. Keeley V, et al. A quality of life measure for limb lymphoedema (LYMQOL). J Lymphoedema. 2010;5(1):26–37.
35. Koide S, Lin CY, Cheng MH. Delayed primary retention suture for inset of vascularized submental lymph node flap for lower extremity lymphedema. J Surg Oncol. 2020;121(1):138–43.

Step-by-Step Instruction: Supraclavicular Vascularized Lymph Node Transplant Procedure

16

Rebecca M. Garza and David W. Chang

Introduction

As vascularized lymph node transplantation (VLNT) grew in popularity, a more desirable lymph node donor site was needed. In 2013, the senior author described harvest of the supraclavicular lymph nodes as a VLN flap [1], and others began to publish on their experience using these lymph nodes in 2014 [2]. Since then, the supraclavicular flap has been shown to be effective in treating both upper and lower extremity lymphedema [3, 4]. Furthermore, it is characterized by a low complication profile, particularly when compared to the groin or lateral thoracic lymph nodes [5], and favorable scar when compared to the submental lymph nodes [4]. Initially, the flap was harvested with an overlying skin paddle, but the senior author's practice has evolved to no longer include the skin, and instead, to bury the flap at the recipient site. Increasingly, simultaneous lymphovenous bypass (LVB) is performed with supraclavicular VLNT [6].

Typical Indications

- Primary lymphedema of the lower extremity with transfer either proximally or distally in the affected limb(s) – bilateral flaps for dual-level transfer can be considered.
- Secondary lymphedema of the upper extremity – neck donor site is selected contralateral to the affected upper extremity, with transfer often performed to a proximal recipient site within the affected arm.
- Secondary lymphedema of the lower extremity – right neck donor site is preferred, with transfer either proximally or distally in the affected limb.

Supplementary Information The online version of this chapter (https://doi.org/10.1007/978-3-030-93039-4_16) contains supplementary material, which is available to authorized users.

R. M. Garza (✉) · D. W. Chang (✉)
Department of Surgery, Section of Plastic and Reconstructive Surgery, University of Chicago, Chicago, IL, USA
e-mail: rgarza@surgery.bsd.uchicago.edu; dchang@surgery.bsd.uchicago.edu

Anatomy

The supraclavicular lymph nodes are located in the neck within level Vb. These lymph nodes are responsible for intrathoracic drainage of the lung and esophagus, as well as drainage of the thyroid and breast [7]. There may be up to an average of eight lymph nodes harvested [8], but the number can vary significantly, with several reports of an average one to three lymph nodes included [9–11]. The arterial pedicle arises 3–4 cm from the origin of the transverse cervical artery (TCA), off of the thyrocervical trunk that branches from the first portion of the subclavian artery (Fig. 16.1) [12]. Less commonly, the vessel may arise directly from the subclavian artery, and rarely, from the internal mammary artery [2]. The arterial pedicle size is typically 1–1.5 mm in diameter. Venous drainage of the flap may be established either through an accompanying transverse cervical vein or by including a branch of the external jugular vein (EJV). A skin paddle may be harvested with the flap when a skin perforator of the transverse cervical vessels is included, but the reliability of skin perfusion varies.

Patient Selection and Preoperative Investigations

Patients with either primary lower extremity lymphedema or secondary upper or lower extremity lymphedema may be considered appropriate candidates for this lymph node trans-

M. V. Schaverien, J. H. Dayan (eds.), *Multimodal Management of Upper and Lower Extremity Lymphedema*,
https://doi.org/10.1007/978-3-030-93039-4_16

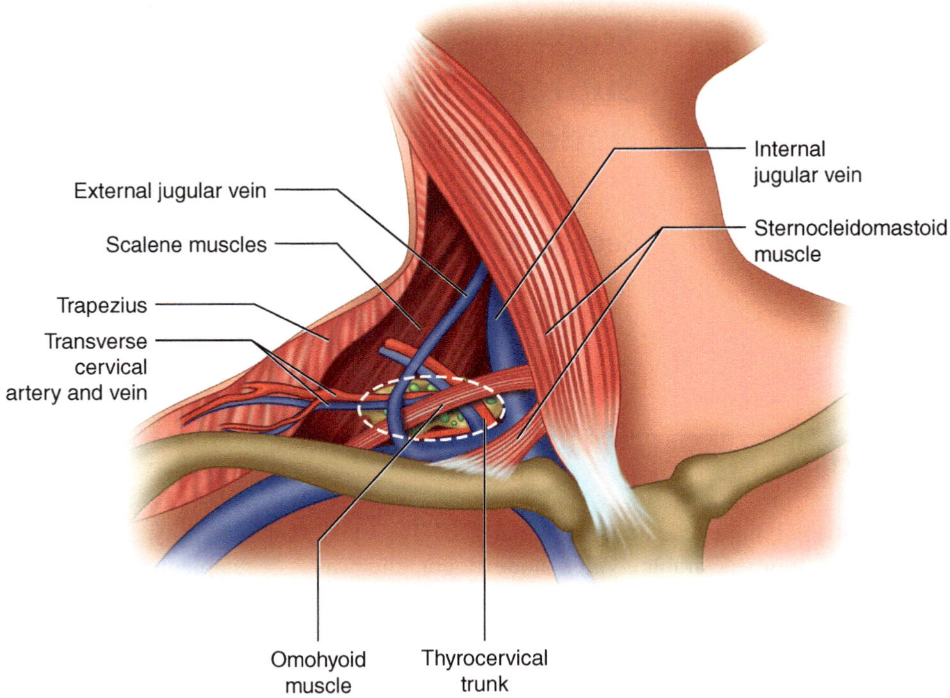

Fig. 16.1 Anatomy of the supraclavicular vascularized lymph node flap. [Illustration provided courtesy of Springer]

plant. In the case of malignancy, patients with active nodal disease at the proposed recipient site are not considered as surgical candidates.

The right or left neck may be used as the donor site, but the right is preferred due to the avoidance of the thoracic duct. In cases of secondary upper extremity lymphedema, the donor site is selected contralateral to the affected upper extremity to prevent disruption of any remaining lymphatic drainage on the affected side. Reverse lymphatic mapping is not routinely used, as no cases of iatrogenic upper extremity lymphedema have been observed with harvest of supraclavicular nodes in our experience.

In cases of previous trauma or surgical resection where soft tissue deficit and scar are present, extensive scar release is recommended. In such cases, other bulkier lymph node flaps may be preferred over the supraclavicular flap in order to provide a larger amount of vascularized tissue to bridge the defect.

Presurgical Markings

A triangle bordered by the clavicle inferiorly, the lateral border of the sternocleidomastoid (SCM) muscle medially, and the EJV laterally is marked. If no skin paddle is planned for inclusion in the flap, a transverse skin incision 1–2 cm above the clavicle is marked within this triangle (Fig. 16.2). If a skin paddle is planned, the paddle should be centered within the triangle with a skin perforator vessel confirmed by Doppler within the flap markings.

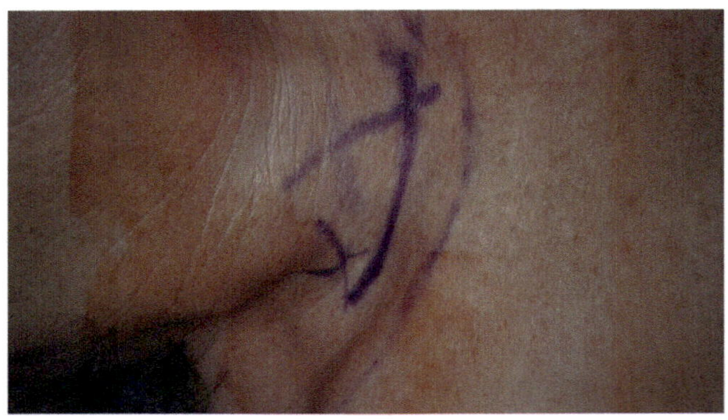

Fig. 16.2 The planned skin incision is marked as a transverse line, 1–2 cm above and parallel to the clavicle, within the triangle bordered by the clavicle, sternocleidomastoid, and external jugular vein

Operative Technique (see supplementary material)

Principles

The neck donor site affords surgeons the ability to perform simultaneous flap harvest and recipient site preparation, and thus decreases operative time. No position changes are required, and patients remain in the supine position. For upper extremity lymphedema, the patient's arms are abducted to 90 degrees and placed on arm boards. The primary surgeon stands below the arm on the donor neck side, and the assistant stands above the patient's contralateral arm. Another surgeon is then able to prepare the recipient site on the affected arm, either in the axilla or more distally. For lower extremity lymphedema, the primary surgeon and assistant work at the neck, while another surgeon prepares the recipient site in the groin or more distal thigh/leg. Surgical loupes are used during harvest and recipient preparation, and the operating microscope is used for micro-anastomosis.

Recipient Site Preparation

Generally, more proximal recipient sites are preferred, as they allow for better camouflage of scars, and, for secondary lymphedema, allow for release of scar tissue within the previously dissected or radiated tissue. Still, a more distal recipient site may be selected if edema is limited to the distal extremity (i.e., recipient site near distal thigh for a patient with only calf and foot swelling with no thigh swelling). If there is insufficient tissue or significant fibrosis that would preclude primary closure over the supraclavicular flap, a flap skin paddle may be included. However, with the small size of the supraclavicular flap, this rarely is required. Vessels that match the caliber of the flap pedicle are identified.

Supraclavicular Flap Harvest Technique

1. The patient's head is turned approximately 45 degrees away from the donor site.
2. A 4–5 cm length skin incision is made 1–2 cm above and parallel to the clavicle within the triangle bordered by the clavicle, SCM, and EJV.
3. The dermis and subcutaneous tissue are divided sharply. Cautery is used to divide the platysma muscle parallel to the incision, and a self-retaining retractor is placed to hold the skin/platysma layer. Fat begins to protrude centrally (Fig. 16.3).
4. Dissection is performed through the fascial/adipose tissue at the medial aspect of the incision to identify the SCM lateral border. Vertical dissection is then carried out while keeping the dissection close to the lateral border of the SCM (Fig. 16.4).

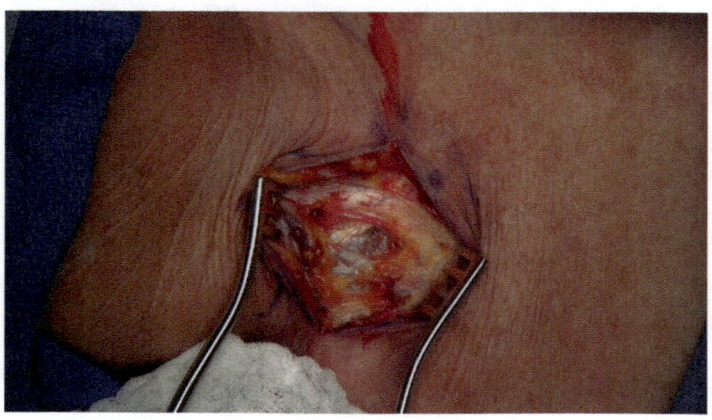

Fig. 16.3 After the skin incision is made, the platysma muscle is divided, and a self-retaining retractor is placed. [With permission [12]]

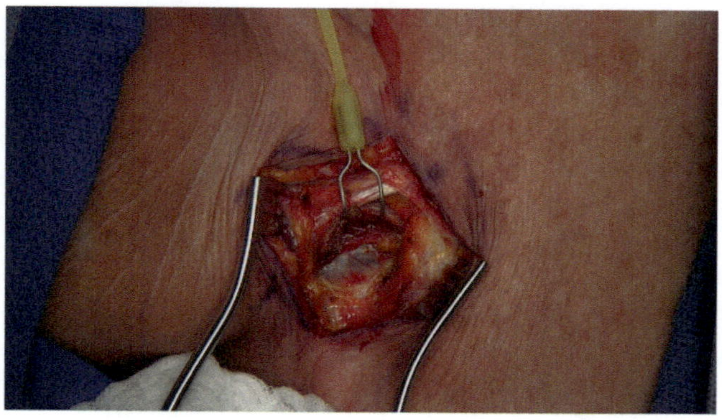

Fig. 16.4 Dissection is carried out medially, along the lateral border of the sternocleidomastoid (retracted), revealing the internal jugular vein. [With permission [12]]

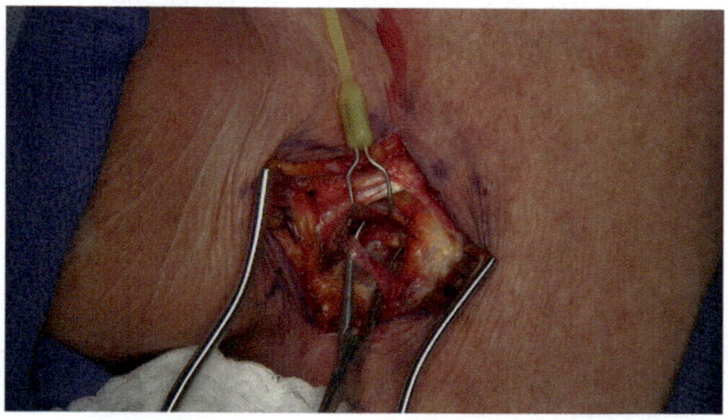

Fig. 16.5 The omohyoid muscle is identified and divided. [With permission [12]]

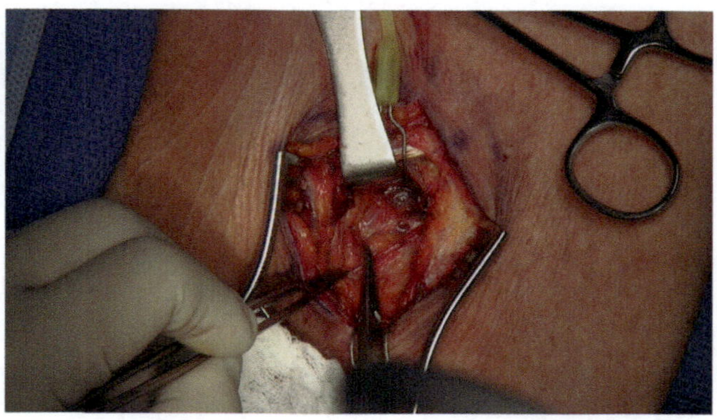

Fig. 16.6 A retractor is used to protect the internal jugular vein, and dissection is continued medially and inferiorly, toward the origin of the transverse cervical artery. [With permission [12]]

5. The omohyoid muscle is identified running obliquely in the fatty tissue deep to platysma and adjacent to the SCM. The belly of the omohyoid is dissected free from surrounding tissue and then transected with cautery (Fig. 16.5).
6. After division of the omohyoid, dissection continues medially and deep to the lateral edge of the SCM. Here, the internal jugular vein (IJV) is identified. Its lateral edge is dissected vertically, and an Army-Navy retractor is then placed to move the vein medially and protect it beneath the SCM (Fig. 16.6).

7. Dissection is carried deep medially, through adipose tissue that surrounds the supraclavicular lymph nodes, until the anterior scalene muscle is visualized. The phrenic nerve lays on the anterior scalene and should be protected.
8. Starting at the medial, deep aspect of the field, the proximal TCA is identified, along with accompanying veins. If the proximal vessel is difficult to identify, you may move more superficially and laterally in the surgical field to identify the distal end of the vessels. It is important to maintain the central connections between the vascular pedicle and nodes (Fig. 16.7).
9. A cluster of deep cervical lymph nodes and surrounding adipose tissue is dissected. Lymphatic vessels are clipped on the "stay" side to prevent leak and left open on the flap side. The distal pedicle artery and vein are clipped and divided (Fig. 16.8).
10. The proximal TCA and vein are ligated and transferred to the recipient site for microvascular anastomosis.
11. Hemostasis is confirmed, and a 10Fr round closed-suction drain is placed, exiting just lateral to the incision through a separate skin site. The platysma and skin layers are closed with absorbable sutures (Fig. 16.9).

Revascularization and Inset

After ligation of the pedicle, the flap is transferred to the recipient site. Arterial anastomosis may be performed first, particularly if multiple veins are included. This allows for identification of the most dominant venous drainage. Venous anastomosis is typically done with a coupler (for veins larger than 1.5 millimeters) or is hand-sewn. An implantable Doppler is placed on the artery, distal to the anastomosis. The flap is secured with 3-0 absorbable sutures to the surrounding tissue and to avoid any kinking of the pedicle. The extremity may be put through a range of motion to be sure the inset/pedicle is not disrupted by movement. A closed-suction drain is placed away from the anastomosis.

Postoperative Care

Patients are admitted for flap monitoring, typically for 3 days. Intravenous antibiotics are given for 24 hours, and patients are kept on bed rest until postoperative day 1 with the affected extremity elevated. For buried flaps, the implantable Doppler is continuously monitored. If LVB is performed

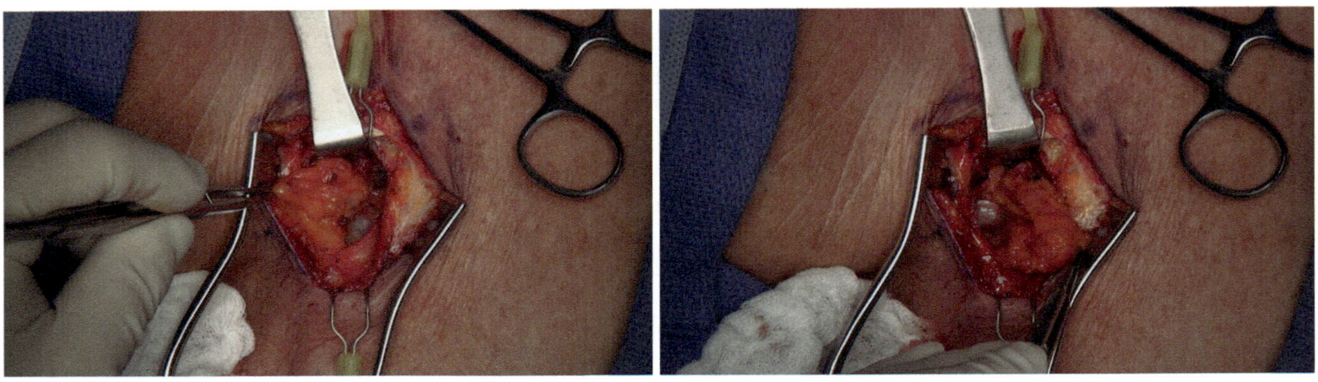

Fig. 16.7 Once the proximal vessel is identified, adipose tissue containing the nodes is peeled off the underlying scalene muscles and dissected from lateral to medial, and superior to inferior, keeping the tissue attached to the vascular pedicle. [With permission [12]]

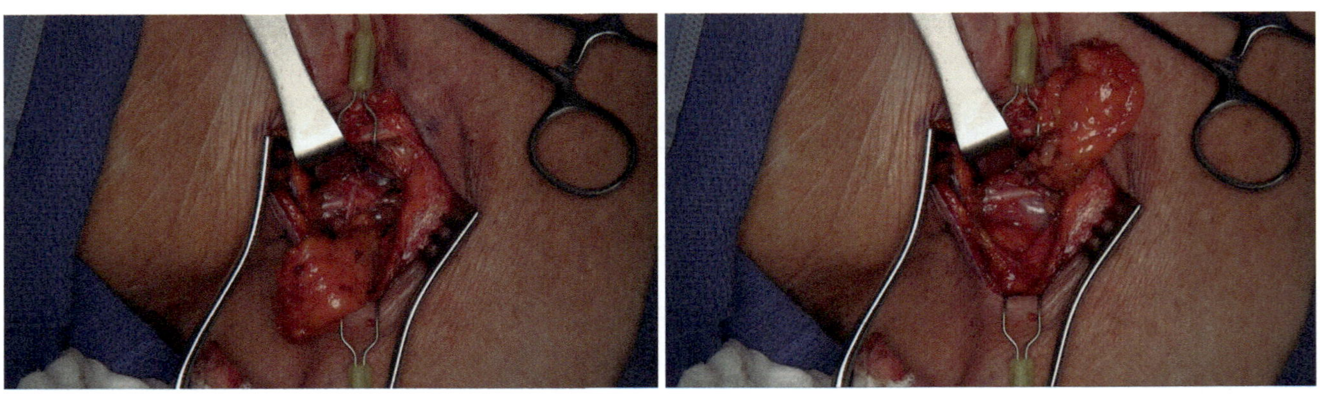

Fig. 16.8 The distal transverse cervical vessels are ligated, as are afferent lymphatic vessels, and the flap is isolated on the proximal pedicle

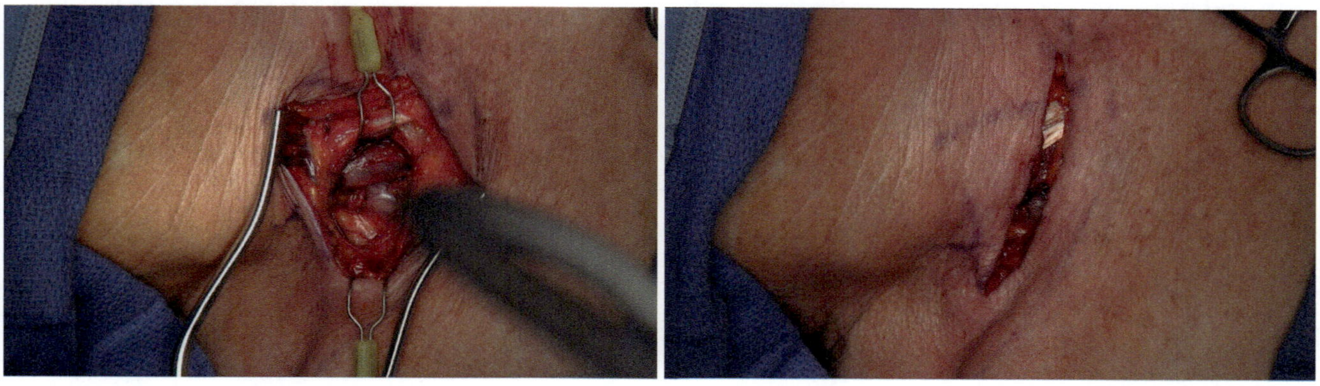

Fig. 16.9 At the deep margin, the anterior scalene muscle with overlying phrenic nerve is visualized (left). [With permission [12]]. Donor site following flap harvest (right)

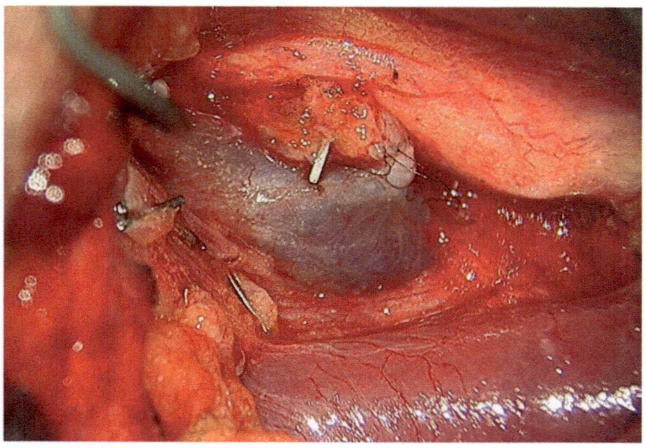

Fig. 16.10 Repair of a thoracic duct injury by lymphovenous anastomosis to a branch of the external jugular vein has been performed

simultaneously, the patient's affected extremity is wrapped by the physical therapist, and this is continued for 1 month postoperatively. If no LVB is performed, the patient's compression garment may be applied postoperatively, provided the wrap will not compress the flap. For a distal flap, no compression garment is used until 1 month postoperatively.

Complications

One of the benefits of the supraclavicular transplant is a low complication profile, particularly when compared to other donor sites. The supraclavicular nerve may be injured during harvest, leading to paresthesia in this distribution on the upper anterior chest. Hematoma, seroma, or cellulitis/abscess may also occur. Chyle leak, particularly if the left neck is used with iatrogenic injury to the thoracic duct, is one of the more challenging complications to manage. Patients with suspected chyle leak are given a low-fat diet. For intractable cases, surgical exploration may be required for ligation of lymphatics or repair of a thoracic duct injury (Fig. 16.10).

Pearls and Pitfalls

- The supraclavicular VLNT, characterized by a low complication profile and inconspicuous donor site, is an effective surgical option for patients with either primary or secondary upper or lower extremity lymphedema.
- A good understanding of the donor site anatomy and variability in flap design/size and course of the pedicle is critical to successfully harvesting this flap. A retrograde dissection of the flap artery may be required if the proximal vessel is not easily visualized.
- Care must be taken to avoid injury to the thoracic duct (when the left neck is used) and other critical neurovascular structures in the neck during harvest.

References

1. Althubaiti GA, Crosby MA, Chang DW. Vascularized supraclavicular lymph node transfer for lower extremity lymphedema treatment. Plast Reconstr Surg. 2013;131:133e–5e.
2. Sapountzis S, Singhal D, Rashid A, Ciudad P, Meo D, Chen H. Lymph node flap based on the right transverse cervical artery as a donor site for lymph node transfer. Ann Plast Surg. 73:398–401.
3. Akita S, Mitsukawa N, Kuriyama M, Kubota Y, Hasegawa M, Tokumoto H, et al. Comparison of vascularized supraclavicular lymph node transfer and lymphaticovenular anastomosis for advanced stage lower extremity lymphedema. Ann Plast Surg. 2015;74:573–9.
4. Maldonado AA, Chen R, Chang DW. The use of supraclavicular free flap with vascularized lymph node transfer for treatment of lymphedema: a prospective study of 100 consecutive cases. J Surg Oncol. 2017;115:68–71.
5. Scaglioni MF, Arvanitakis M, Chen Y-C, Giovanoli P, Chia-Shen Yang J, Chang EI. Comprehensive review of vascularized lymph node transfers for lymphedema: outcomes and complications. Microsurgery. 2018;38:222–9.
6. Beederman M, Garza RM, Agarwal S, Chang DW. Outcomes for physiologic microsurgical treatment of secondary lymphedema involving the extremity. Ann Surg. 2020; Epub ahead of print.

7. Shah JP, Patel SG, Singh B. Head and neck surgery and oncology. Philadelphia: Elsevier health sciences; 2012. Philadelphia: Elsevier Health Sciences; 2012.
8. Liu H, Chung JC. The lymph node content of supraclavicular lymph node flap: a histological study on fresh human specimens. Lymphat Res Biol. 2019;17:537–42.
9. Steinbacher J, Tinhofer IE, Meng S, Reissig LF, Placheta E, Roka-Palkovits J, et al. The surgical anatomy of the supraclavicular lymph node flap: a basis for the free vascularized lymph node transfer. J Surg Oncol. 2017;115:60–2.
10. Patel KM, Chu S-Y, Huang J-J, Wu C-W, Lin C-Y, Cheng M-H. Preplanning vascularized lymph node transfer with duplex ultrasonography: an evaluation of 3 donor sites. Plast Reconstr Surg Glob Open. 2014;2:e193.
11. Gerety PA, Pannucci CJ, Basta MN, Wang AR, Zhang P, Mies C, et al. Lymph node content of supraclavicular and thoracodorsal-based axillary flaps for vascularized lymph node transfer. J Vasc Surg Venous Lymphat Disord. 2016;4:80–7.
12. Ooi ASH, Chang DW. 5-step harvest of supraclavicular lymph nodes as vascularized free tissue transfer for treatment of lymphedema. J Surg Oncol. 2017;115:63–7.

Step-by-Step Instruction: Lateral Thoracic Vascularized Lymph Node Transplant Procedure

17

Joseph H. Dayan

Introduction

The lateral thoracic donor site is a highly versatile option when skin replacement is required or when alternative donor sites are unavailable. Vascularized lymph node transplants (VLNT) in this region can be based on the thoracodorsal vessels, the lateral thoracic vessels, or both [1–3]. The lateral thoracic donor site arguably provides the most abundant skin and soft tissue compared to other lymph node donor sites. Consequently, it is our go-to for the most severely radiated and contracted axilla or groin where skin and soft tissue replacement are required. We also routinely use this for lower extremity lymphedema by burying these lymph nodes into the calf if the omentum is not available. The donor site is well hidden and well tolerated by patients. Using reverse lymphatic mapping, an abundance of lymph nodes can be safely harvested by avoiding any lymph nodes draining the adjacent limb. The author has been using this technique for over the past 10 years without causing donor site lymphedema [4].

Typical Indications

- Upper or lower extremity lymphedema when other options are unavailable
- Severely radiated or contracted defects requiring extensive skin and soft tissue replacement

Supplementary Information The online version of this chapter (https://doi.org/10.1007/978-3-030-93039-4_17) contains supplementary material, which is available to authorized users.

J. H. Dayan (✉)
Division of Plastic and Reconstructive Surgery, Memorial Sloan Kettering Cancer Center, New York, NY, USA
e-mail: dayanj@mskcc.org

Anatomy

Lymph nodes can be harvested from either the lateral thoracic or thoracodorsal vessels or both [5, 6]. The lateral thoracic artery and vein lie along the lateral chest wall (Fig. 17.1). The artery is typically small and has been reported to be absent around 12.5% of the time [7]. Based on the author's series at 1-year imaging follow-up, between seven and 13 lymph nodes can be safely harvested with proper technique [7, 8]. However, there are cases where the artery is absent or tiny along with a paucity of lymph nodes. In these cases, the thoracodorsal artery and vein will reliably supply adequate lymph nodes for transplant. The thoracodorsal vessels are easily identified on the undersurface of the latissimus dorsi muscle. The descending branch of the thoracodorsal nerve runs with the pedicle and can usually be

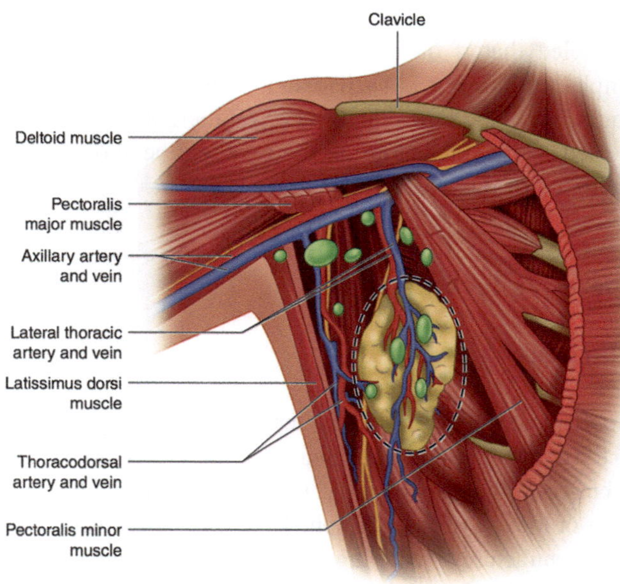

Fig. 17.1 Anatomy of the lateral thoracic/thoracodorsal vascularized lymph node transplant (VLNT) (Illustration provided courtesy of Springer)

M. V. Schaverien, J. H. Dayan (eds.), *Multimodal Management of Upper and Lower Extremity Lymphedema*, https://doi.org/10.1007/978-3-030-93039-4_17

spared. Occasionally, the nerve traverses between the artery and vein and must be divided and then repaired after flap harvest. In some cases, both lateral thoracic and thoracodorsal lymph nodes can be harvested on one vessel, but vascular perfusion is unreliable. Perfusion can easily be confirmed with indocyanine green (ICG) fluorescence angiography or by visualizing back-bleeding in the artery that is not selected as the main pedicle.

Knowledge of the lymphatic drainage of the upper extremity is critical to safely performing this procedure and requires reverse lymphatic mapping [9]. The sentinel lymph nodes (SLNs) draining the upper limb are typically located anteriorly within the axillary limb node cluster, just deep to the lateral border of the pectoralis major muscle [10, 11]. The posterior axillary lymph nodes based on the thoracodorsal vessels or the lateral thoracic lymph nodes can safely be harvested with careful navigation using reverse mapping [4].

Patient Selection

The lateral thoracic donor site is preferable in thinner patients as exploration of the axilla can be challenging in patients with a high body mass index (BMI). If there was a prior supraclavicular lymph node harvest or neck dissection, the ipsilateral axillary donor site should be avoided. This donor site is fairly inconspicuous and provides an abundance of lymph nodes and skin, making it ideal for situations requiring significant skin replacement. Contraindications include prior axillary surgery, radiation therapy, or preexisting limb swelling. Patients should be counseled that if during reverse lymphatic mapping the lymphatic drainage is such that it is not safe to harvest lymph nodes from this donor site, an alternate option will be used such as omentum, or the case will be aborted; the likelihood of this event in our series is under 3%.

Operative Technique

Principles

We often use this option in two separate patient populations: (1) lower extremity lymphedema where the lymph nodes will be buried in the calf (Fig. 17.2) and (2) patients with either upper or lower extremity lymphedema who have severe radiated contractures requiring extensive skin replacement (Fig. 17.3). The key to safe and successful harvest is reverse lymphatic mapping. Various approaches have been described using different agents. The author prefers using filtered technetium 0.2 millicuries injected into the first and third web spaces of the ipsilateral hand the morning of surgery. Our preference is for technetium because the location of the lymph nodes we wish to avoid can be identified prior to skin incision and throughout exploration using a gamma probe.

Recipient Site Preparation

In cases where the flap is being buried in the calf, the medial sural vessels are used. The patient is positioned supine and frog-legged. The border of the medial gastrocnemius muscle is marked, and a longitudinal incision is made over the center mass of the gastrocnemius from the popliteal crease downward for approximately 8–10 cm. The incision extends down through the deep investing muscle fascia. The subfascial plane is explored, and once a perforator is identified, a retrograde intramuscular dissection is performed down to the medial sural vessels. These recipient vessels are prepared for anastomosis and typically consist of large venae comitantes and a small but reliable artery. A portion of the subcutaneous tissue and muscle fascia are excised to allow for space to place the buried flap. Care is taken not to injure the sural nerve posteriorly, or the greater saphenous vein at the anterior margin of the gastrocnemius.

Flap Harvest Technique (see supplementary material)

- Once the location of the SLNs draining the upper limb is identified with a gamma probe, a transverse incision is marked, approximately 4 cm below the axillary crease.
- If a large amount of skin replacement is required, the thoracodorsal vessels will be included in the flap to allow for inclusion of a latissimus dorsi or a thoracodorsal artery perforator (TDAP) flap.
- The transverse incision is made, and then a subcutaneous flap is elevated to expose the clavipectoral fascia.
- A gamma probe is used to locate the critical lymph nodes draining the upper limb and to determine how high in the axilla they are located. Care is taken to stay below this level. However, at some point in the dissection, one can harvest more superiorly and posteriorly once the anterior axillary nodes are clear.
- Dissection begins along the border of the pectoralis major muscle and continues directly to the lateral chest wall. It is easy to be too posterior and miss the lateral thoracic vessels, so it is safest to hug the undersurface of the pectoralis until the chest wall is encountered.
- A plane between the lateral thoracic lymph node packet and the chest wall is created.
- The distal lateral thoracic artery and vein are divided but kept long in case of a need to turbocharge.
- Using the gamma probe, the superior extent of dissection is determined to be the point where there is no "hot" signal from the probe. Dissection proceeds straight down to

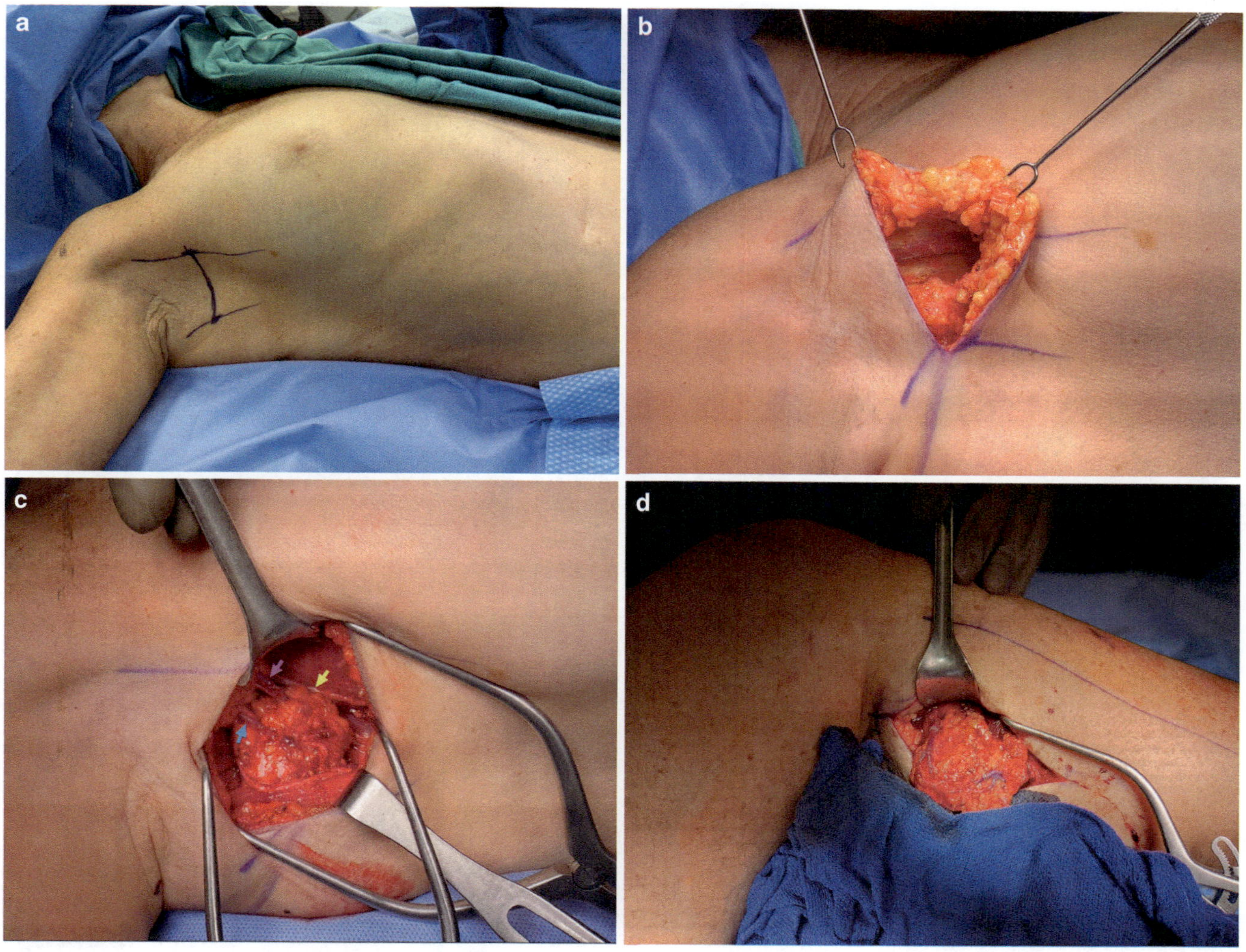

Fig. 17.2 (**a**) Marking for lateral thoracic vascularized lymph node transplant. (**b**) Elevation of subcutaneous flaps exposing clavipectoral fascia. (**c**) Final flap elevation based on both lateral thoracic (purple arrow) and thoracodorsal (blue arrow) vessels. Long thoracic nerve is highlighted with the yellow arrow. (**d**) Flap inset with anastomosis to medial sural vessels. As there was only one usable recipient artery and vein, the lateral thoracic artery and vein were chain-linked and anastomosed to the distal thoracodorsal pedicle

the proximal pedicle. It is critical not to skeletonize the vessels or the lymph nodes may become devascularized and soon you realize you are harvesting mostly a pedicle without lymph nodes.

- The intercostal brachiocutaneous nerve should be preserved to avoid loss of sensation. As a general rule, dissection should not be superior to this nerve as you will be in the territory of the critical lymph nodes draining the upper limb.
- In the event that the lateral thoracic artery is absent or there are too few lymph nodes based on this system, or a large skin flap is required, the thoracodorsal vessels are used.
- To include the thoracodorsal vessels, dissection simply continues in the same plane down to the latissimus muscle.
- The thoracodorsal pedicle is easily identified by exposing the anterior border of the latissimus muscle and hugging the muscle until the pedicle is seen on its undersurface.
- The distal thoracodorsal vessels are divided, and the lymph node flap is elevated from the underlying muscle, carefully dividing the many branches present.
- Particular care is taken when encountering the serratus branch of the thoracodorsal vessels that runs alongside the long thoracic nerve.
- Finally, using the gamma probe, the superior extent of the flap is where the gamma probe signal is no longer "hot". Dissect directly to the proximal thoracodorsal pedicle without skeletonizing it.
- The thoracodorsal nerve should be preserved, but if it runs between the artery and vein, it may need to be divided and then repaired.
- ICG angiography is used to confirm adequate perfusion of the lymph node flap.
- Liposomal bupivacaine is injected for pain relief, and a layered closure is performed over a closed suction drain.

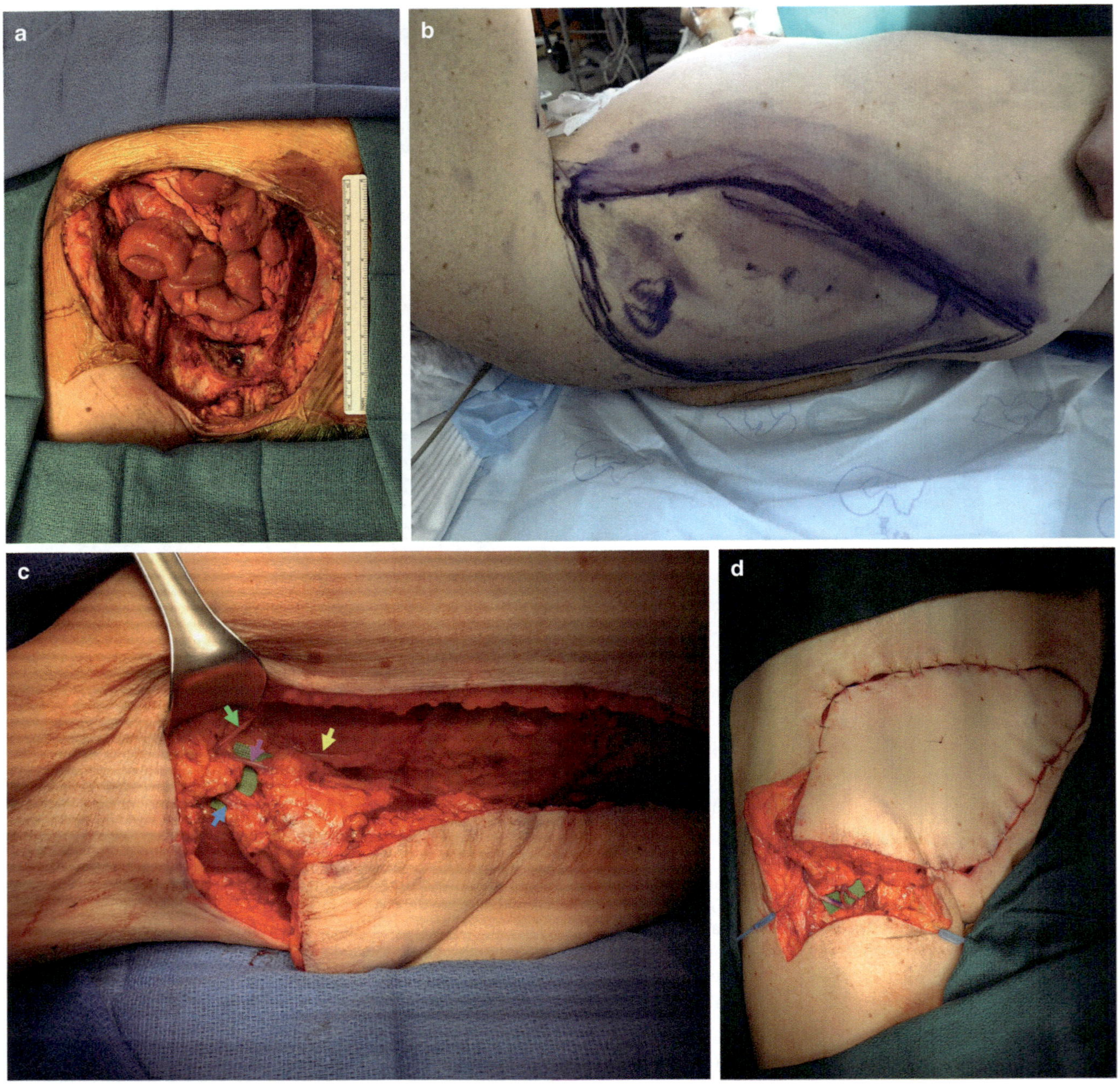

Fig. 17.3 (**a**) Large radiated inguinal and abdominal defect with lower extremity lymphedema. (**b**) Flap marking for combined latissimus dorsi and lateral thoracic lymph node transplant. (**c**) Flap containing both lymph nodes and large skin paddle based on both the lateral thoracic (purple arrow) and thoracodorsal vessels (blue arrow). Intercostobrachial cutaneous nerve (green arrow); long thoracic nerve (yellow arrow). (**d**) Flap inset

Revascularization and Inset

Revascularization is straightforward if one pedicle is used. In cases where both pedicles are used, there may not be an adequate communication, and both thoracodorsal and lateral thoracic arteries as well as thoracodorsal and lateral thoracic veins will need to be anastomosed. If there are not enough recipient vessels to accommodate this, then the flaps can be daisy-chained—a reason to harvest the flaps with adequate length on the distal pedicles.

Postoperative Care

Flaps are monitored via Doppler probe, and in the case of buried flaps, handheld Doppler can be performed through the overlying skin. Enoxaparin is given prior to the start of surgery for deep vein thrombosis prophylaxis: a 7-day course is used for upper extremity lymphedema, and a 30-day course is used for lower extremity lymphedema. The typical antibiotic course is 2 weeks, but if the patient is already on prophylactic antibiotics or has frequent bouts of cellulitis, this may be increased. Patients with lower extremity lymphedema are non-weight bearing for 2 weeks with a walker. After 2 weeks, compression wrapping is applied by a lymphedema therapist, and weight-bearing restrictions are removed.

Complications

Complications for this donor site are uncommon, but the most serious potential complication is donor site lymphedema. This is why reverse lymphatic mapping is critical to patient safety. Other potential complications are the need to divide and repair the thoracodorsal nerve and injury to the long thoracic nerve (although rare). Patients are also at risk for injury to the intercostal brachiocutaneous nerve, which can lead to loss of sensation in the axilla.

Pearls and Pitfalls

- The lateral thoracic/thoracodorsal donor site is ideal for both a minimally morbid and concealed donor site as well as a go-to option for the most challenging defects requiring skin replacement.
- It is a safe donor site option as long as reverse lymphatic mapping with the gamma probe is used throughout the procedure.
- Do not assume that the thoracodorsal pedicle will perfuse the lateral thoracic lymph nodes.
- Identify and preserve the intercostal brachiocutaneous nerve.
- Avoid this donor site if ipsilateral supraclavicular lymph nodes have already been harvested.

References

1. Barreiro GC, Baptista RR, Kasai KE, et al. Lymph fasciocutaneous lateral thoracic artery flap: anatomical study and clinical use. J Reconstr Microsurg. 2014;30:389–96.
2. Batista BN, Germain M, Faria JC, Becker C. Lymph node flap transfer for patients with secondary lower limb lymphedema. Microsurgery. 2017 Jan;37(1):29–33.
3. Inbal A, Teven CM, Chang DW. Latissimus dorsi flap with vascularized lymph node transfer for lymphedema treatment: technique, outcomes, indications and review of literature. J Surg Oncol. 2017;115:72–7.
4. Dayan JH, Dayan E, Smith ML. Reverse lymphatic mapping: a new technique for maximizing safety in vascularized lymph node transfer. Plast Reconstr Surg. 2015;135:277–85.
5. Harii K, Torii S, Sekiguchi J. The free lateral thoracic flap. Plast Reconstr Surg. 1978;62:212–22.
6. Bhattacharya S, Bhagia SP, Bhatnagar SP, Aabdi SM, Chandra R. The anatomical basis of the lateral thoracic flap. Eur J Plast Surg. 1990;13:238–40.
7. Tinhofer IE, Meng S, Steinbacher J, et al. The surgical anatomy of the vascularized lateral thoracic artery lymph node flap-A cadaver study. J Surg Oncol. 2017;116:1062–8.
8. Smith ML, Molina BJ, Dayan E, et al. Heterotopic vascularized lymph node transfer to the medial calf without a skin paddle for restoration of lymphatic function: proof of concept. J Surg Oncol. 2017;115:90–5.
9. Vignes S, Blanchard M, Yannoutsos A, Arrault M. Complications of autologous lymph-node transplantation for limb lymphoedema. Eur J Vasc Endovasc Surg. 2013;45:516–20.
10. Coroneos CJ, Woodward WA, Wong FC, Caudle AS, Shaitelman SF, Kuerer HM, Schaverien MV. Anatomy and physiology of the sentinel lymph nodes of the upper extremity: implications for axillary reverse mapping in breast cancer. J Surg Oncol. 2021;123(4):846–53.
11. Nos C, Clough KB, Bonnier P, et al. Upper outer boundaries of the axillary dissection. Result of the SENTIBRAS protocol: multicentric protocol using axillary reverse mapping in breast cancer patients requiring axillary dissection. Eur J Surg Oncol. 2016;42:1827–33.

Step-by-Step Instruction: Omental Vascularized Lymph Node Transplant Procedure: Laparoscopic and Open Harvest Techniques

18

Carrie K. Chu and Mark V. Schaverien

Introduction

The omental flap was first described to treat lymphedema by Goldsmith in 1967 as a pedicled flap [1]. Despite encouraging clinical outcomes, its use was limited by a high-risk profile [2]. The introduction of laparoscopic techniques enabling minimally invasive free omental vascularized lymph node (VLN) flap harvest has led to renewed interest and widespread adoption of this flap to treat lymphedema using both laparoscopic and mini-laparotomy approaches [3, 4].

The principal advantages of the omental vascularized lymph node transplant (VLNT) include avoidance of any risk of iatrogenic donor site lymphedema and the potential for dual-level transfer, making it the most versatile of the VLNT options available. The omentum is known as the "policeman of the abdomen" because of its immunogenic and angiogenic properties [5]. In addition to the gastroepiploic lymph nodes that lie along the pedicle axis, the free omental vascularized lymphatic flap incorporates additional critical lymphatic structures, including lymphoreticular bodies known as "milky spots" that form the omentum-associated lymphoid tissue (OALT) [6–8]. Further, the omental tissue promotes lymphangiogenesis mediated by vascular endothelial growth factor (VEGF) [9]. Given these properties, the omentum has been described as a large flattened-out lymph node [10].

Supplementary Information The online version of this chapter (https://doi.org/10.1007/978-3-030-93039-4_18) contains supplementary material, which is available to authorized users.

C. K. Chu (✉) · M. V. Schaverien (✉)
Department of Plastic Surgery, The University of Texas MD Anderson Cancer Center, Houston, TX, USA
e-mail: CKChu@mdanderson.org; mvschaverien@mdanderson.org

Typical Indications

- The omental VLN flap is indicated for the treatment of established lymphedema, in particular where there is a history of cellulitis.
- Indicated for orthotopic transplantation into the axilla following radical scar release using recipient vessels from the subscapular axis; the bulk is useful for correcting the axillary contour deformity following axillary lymphadenectomy and radiation therapy, as well as ablative breast deformities.
- The right or left gastroepiploic VLNT may be harvested as a low volume flap while maintaining the lymph nodes about the pedicle and associated lymphatic tissue, suitable for heterotopic (non-anatomic) transplantation.
- The flap can be divided predictably into right and left gastroepiploic systems for dual level transfer.

Anatomy

The greater omentum is a doubly peritoneum-lined fibroadipose structure that hangs in apron-like fashion from the greater curvature of the stomach. Inferiorly it drapes over the intestinal viscera and then folds under itself to attach to the transverse colon and mesocolon. The lateral boundaries are the gastrosplenic ligament on the left and the duodenum and hepatic flexure on the right. There is a bipedicled vascular supply; the right gastroepiploic artery arises from the gastroduodenal artery off of the common hepatic artery, while the left gastroepiploic artery originates from the splenic artery. The right and left gastroepiploic vessels then converge along the greater curvature of the stomach. The right and left gastroepiploic veins drain into the superior mesenteric vein and the splenic vein, respectively.

The gastroepiploic lymph nodes lie along the greater curvature of the stomach in continuity with the omentum [11] (Fig. 18.1). The gastroepiploic nodal basins have been well

M. V. Schaverien, J. H. Dayan (eds.), *Multimodal Management of Upper and Lower Extremity Lymphedema*,
https://doi.org/10.1007/978-3-030-93039-4_18

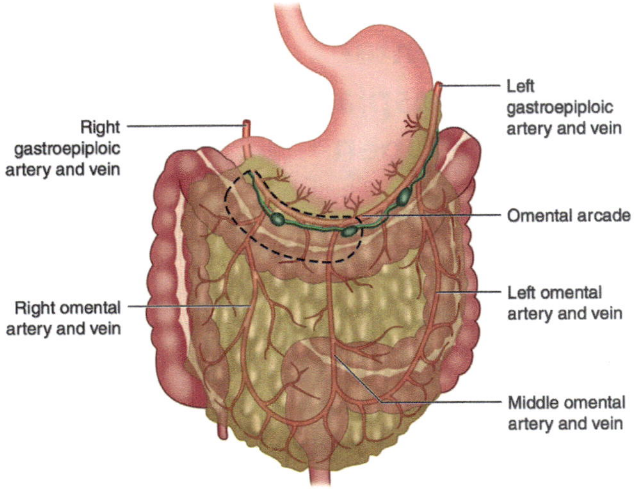

Fig. 18.1 Vascular anatomy of the omental/right gastroepiploic vascularized lymph node flap. (Illustration provided courtesy of Springer)

defined through gastric cancer staging. Along the greater curvature of the stomach, there are an average of 6.4 (±7.3) lymph nodes in association with the right gastroepiploic pedicle and 8.3 (±7.9) with the left gastroepiploic pedicle [12]. Beyond the discrete nodes, there are numerous "micro" lymph nodes less than 1.5 mm in size [13], as well as lymphoreticular bodies ("milky spots") and OALT. The gastroepiploic VLN flap is limited to the area adjacent to the gastroepiploic vascular arcade, since the lymph nodes are located around these vessels [11]. This allows for the creation of a relatively small lymph node flap that allows heterotopic placement in the distal extremity with acceptable cosmetic outcome. The gastroepiploic VLNT is often harvested using the right gastroepiploic artery due to relative ease of access compared to the left side while avoiding the pancreatic tail and spleen. For the free omental VLNT, the pedicle length varies between 4 and 10 cm, and the diameters of the artery and vein are typically 2–2.5 mm and 2.5–4 mm, respectively. While a small lymph node flap may be procured, a fully harvested omental flap may provide a surface area in excess of 900 cm^2, rendering significant flexibility for flap tailoring as dictated by recipient site needs. However, there is substantial individual variability in omental dimensions including thickness, in part as a function of body habitus.

Patient Selection

Intra-abdominal flap harvest has rare but potential risks including visceral injury, intestinal ileus/obstruction, and bulge/hernia, and, therefore, appropriate patient selection is critical to minimize the occurrences of complications. Consideration of previous abdominal medical and surgical history will reveal factors associated with adhesions that increase the difficulty of laparotomy/laparoscopy. Relative contraindications include a history of previous open laparotomies, intra-abdominal radiation, disseminated intra-abdominal infections, or ventral hernia repair. Examples of absolute contraindications include prior omentectomy, previous adhesive bowel obstruction, and recurrent hernia repairs. Particular attention should be paid to foregut or colonic procedures that may have disrupted the anatomy of the omentum or superior mesenteric axis. Increased body mass index correlates positively with abdominal wall morbidity risk, and these patients may be better suited for a minimally invasive approach if an intra-abdominal donor site is required. Recurrent episodes of cellulitis are a strong indication for the use of the omental VLN flap. It is imperative that patients undergoing a laparoscopic approach be counseled about the potential need for open conversion.

Surgical Techniques

Principles

Harvest of the gastroepiploic VLNT may be undertaken via an open mini-laparotomy or laparoscopic technique. These minimally invasive approaches to intra-abdominal surgery confer advantages including reduced postoperative pain, shorter surgical scars, faster time to return of bowel function, reduced adhesions, and decreased abdominal wall morbidity [14]. A two-team approach may be preferable. At our center, the laparoscopic procedure is often performed by a two-surgeon microsurgical team including a specialist with dual training in general and microvascular surgery. Although either the right or left gastroepiploic pedicle may be selected, the right gastroepiploic pedicle is preferentially used if only a single flap is required due to its more favorable regional anatomy [15].

Recipient Site Preparation

The affected extremity recipient site, proximally or distally, is chosen based on the imaging and physical examination findings. The most common indication is for orthotopic (proximal) transfer to the axilla, and this may be performed via the preexisting axillary lymphadenectomy scar. Radical axillary scar release is performed. Subsequently, branches of the subscapular axis are prepared with lysis of perivascular scar, preserving the thoracodorsal pedicle, and therefore the latissimus dorsi flap, if possible. Care is taken to select veins without venous backflow.

For heterotopic (distal) extremity transfer, a right gastroepiploic lymph node flap is preferred. An incision is made over the chosen recipient vessels, and then surgical debulking of the deep subcutaneous tissue and deep fascia is performed to create an unscarred recipient pocket approximating the dimensions of the flap, preserving superficial veins and cutaneous nerves. In the forearm, either the radial or ulnar artery is used, and in the lower leg, the posterior tibial artery is typically preferred. Preoperative vascular imaging of the lower extremity using computed tomography angiography (CTA) can be helpful in patients with primary lymphedema where there may be anatomical variabilities in the presence and caliber of the posterior tibial artery.

Algorithm for Flap Harvest Technique (see supplementary material)

Patients without an abdominal history are well suited to laparoscopic flap harvest. Where prior free abdominal flap breast reconstruction has been performed, the abdominoplasty flap can be elevated to allow a supra-umbilical mini-laparotomy or hybrid laparoscopic approach without creation of additional skin-level scars. In selected patients where a combined free abdominal flap with superficial inguinal (groin) VLNT is not possible or not desired, this can be performed at the time of breast reconstruction.

Laparoscopic Flap Harvest Technique

- The peritoneal cavity is insufflated after peri-umbilical access with a 10-mm trocar. After entry, three additional 5-mm trocars are placed under direct vision.
- Abdominal exploration and critical structures are identified. We prefer utilizing atraumatic, non-locking instruments as meticulous traction and minimal touch technique is required to limit lymphatic disruption throughout the critical lymphatic structures of the flap. Mapping of the lymphosome of the right gastroepiploic lymph nodes using indocyanine green (ICG) and Technetium-99m injection via upper endoscopy has been described to allow flap harvest separately along anatomic planes, leaving the left lymphosome in situ [4].
- Flap dissection utilizes monopolar cautery, a bipolar energy-assisted tissue sealing device, and vascular clips when appropriate to minimize thermal injury to the vascular pedicle and critical lymphatic structures.
- The sequence of dissection starts with the release of the omentum off the transverse colon and hepatic flexure followed by development of the avascular plane between the transverse colonic mesentery and the posterior surface of the omentum. Care is taken to avoid injury to the mesenteric vessels (Fig. 18.2).
- The lesser sac posterior to the stomach is entered.
- Based on flap size requirement, the omentum is divided in the vertical axis toward the stomach.
- The left gastroepiploic vessels are identified and then ligated.
- The gastric branches arising perpendicular to the gastroepiploic vascular arcade are sequentially divided off of the greater curvature of the stomach carefully using a bipolar energy-assisted sealing device where safe and by vascular clips where necessary, taking care to avoid injury to the pedicle and lymph nodes (Fig. 18.3).
- Just proximal to the pylorus, the right gastroepiploic artery and vein are identified and isolated (Fig. 18.4).
- The pedicle is rendered ischemic after double clip ligation on the patient side followed by sharp transection.
- The peritoneal cavity is inspected for hemostasis. The ports are removed under visualization, and the abdomen is desufflated.
- Depending upon flap size, the umbilical port incision is extended to 3–5 cm to facilitate gentle, atraumatic flap extraction (Figs. 18.5 and 18.6).

Open Flap Harvest Technique

This approach is via a supra-umbilical mini-laparotomy incision around 5 cm in length. The abdominal cavity is accessed with the assistance of Bookwalter retractors. Similar to the

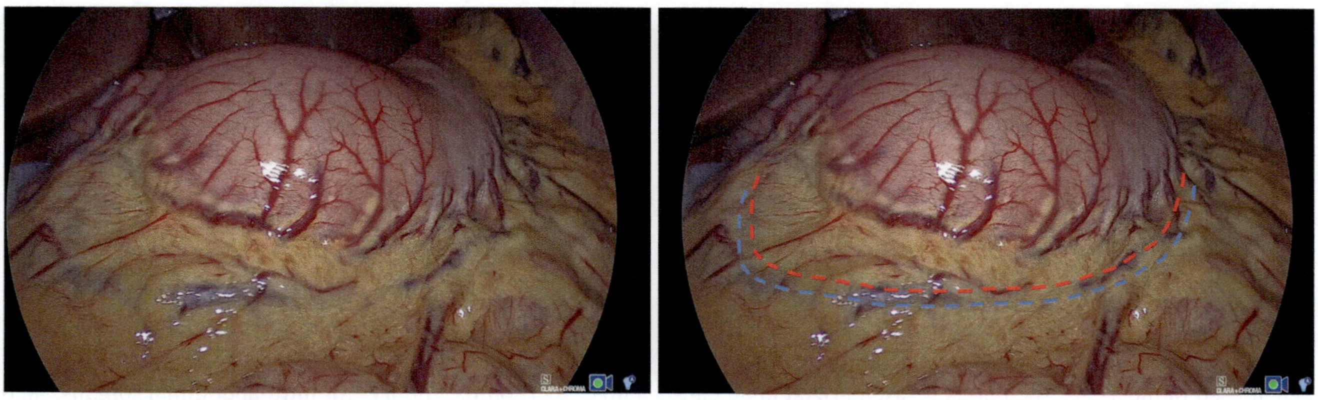

Fig. 18.2 Laparoscopic visualization of the omentum. Red and blue dotted lines (right) represent the convergent courses of the right and left gastroepiploic arterial and venous arcades along the greater curvature of the stomach

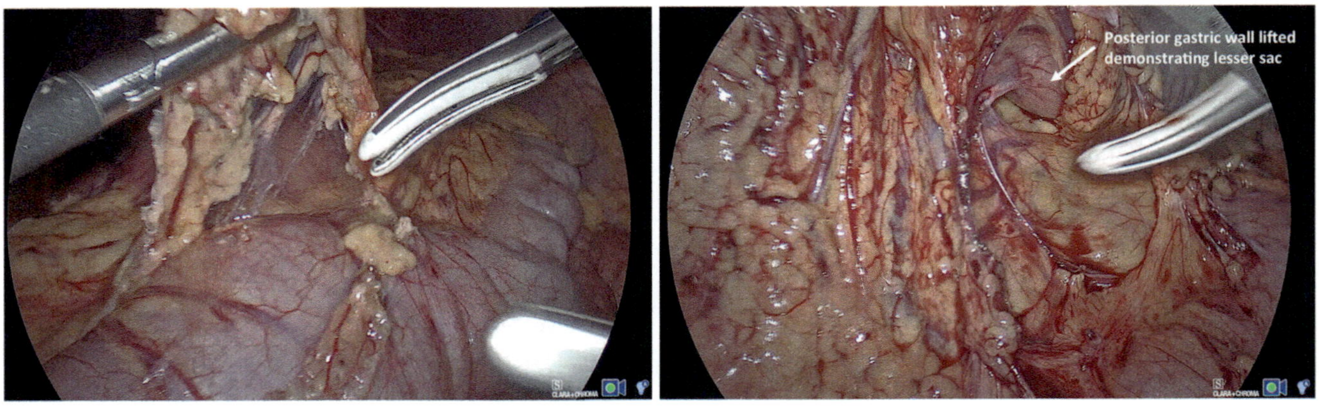

Fig. 18.3 The greater omentum is freed from its attachments along the transverse colon and hepatic flexure (left). The plane between the omentum and the transverse mesocolon is developed, and the lesser sac posterior to the stomach is entered (right)

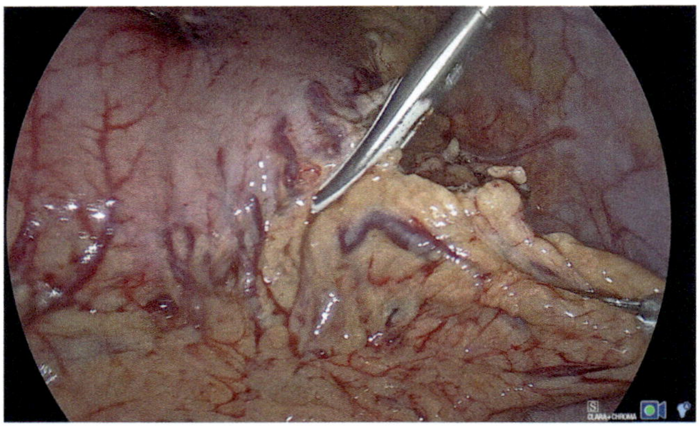

Fig. 18.4 The omentum is divided off of the greater curvature of the stomach with ligation of the perpendicular gastric branches. The left gastroepiploic vessels have been divided

laparoscopic approach, the sequence is releasing the greater omentum from its attachments along the transverse colon and hepatic flexure, and then the lesser sac is entered with finger dissection to protect the middle colic vessels. The pedicle is identified, then the left gastroepiploic vessels are ligated, and next the omentum is freed staying close to the greater curve of the stomach to avoid injury to the pedicle with ligation of the short gastric vessels using an energy-assisted tissue sealing device, suture ties, or vascular clips, as appropriate. Just proximal to the pylorus, the right gastroepiploic artery and vein are isolated and divided. A transversus abdominis plane (TAP) block is then performed under direct vision.

Revascularization and Inset

Following harvest, the flap is reperfused at the recipient site. When used in the axilla, the flap is revascularized in an end-to-end fashion to a branch of the subscapular axis. The gastroepiploic vein has bidirectional venous outflow due to the absence of valves, and anastomosis to one or two recipient veins is performed [16]. In the distal extremity, the preference is for a flow-through configuration for the artery or end-to-side, with venous anastomosis to one or two veins from the superficial and/or deep venous system.

Flap final volume is tailored based on recipient site characteristics with assistance using ICG lymphography perfusion mapping following reperfusion with excision of marginally vascularized portions of the flap while maintaining hemostasis. In particular, the omentum suitably fills the concavity and contour deformity often created by axillary lymphadenectomy. Our preference is to avoid the use of a skin graft.

Postoperative Care

Postoperatively, flaps are initially monitored hourly on a hospital free flap floor. Diet is advanced as tolerated. Deep venous thrombosis prophylaxis is given postoperatively until discharge. Patients are discharged on postoperative day 3 or 4. Antibiotics are given for 2 weeks postoperatively.

For lower extremity distal flap placement, patients begin a dangling protocol on postoperative day 3. Patients resume compression garments at 4 weeks postoperatively.

Complications

Although complications are rare, the patient needs to be counselled preoperatively regarding the potential risks inherent with these approaches, including incisional hernia or bulge, peritonitis, injury to intra-abdominal organs, and bowel obstruction.

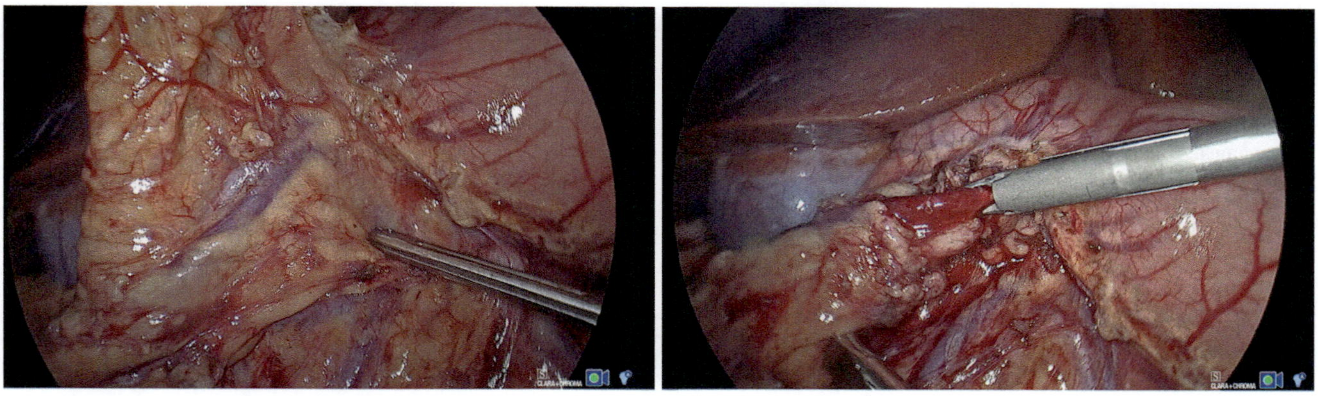

Fig. 18.5 Just proximal to the pylorus, the right gastroepiploic artery and vein are identified (left). The pedicle is clipped and transected (right)

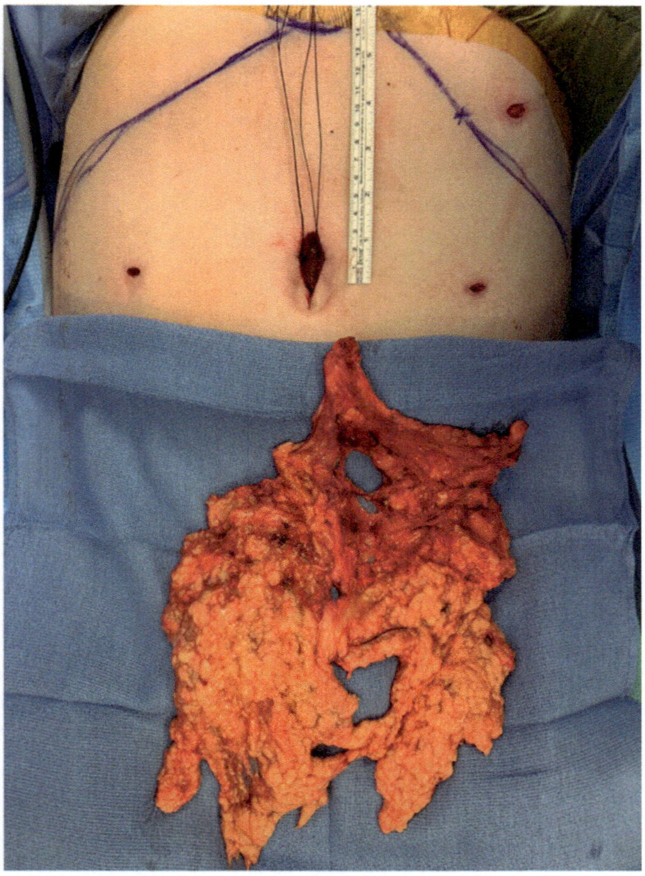

Fig. 18.6 The omental vascularized lymph node flap is then retrieved by extension of the midline incision to 3–5 cm with care taken not to injure the flap by shear

Future Directions

Although well established for the treatment of established lymphedema, the role of the omental VLN flap at the time of lymphadenectomy to reduce the risk of developing lymphedema is being investigated.

Pearls and Pitfalls

- Minimally invasive approaches have minimized the morbidity associated with the procedure; laparoscopic techniques should be considered for suitable patients in centers with this expertise.
- The omental vascularized lymphatic flap is an excellent option for orthotopic transfer to the axilla, reconstructing the three-dimensional deadspace following radical axillary scar release and correcting the contour deformity resulting from axillary lymphadenectomy; dual-level transfer should be considered where the entire extremity is affected.
- Performing dual venous outflow for the gastroepiploic vein to restore physiological drainage can reduce venous hypertension secondary to the avalvular system with bidirectional flow.

References

1. Goldsmith HS, De los Santos R, Beattie EJ Jr. Relief of chronic lymphedema by omental transposition. Ann Surg. 1967;166(4):573–85.
2. Goldsmith HS. Long term evaluation of omental transposition for chronic lymphedema. Ann Surg. 1974;180(6):847–9.
3. Nguyen AT, Suami H. Laparoscopic free omental lymphatic flap for the treatment of lymphedema. Plast Reconstr Surg. 2015;136(1):114–8.
4. Nguyen AT, Suami H, Hanasono MM, Womack VA, Wong FC, Chang EI. Long-term outcomes of the minimally invasive free vascularized omental lymphatic flap for the treatment of lymphedema. J Surg Oncol. 2017;115(1):84–9.
5. Morrison R. Functions of the omentum. BMJ. 1906;1:76–8.
6. Kinami S, Fujimura T, Ojima E, et al. PTD classification: proposal for a new classification of gastric cancer location based on physiological lymphatic flow. Int J Clin Oncol. 2008;13:320–9.
7. Liebermann-Meffert D. The greater omentum: anatomy, embryology, and surgical applications. Surg Clin North Am. 2000;80:275–293, xii.
8. Shimotsuma M, Shields JW, Simpson-Morgan MW, et al. Morpho-physiological function and role of omental milky spots as omentum-associated lymphoid tissue (OALT) in the peritoneal cavity. Lymphology. 1993;26:90–101.

9. Zhang QX, Magovern CJ, Mack CA, et al. Vascular endothelial growth factor is the major angiogenic factor in omentum: mechanism of the omentum-mediated angiogenesis. J Surg Res. 1997;67:147–54.
10. Ranvier I. Du développement et de l'accroissement des vaisseaux sanguins. Arch Physiol Norm Path. 1874;6:429–49.
11. Howell AC, Gould DJ, Mayfield C, Samakar K, Hassani C, Patel KM. Anatomical basis of the gastroepiploic vascularized lymph node transfer: a radiographic evaluation using computed tomographic angiography.
12. Borchard F, Betz P. Number and size of perigastric lymph nodes in human adults without gastric cancer. Surg Radiol Anat. 1991;13:117–21.
13. Agko M, Ciudad P, Chen HC. Histo-anatomical basis of the gastroepiploic vascularized lymph node flap: the overlooked "micro" lymph nodes. J Plast Reconstr Aesthet Surg. 2017;17:S1748–6815.
14. Ciudad P, Kiranantawat K, Sapountzis S, et al. Right gastroepiploic lymph node flap. Microsurgery. 2015;35:496–7.
15. Kenworthy EO, Nelson JA, Verma R, Mbabuike J, Mehrara BJ, Dayan JH. Double vascularized omentum lymphatic transplant (VOLT) for the treatment of lymphedema. J Surg Oncol. 2018;117(7):1413–9.
16. Dayan JH, Voineskos S, Verma R, Mehrara BJ. Managing venous hypertension in vascularized Omentum lymphatic transplant: restoring bidirectional venous drainage. Plast Reconstr Surg. 2018;141(2):326e–327e.

Step-by-Step Instruction: Jejunal Mesenteric Vascularized Lymph Node Transplant Procedure

19

Duane Wang and Roman Skoracki

Introduction

Intra-abdominal vascularized lymph node transfer (VLNT) has been utilized to try to avoid the risks of donor site lymphedema that are associated with other lymph node donor sites. The most common donor site is the omentum with documented favorable outcomes [1]. Unfortunately, the omentum itself has few actual lymph nodes, and these are mostly clustered along the greater curvature of the stomach. Rather, the majority of the omentum proper is composed of lymphoid lakes [2, 3]. The mesoappendix was also considered as a donor site due to its abundant lymphoid tissue; however, anatomical studies demonstrated a single lymph node in only 8% of patients, making it an inconsistent donor site for lymph nodes [4]. A third intra-abdominal site, rich in lymphatics and clusters of lymph nodes, is the mesentery, which sparked interest in it as a potential donor site for lymph node transfer.

The vascularized jejunal mesenteric lymph node flap has been described by Coriddi et al. and Schaverien et al. [5, 6]. Like the omental flap, the principal advantage of using the jejunal mesenteric lymph nodes is the avoidance of iatrogenic donor site lymphedema. The scar is typically small and well hidden, and multiple clusters of nodes can be harvested simultaneously if needed. The vascular anatomy is reliable and usually can be identified prior to flap elevation, allowing for examination of the entire mesentery to identify the optimal combination of the lymph node cluster and associated vascular pedicle before committing to flap harvest. The recipient site can be in the distal leg, groin, distal forearm, or axilla. The first reported case series of 15 patients demonstrated no donor site lymphedema, and 85.7% reported a subjective improvement with a follow-up range of 1–19 months [7]. A subsequent follow-up study of 29 patients demonstrated an acceptable complication profile, with only one flap loss (3.3%) [8].

Supplementary Information The online version of this chapter (https://doi.org/10.1007/978-3-030-93039-4_19) contains supplementary material, which is available to authorized users.

D. Wang
Division of Plastic and Reconstructive Surgery, Department of Surgery, University of Washington School of Medicine, Seattle, WA, USA
e-mail: Dwang6@uw.edu

R. Skoracki (✉)
Department of Plastic Surgery, Arthur G. James Cancer Hospital and Richard J. Solove Research Institute and Comprehensive Cancer Center, The Ohio State University Wexner Medical Center, Columbus, OH, USA
e-mail: Roman.skoracki@osumc.edu

Typical Indications

The vascularized jejunal mesenteric lymph node flap is indicated for heterotopic transplantation into distal extremities or the head and neck region for lymphedema, most commonly following lymphadenectomy and radiation therapy. It can be viewed as a complementary procedure to the omental transfer procedure, when an additional node-containing flap smaller in overall size and volume is preferred, such as for the distal extremity. The mesenteric lymph node packets are typically only 3–5 cm in length, making them less suited for the larger more proximal recipient sites such as the axilla and groin that require scar release – these benefit from larger flaps to place into the wound beds to avoid recurrence of the scaring; an omental flap is more suited for these locations. However, this flap can still be utilized in more proximal sites if an extensive scar release is not indicated and only a small flap is required.

A major advantage of mesenteric lymph node flap harvest is the ability to harvest multiple packets of nodes simultaneously from the same donor site to address multiple sites of lymphedema.

M. V. Schaverien, J. H. Dayan (eds.), *Multimodal Management of Upper and Lower Extremity Lymphedema*,
https://doi.org/10.1007/978-3-030-93039-4_19

Anatomy

The small intestine extends from the pylorus to the ileocecal valve. After the first 25 cm of duodenum, the remaining 3–7 m of intestine is divided into the jejunum and ileum. Because the duodenum is a retroperitoneal structure and the jejunum is intraperitoneal, the beginning of the jejunum is easily recognized at the ligament of Treitz. The jejunum and ileum are attached to the posterior abdominal wall by mesentery and arranged in a series of loops. The mesentery is fan shaped and consists of two layers of peritoneum containing the jejunum and ileum. The mesentery is attached superiorly to the posterior abdominal wall along an oblique line running from the left side of the body of the second lumbar vertebra to the right sacroiliac joint. This attachment line is called the mesenteric root. The blood supply to the jejunum arises from the superior mesenteric artery that comes directly out of the aorta 1 cm inferior to the celiac trunk. The blood supply to the jejunum is a highly organized branching network consisting of multiple tiered vascular loops called arcades.

The mesenteric lymph nodes lie within the folds of the mesentery itself. Based on cadaveric studies, the average total number of lymph nodes in the proximal segment is 19.2, in the middle segment 13.8, and in the distal segment 9.6. Blood flow to these lymph nodes is provided by adjacent vascular arcades. The majority of the lymph node clusters are located toward the root of the mesentery with fewer at the periphery of the mesentery near the jejunum. For the free jejunal mesenteric flap, the pedicle length is typically 3–5 cm with diameters of the artery and vein being 1–3 mm and 2–5 mm, respectively [7]. The significant variation in diameter reflects the considerable difference in the diameter of the vasculature at the root of the mesentery as opposed to that in the periphery (Fig. 19.1).

Patient Selection

Patient selection primarily focuses on prior medical and surgical (especially intra-abdominal) history. This minimizes the potential complications of viscera injury, hernia, and intestinal ileus/obstruction. A history of prior abdominal surgery with any adhesions increases the level of difficulty of the procedure and increases the risk of bowel injury. Relative contraindications include history of multiple previous open laparotomies, intra-abdominal radiation, disseminated intra-abdominal infections, and/or ventral hernia repair. Absolute contraindications include previous adhesive bowel obstruction, multiple previous hernia repairs with or without recurrence, and history of mesenteric ischemia [9]. Particular attention should be paid to foregut and colonic procedures that may disrupt the anatomy of the superior mesenteric axis.

Operative Technique

Principles

A two-team approach is preferable. At our center, this procedure is performed by a microsurgical team including a plas-

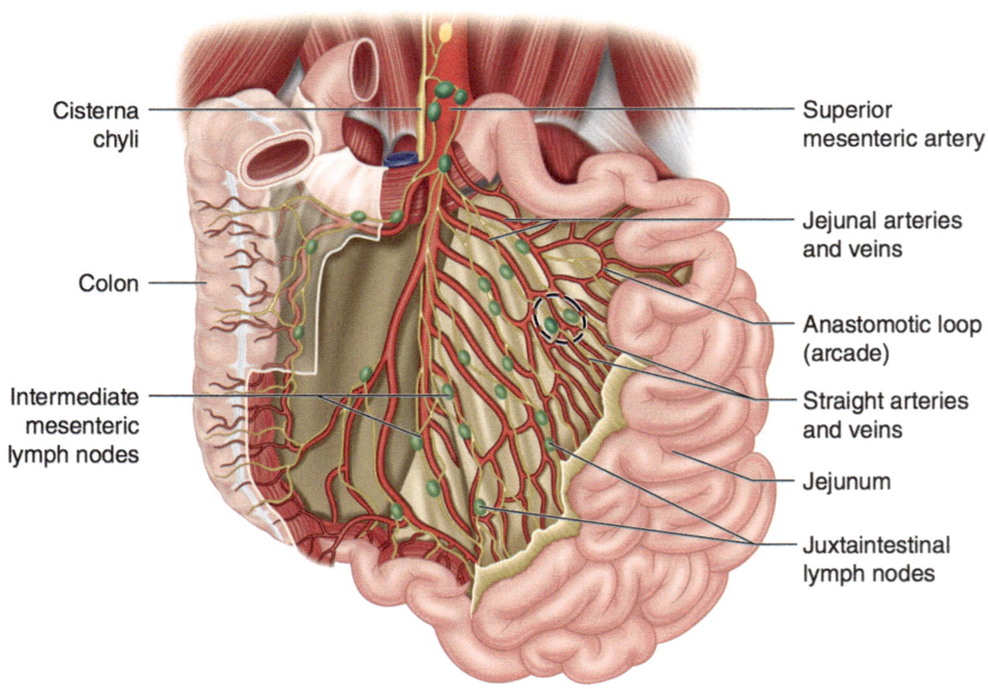

Fig. 19.1 Anatomy of the jejunal mesenteric vascularized lymph node flap. The mesenteric lymph nodes lie both next to the intestines and along the vascular arcades supplying the jejunum. There are arcades of primary, secondary, and third order. Typical mesenteric lymph node harvest will be at the periphery while being careful not to damage the jejunum. (Illustration provided courtesy of Springer)

tic surgeon and a general surgeon. The night prior to the procedure, we recommend that the patient ingest a milkshake or other fatty drink. This makes direct visualization of the individual lymphatic channels in the mesentery more straightforward and also allows for easier direct lymphatic coaptation at the recipient site if desired.

Harvest of the vascularized jejunal mesenteric lymph node flap is through a midline supraumbilical mini-laparotomy incision that is 3–7 cm in length, with the incision length correlating with the patient's body mass index (BMI). Lymph node clusters may be harvested from the root of the mesentery, taking care to avoid sacrifice of any major blood vessels to the bowel, ensuring redundancy of a vascular supply to any given jejunal segment before harvest. The vascular supply of the jejunum has enough redundancy with multiple anastomotic loops or arcades that the sacrifice of a single arcade is usually safe. A flow-through flap design is recommended to maintain optimal arterial inflow and venous outflow of the flap itself as the capillary network connecting the arterial and venous sides will be very limited at this level of the mesentery. A lymph node flap harvested from the periphery of the mesentery usually includes a greater capillary network, especially in relation to the source flap vessels, which are only about 1–1.5 mm for the arterial diameter and 2–2.5 mm for the venous diameter at this level. Therefore, a traditional end-to-side anastomotic technique of the flap to the extremity vessels is preferred. Greater caution must be exercised at the periphery of the mesentery to ensure preservation of adequate blood flow to the adjacent bowel as there is less redundancy at this level than at the root of the mesentery.

The process of lymph node selection is done with transillumination and palpation. For this reason, the bowel must be delivered extracorporally. While the flap harvest can be performed laparoscopically, the identification of the most optimal combination of nodes with their associated blood supply and avoidance of bowel ischemia requires transillumination and cannot be adequately accomplished laparoscopically, in our experience.

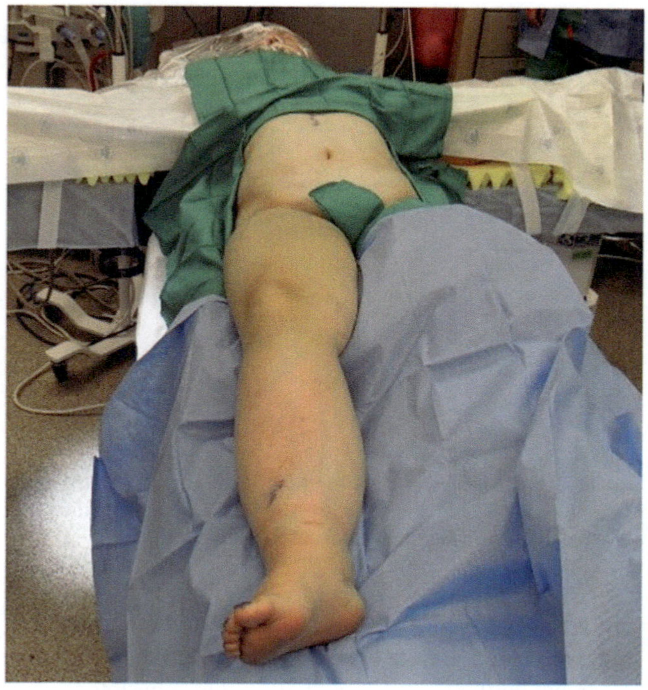

Fig. 19.2 Small midline laparotomy incision. The affected extremity is also prepped and draped

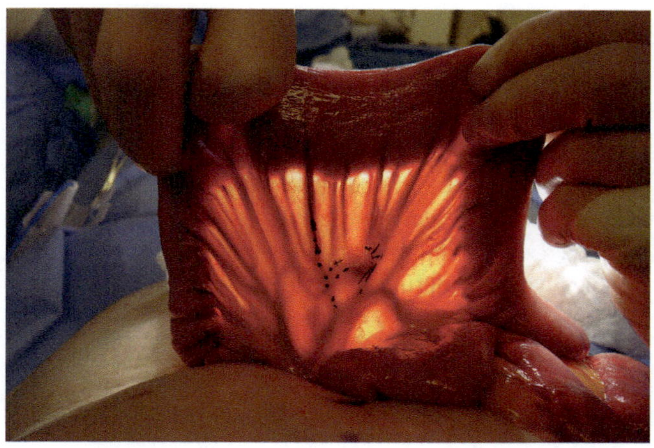

Fig. 19.3 Jejunum is delivered through the incision and transilluminated. Cluster of lymph nodes and vascular arcades are identified

Flap Harvest Technique (see supplementary material)

- The approach is via a mini-laparotomy incision around 3–5 cm in length (Fig. 19.2). An orogastric tube is placed to decompress the stomach. The desired section of jejunum, usually the first segment just beyond the ligament of Treitz as this contains the greatest number of nodes, is identified and then delivered from the abdomen extracorporally onto the surgical field (Fig. 19.3).
- Lymph nodes, flap donor vessels, and remaining blood supply to the jejunum are identified using transillumination and confirmed using palpation and inspection. The flap is raised en bloc with a cluster of lymph nodes and the mesenteric vascular pedicle.
- Once a favorable cluster of nodes with adequately sized vessels are identified, one side of the peritoneum is scored around the distal periphery of the flap.
- Distal vascular branches are ligated. An arcade immediately adjacent to the intestine is preserved to ensure vascularity of the jejunum. The bowel is preserved throughout.
- Harvest of the nodes at the periphery is preferred. When possible, we avoid lymph node clusters located at the root of the mesentery to avoid sacrifice of the major blood sup-

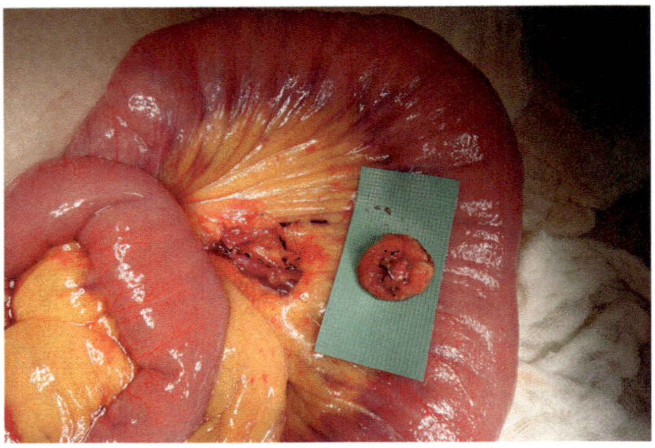

Fig. 19.4 Jejunal mesenteric lymph node flap dissected leaving the posterior leaflet of peritoneum intact. Lymph nodes are identified with a combination of transillumination and palpation

ply to the bowel. Flaps harvested from the periphery of the mesentery have a better balance of arterial inflow and venous outflow as they contain a more physiologic balance of capillary network to blood flow rate as a function of donor vessel diameter when compared with flaps raised closer to the root where the vascular supply largely bypasses the nodes. That is why we recommend designing flaps from the root of the mesentery as flow-through flaps with two arterial and venous anastomoses each (at the distal and proximal end of the flap) at the recipient site.

- The flap is then elevated from the periphery toward the root of the mesentery, preserving the posterior peritoneal layer. Leaving this peritoneum intact or repairing any holes created during dissection prevents an internal hernia.
- Dissection continues until vessel caliber is adequate for microvascular anastomosis and pedicle length is as desired while preserving all major vessels to the jejunum. Pedicle length is generally 3–5 cm. The average size of the flap is also around 3–5 cm (Fig. 19.4).
- After flap elevation, the anterior layer of peritoneum is repaired with a running silk suture as an additional precaution against an internal hernia. The abdominal incisions are then closed in a standard fashion.

Recipient Site Preparation, Flap Revascularization, and Inset

The recipient site is chosen according to the location of the lymphedema and previous treatment history. It includes scar removal when applicable from previous lymph node dissection. Our preference is to perform a proximal scar release and flap placement in cases of Grade 3 (Ohio Scar Scale; Table 19.1), or greater, scarring and the indications are as outlined below for the upper and the lower extremity [10]. For the upper extremity, the wrist/forearm is chosen if the lymphedema is more severe in the hand and forearm than the upper arm. The axilla is chosen if the complete upper extremity is involved or excess scarring is present in the axilla. The distal leg is chosen if the patient has had a previous peri-aortic or deep pelvic lymph node dissection and inguinal nodes are intact. The groin is chosen if there has been a previous inguinal lymph node dissection and the patient has significant thigh swelling. However, if these proximal sites have a large area of scarring and require more bulk of vascularized tissue, the omental flap may be a better option. In these cases, we will consider a dual-level node transfer with an omental flap placed proximally and a mesenteric flap distally.

Table 19.1 Ohio Scar Scale – examination and quantification of lymph node resection scar

Grade	Description
0	No scar, no surgical intervention to area
1	Superficial scar, mobile (no tethering, adequate subcutaneous fat layer)
2	Scar extending into subdermal structures, deep palpable scar, remains mobile against deeper structures (i.e., chest wall, groin, fascia/musculature)
3	Visible tethering of skin, scar tethering skin to underlying deeper structure (i.e., chest wall, deep fascia of the groin), scar is usually depressed/dimpling
4	Painful tethered scar

Typically, a recipient artery and one vein are prepared for anastomosis. In the forearm, either the radial or ulnar artery is used, and in the lower leg, the anterior or posterior tibial artery is typically preferred. Preoperative vascular imaging of the lower extremity can be helpful in patients with primary lymphedema where there may be anatomic variabilities in the presence and caliber of the vasculature. If a partial venous outflow obstruction is suspected due to the prior proximal node dissection, a venogram should be performed preoperatively as venous hypertension will place the flap at risk.

Following harvest, the flap is then reperfused at the recipient site (Fig. 19.5). The mesenteric vessels closer to the root can be larger. If the flap was taken at this level, there can be a mismatch between the arterial inflow and the outflow possible based on the capillary bed alone. For this reason, we will inset the flap vessels as a flow-through flap with anastomoses at the distal and proximal ends of the flap artery and vein either in an end-to-side or end-to-end fashion, or if this is not an option, we will perform a direct end-to-end anastomosis between distal flap artery and vein to create an arteriovenous (AV) loop and alleviate this problem (Fig. 19.5).

Primary skin closure can be achieved if some of the subcutaneous tissue at the recipient site is removed with electro-

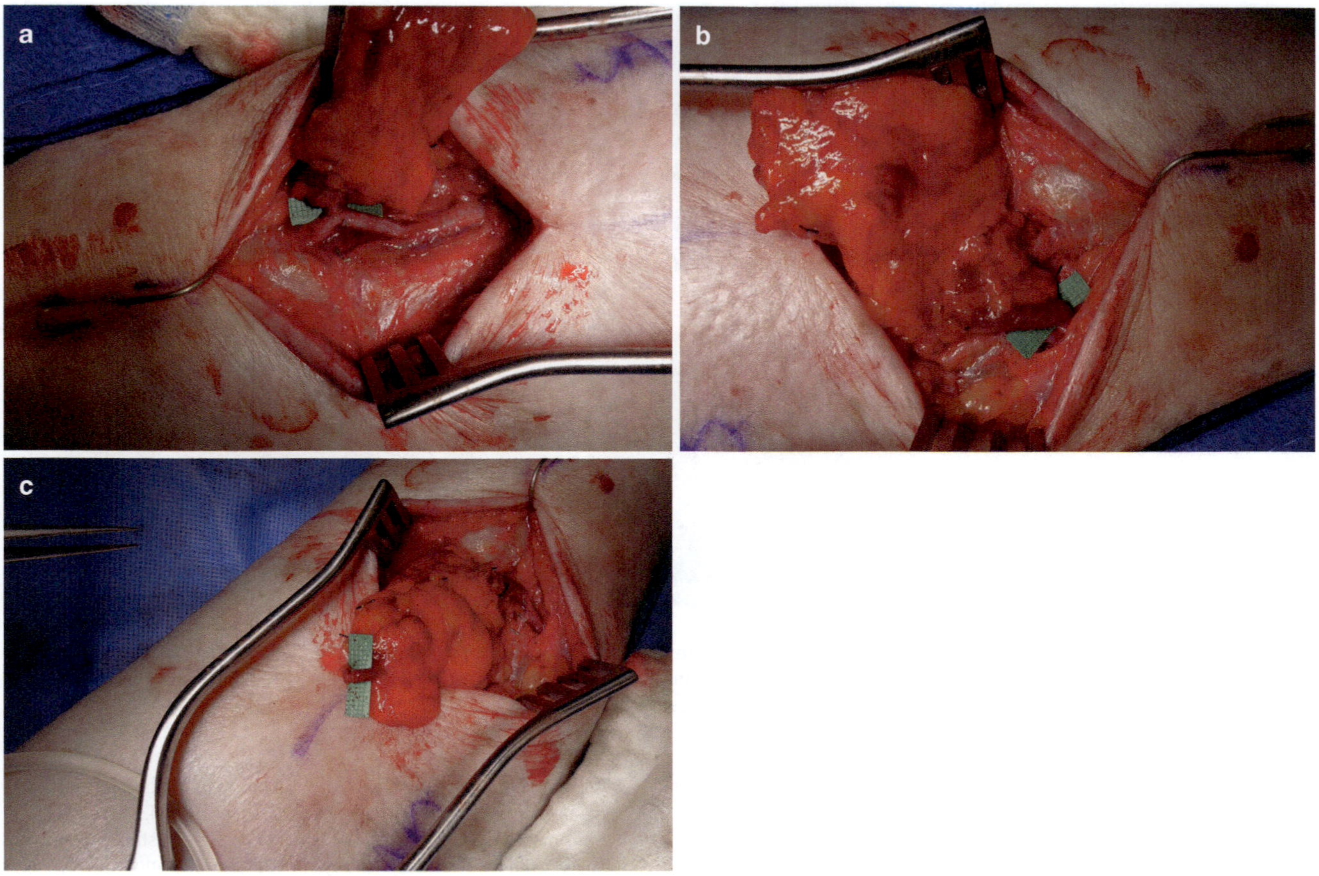

Fig. 19.5 Jejunal mesenteric artery and vein anastomosed to the recipient vessels: (**a**) arterial anastomosis; (**b**) venous anastomosis; (**c**) here, an arteriovenous (AV) loop has also been performed at the distal flap end to optimize the balance between arterial inflow and venous outflow for the larger donor vessels included in this flap harvested from the root of the mesentery

cautery. In cases when this would place too much pressure on the flap, a small full-thickness skin graft harvested adjacent to the laparotomy incision can be placed over the mesenteric lymph node packet (Fig. 19.6). This can be excised at a later date if it is cosmetically displeasing to the patient. Flap monitoring can be performed percutaneously with a handheld Doppler over the skin graft or the primarily closed dermis. We have also successfully used an implantable Doppler with the piezoelectric crystal removed from the silastic cuff and inserted directly into the fat of the flap adjacent to the vasculature.

Postoperative Care

Patients are typically admitted to the hospital to the free flap floor with the flap monitored with standard Doppler checks. The orogastric tube is removed during extubation. Diet is advanced from clears as tolerated. Occasionally, Reglan may be prescribed to help bowel motility. We use this commonly for omental flap harvests to encourage gastric emptying after manipulation of the greater curvature of the stomach intraoperatively. Antibiotics are prescribed for 1 week postoperatively, as patients with lymphedema are at increased risk of infection to the affected limb.

There are also site-specific considerations. For flaps to the axilla, the arm should be abducted with an abduction pillow for 1 week postoperatively to avoid flap compression, followed by gradual return to full shoulder range of motion. The forearm/wrist requires extremity elevation. For the groin, the patient is instructed to avoid hip flexion beyond 45 degrees for 3–4 weeks postoperatively. Distally placed flaps in the lower extremity undergo a strict dangle protocol. Patients resume their compression garments 6–8 weeks postoperatively. The patients will see maximal benefit at 1–2 years postoperatively and will be followed in clinic for physical therapy and measurements for the rest of their lives.

Complications

A study of 29 patients demonstrated an acceptable complication profile of one flap loss (3.3%), four postoperative hernias (13.8%), and three nonoperative small bowel

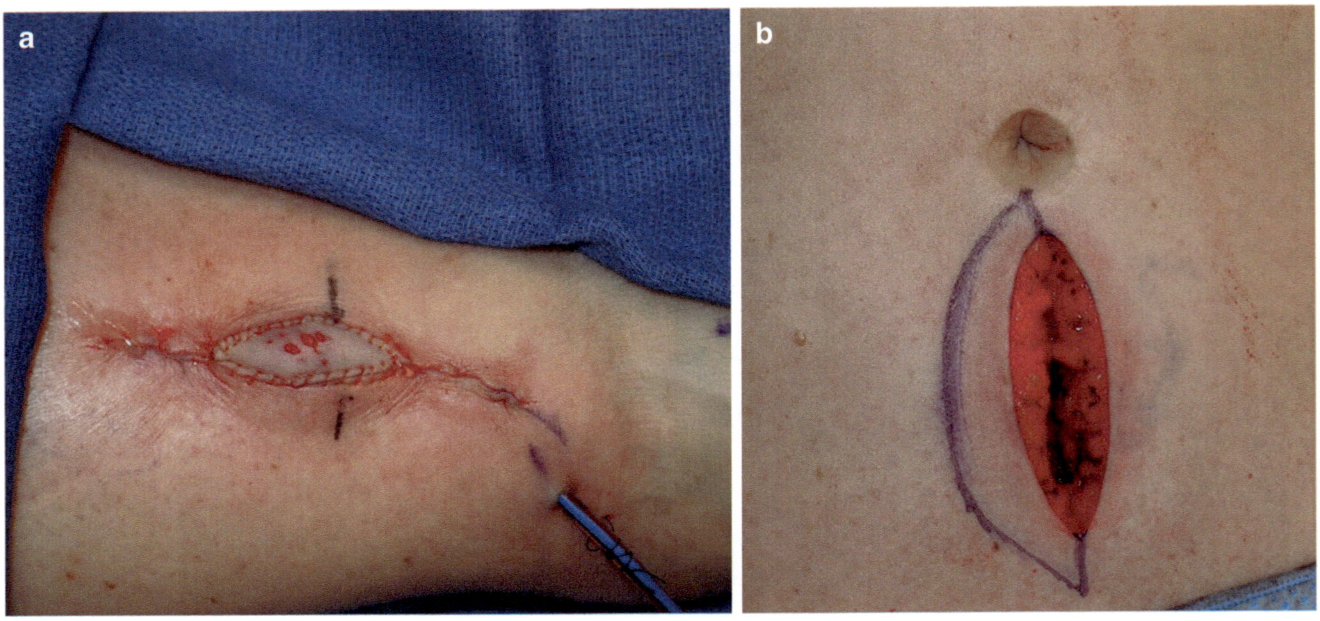

Fig. 19.6 (a) Inset of the flap in the distal extremity. Subcutaneous tissue can be excised to accommodate the flap, or alternatively a skin graft can be placed over the flap and later excised. Monitoring can be performed either by an implantable Doppler or through percutaneous Doppler checks. (b) Skin graft is harvested adjacent to the laparotomy site to avoid an additional scar

obstructions (10.3%) [8]. Patients should also be counseled about the inherent risks of this approach including incisional hernias, peritonitis, bowel ischemia, adhesions, and injury to other abdominal organs.

Pearls and Pitfalls

- The mesenteric lymph node donor site allows for the harvest of multiple packets of lymph nodes from the mesentery and/or the omentum to address multiple recipient sites if necessary. The donor site can also be used again at a later time from the original transfer surgery.
- The mesenteric lymph node flap is a good option for heterotopic transfer to the distal extremity due to its small size and high lymph node density.
- Consider performing a flow-through flap inset or distal AV loop when the flap is taken more toward the root of the mesentery to optimize inflow and outflow balance for a flap with large (3 mm artery and ≥4 mm vein) donor vessels and a relatively small capillary network connecting these.
- For flaps harvested from the mesenteric periphery, ensure preservation of blood flow to the adjacent small bowel by careful flap location choice and design.

References

1. Nguyen AT, Suami H, Hanasono MM, Womack VA, Wong FC, Chang EI. Long-term outcomes of the minimally invasive free vascularized omental lymphatic flap for the treatment of lymphedema. J Surg Oncol. 2017;115:84–9.
2. Liebermann DM, Kaufmann M. Utilization of the greater omentum in surgery: a historical review. Neth J Surg. 1991;43:136–44.
3. Shimotsuma M, Simpson-Morgan MW, Takahashi T, Hagiwara A. Activation of omental milky spots and milky spot macrophages by intraperitoneal administration of a streptococcal preparation, OK-432. Cancer Res. 1992;52:5400–2.
4. Ruter D, Chen W, Garza R 3rd, Eiferman D, Skoracki R. Mesoappendix as potential donor site for vascularized lymph node transfer: anatomic study. J Surg Res. 2018;230:143–7.
5. Coriddi M, Wee C, Meyerson J, Eiferman D, Skoracki R. Vascularized jejunal mesenteric lymph node transfer: a novel surgical treatment for extremity lymphedema. J Am Coll Surg. 2017;225:650–7.
6. Schaverien MV, Hofstetter WL, Selber JC. Vascularized jejunal mesenteric lymph node transfer for lymphedema: a novel approach. Plast Reconstr Surg. 2018;141:468e–9e.
7. Coriddi M, Skoracki R, Eiferman D. Vascularized jejunal mesenteric lymph node transfer for treatment of extremity lymphedema. Microsurgery. 2017;37:177–8.
8. Kraft CT, Eiferman D, Jordan S, Skoracki RJ. Complications after vascularized jejunal mesenteric lymph node transfer: a 3-year experience. Microsurgery. 2019;39:497–501.
9. Chu CK, Schaverien MV, Chang EI, Hanson SE, Hanasono MM, Selber JC. Intra-abdominal lymph nodes: a privileged donor site for vascularized lymph node transfer. Plast Reconstr Surg Glob Open. 2020;8:e2673.
10. Coriddi MR, Eiferman DS, Skoracki RJ. Double-level vascularized lymph node transfer for treatment of extremity lymphedema. J Reconstr Microsurg Open. 2017;2:75–7.

Step-by-Step Instruction: Suction-Assisted Lipectomy Procedure with Controlled Compression Therapy

20

Håkan Brorson

Introduction

Our first liposuction procedure for lymphedema was undertaken in 1987, but it was not until 1993 that a more detailed treatment protocol was established for arm lymphedema [1, 2]. Liposuction for leg lymphedema was established 5 years later. Initially, the "dry" technique was used; the introduction of the use of a tourniquet and tumescence has made liposuction a safe procedure, and there is no longer any need for blood transfusions [3]. Liposuction is the only method to completely reduce chronic non-pitting lymphedema. The result is maintained with compression garments.

Typical Indications

- Primary and secondary upper and lower extremity lymphedema with a limb excess volume of 10% or greater
- Minimal pitting: 4–5 mm in arms and 5–6 mm in legs
- No active cancer
- No further improvement with conservative treatment
- No active wounds
- No age limit

Supplementary Information The online version of this chapter (https://doi.org/10.1007/978-3-030-93039-4_20) contains supplementary material, which is available to authorized users.

H. Brorson (✉)
Lymphedema Center, Plastic and Reconstructive Surgery, Skåne University Hospital, Malmö, Sweden

Department of Clinical Sciences, Malmö, Lund University, Lund, Sweden
e-mail: hakan.brorson@med.lu.se

Excess Subcutaneous Adiposity and Chronic Lymphedema

Liposuction in the only method to completely reduce non-pitting chronic lymphedema where the excess volume is dominated by adipose tissue [4–6]. The incidence of post-mastectomy arm lymphedema varies between 13% and 52%, depending in part on whether axillary lymph nodes have been removed and postoperative radiation has been given [7, 8]. The sentinel node technique had decreased the incidence of postoperative lymphedema to an estimated incidence of approximately 6–8% [9]. Risk-reducing surgery using immediate lymphatic reconstruction shows an incidence of lymphedema of 9.1% at short-term follow-up [10].

The outcome of the surgical procedure as well as the radiation to the tissues often results in destruction of lymphatic vessels. When this is combined with the removal of lymph nodes and tissue scarring, the lymphatic vessels that remain are likely to be unable to remove the lymph fluid load. The remaining lymph collectors become dilated and overloaded, and their valves become incompetent, preventing the lymphatics from performing their function. This failure spreads distally until even the most peripheral lymph vessels, draining into the affected system, also become dilated [11]. In a parallel process, the cells of the mononuclear phagocytic system of the mesenchymal tissues begin to lose their capability to remove the protein that accumulates. The accumulated interstitial proteins, as osmotically active molecules, attract fluid to the area. This accumulation of protein and fluid is usually a transient phase, lasting between 1 and 3 weeks [11].

In the latent phase, there may still initially be no clinical signs of any discernible lymphedema. The latent phase normally varies from about 4 months to 10 years. At the end of the latent phase, pitting of the edematous limb on pressure can be observed. This can be objectively measured by plethysmography and by decreased tissue compressibility using a tissue tonometer [11, 12].

M. V. Schaverien, J. H. Dayan (eds.), *Multimodal Management of Upper and Lower Extremity Lymphedema*,
https://doi.org/10.1007/978-3-030-93039-4_20

The enlargement of the extremity leads to discomfort and complaints in the form of heaviness, weakness, pain, tension, and sensory deficit of the limb, as well as anxiety, psychological morbidity, maladjustment and social isolation, and increasing hardness of the limb [13, 14]. Adipose tissue deposition already starts within the first year after lymphedema onset [15–18]. In time, there is also an increase in the adipose tissue content of the swollen limb. The author has observed this clinically since 1987, when the first lymphedema patient was operated on [1, 2]. This phenomenon led to further research, as presented in this chapter [15–19].

There are various possible explanations for the adipose tissue hypertrophy. There is a physiological imbalance of blood flow and lymphatic drainage, resulting in the impaired clearance of lipids and their uptake by macrophages [20, 21]. There is increasing support, however, for the view that the fat cell is not simply a container of fat, but it behaves like an endocrine organ and a cytokine-activated cell [22, 23], and chronic inflammation plays a role here [24, 25]. The same pathophysiology goes for primary and secondary lymphedema. For more detailed information about investigational advances and the relationship between slow lymph flow and adiposity, as well as that between structural changes in the lymphatic system and adiposity, see data from studies published by Harvey et al. [26] and Schneider et al. [27], as well as other studies with contributory evidence [6, 12, 15, 16, 24, 28–33].

A common misunderstanding among clinicians is that the swelling of a lymphedematous extremity, whether it is primary or secondary, is due purely to the accumulation of lymph and/or fibrosis. In one study, preoperative investigation with volume-rendered computed tomography (CT) images showed a significant preoperative increase of adipose tissue in the swollen arm, the excess volume consisting of 81% (range, 68–96%) fat [15]. In another study, analyses with dual x-ray absorptiometry (DXA) that were compared to plethysmography in 18 women with arm lymphedema following mastectomy showed a significant increase of adipose tissue, 73% (range, 43–111%), in the non-pitting swollen arm before surgery [16]. Consecutive analyses of the content of the aspirate removed under bloodless conditions using a tourniquet showed a very high content of adipose tissue in 105 women with postmastectomy arm lymphedema (mean, 94%; range, 58–100%) [6]. Lymph can be removed by the use of noninvasive conservative regimens such as complex decongestive therapy (CDT) and controlled compression therapy (CCT). These therapies work well when the excess swelling consists of accumulated lymph but do not work when the excess volume is dominated by adipose tissue [1, 2, 15–19, 34]. The same may go for microsurgical procedures using lymphovenous shunts [35, 36], lymph vessel transplantation [37, 38], and vascularized lymph node transfer [39].

How to Assess the Efficacy of Liposuction

Today, chronic non-pitting arm lymphedema of more than 4 L in excess can be effectively removed by the use of liposuction without any further reduction in lymph transport. Long-term results have not shown any recurrence of the arm swelling (Figs. 20.1 and 20.2) [1, 2, 5, 6]. Promising results can also be achieved for primary and secondary leg lymphedema, where over 6 L in excess volume can be completely reduced (Figs. 20.3, 20.4, and 20.5) [4, 40].

Preoperative Planning for Arm Liposuction

Made-to-measure compression garments (three sleeves and two gloves) are ordered 2 weeks before surgery. One garment, to be put on the arm at the time of surgery, is sterilized and used for only 2 days since it loses some of its pressure

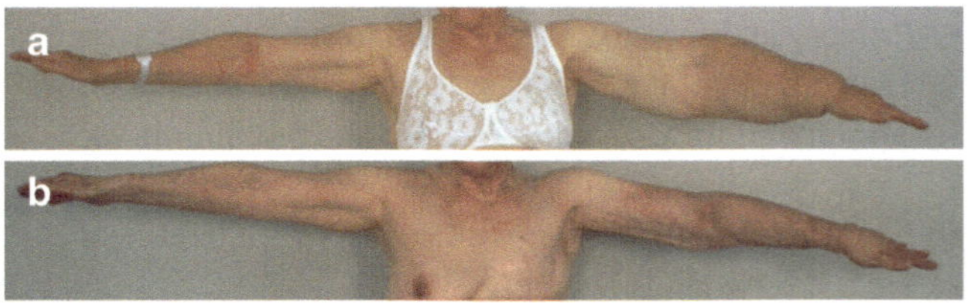

Fig. 20.1 (**a**) A 74-year-old woman with non-pitting arm lymphedema for 15 years. Preoperative excess volume was 3090 mL. (**b**) Postoperative result

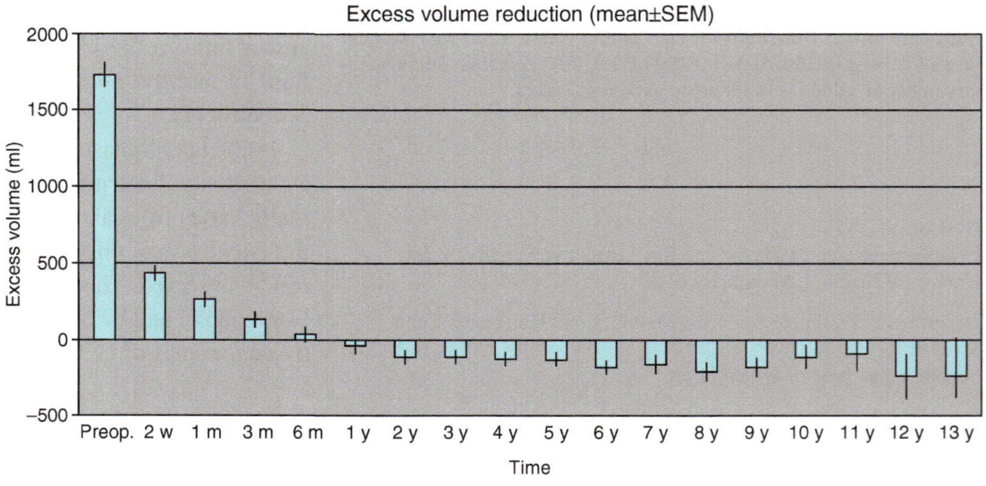

Fig. 20.2 Mean postoperative excess volume reduction in 95 women with arm lymphedema following breast cancer [52]

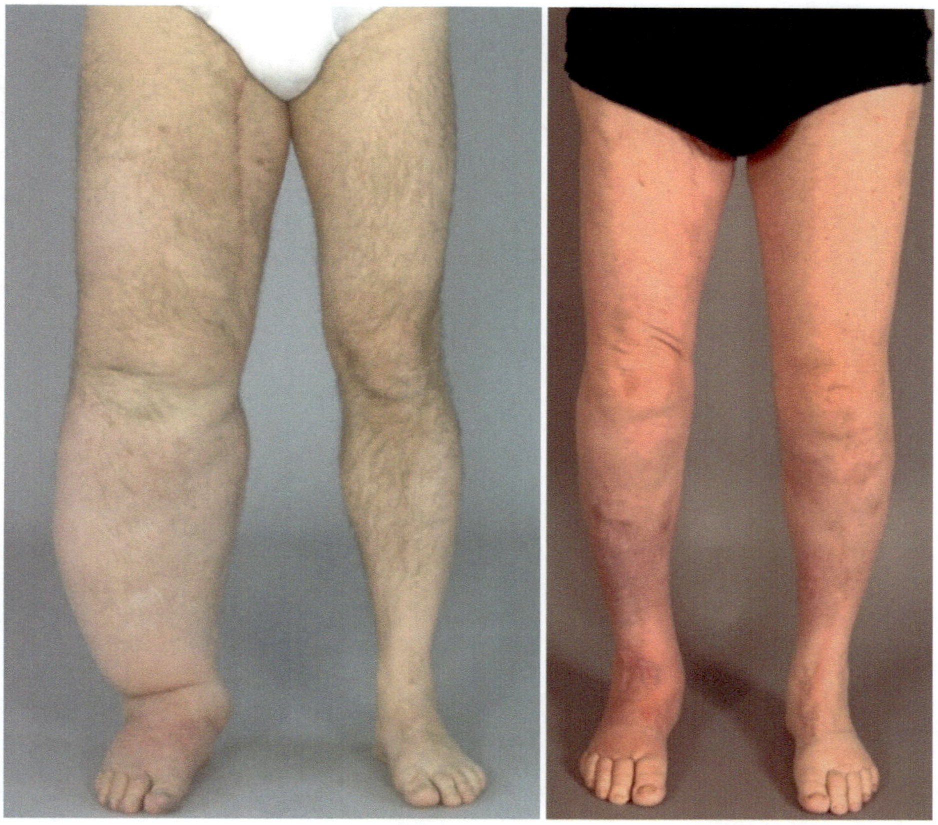

Fig. 20.3 Preoperative excess volume 5380 mL (left). Postoperative result after 3 years where excess volume is -255 mL, i.e., the treated leg is somewhat smaller than the normal one (right)

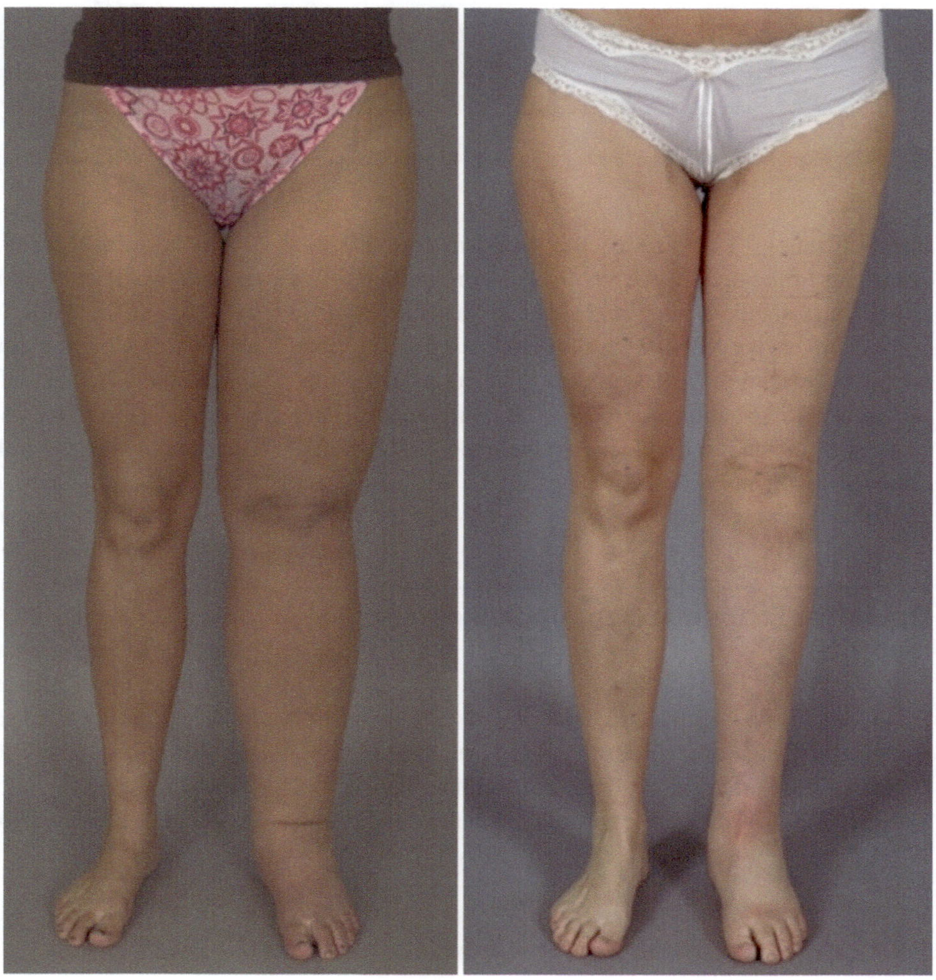

Fig. 20.4 Preoperative excess volume 6630 mL (left). Postoperative result after 2 years with complete reduction (right)

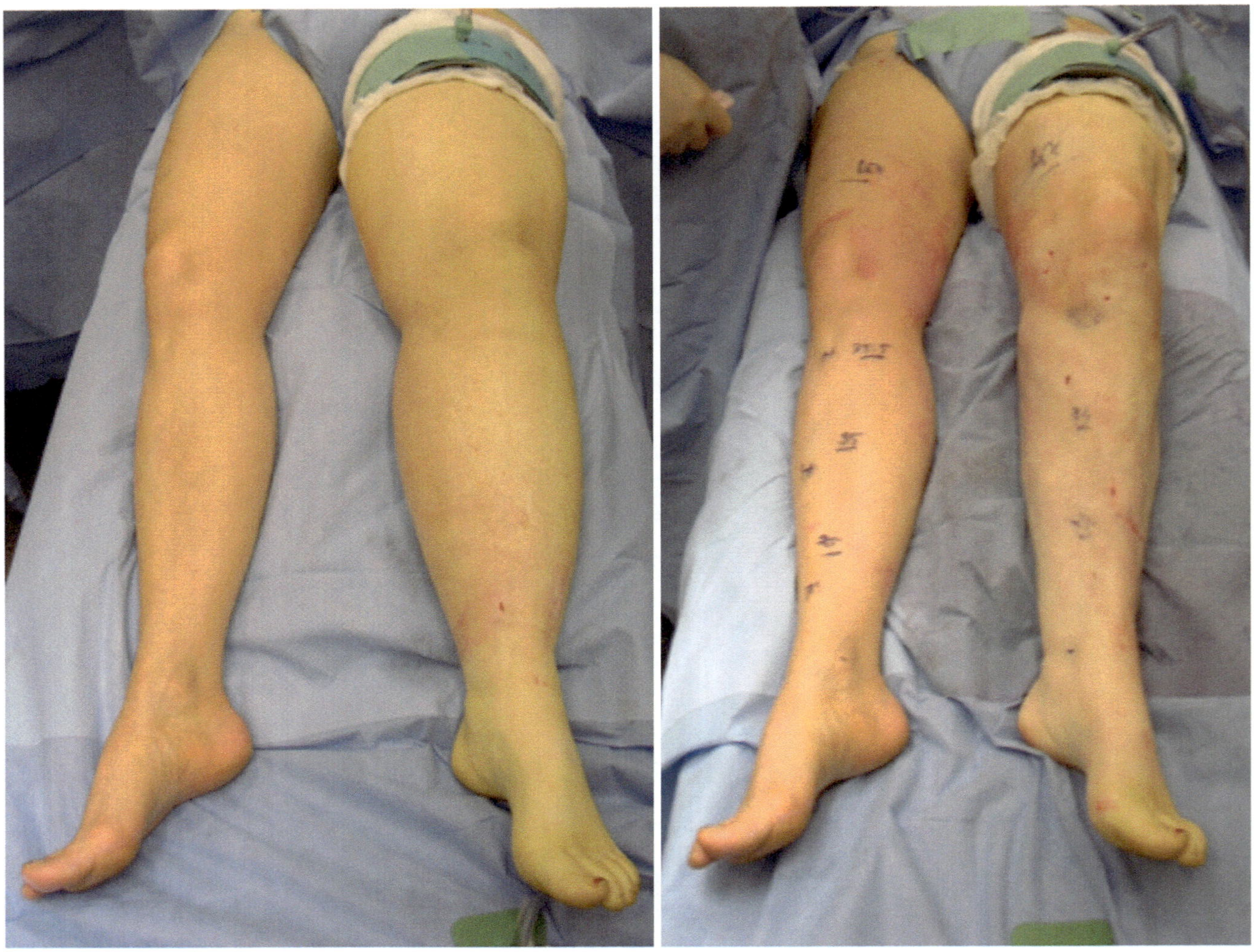

Fig. 20.5 Primary lymphedema, excess volume 4940 mL before liposuction (left). After liposuction up to the tourniquet (right)

by sterilization. The size of the garments is measured according to the size of the unaffected arm and hand. We always have standard interim gloves and gauntlets (a glove without fingers but with a thumb) in stock, used as described later. One interim glove is sterilized to be put on at the time of surgery. Liposuction is executed circumferentially, step by step, from hand to shoulder, and the hypertrophied fat is removed as much as possible (Figs. 20.6, 20.7, 20.8, and 20.9).

Operative Technique (see supplementary material)

For the majority of patients, power-assisted liposuction (Lipomatic, Nutational Infrasonic Liposculpture, Euromi, Andrimont, Belgium) is performed to facilitate liposuction. Around ten 3- to 4-mm-long incisions are made, and liposuction is performed using 15- and 25-cm-long cannulas with diameters of 3 and 4 mm. Initially, the hand was also treated, but since no fat could be aspirated, we ceased to treat this area. Circumferential liposuction is performed from wrist to shoulder and as much of the hypertrophied fat is removed as possible using previously measured circumferences of the healthy arm as a control (Figs. 20.6, 20.7, and 20.8). When the arm distal to the tourniquet has been treated, a sterilized custom-made compression sleeve is applied (Jobst Elvarex, compression class 2) to the arm to minimize bleeding and reduce postoperative edema. A sterilized, standard interim glove (Cicatrex interim, Thuasne Begat, France) is put on the hand. The tourniquet is then removed, and the most proximal part of the upper arm is treated using the tumescent technique, where 1000 ml saline is mixed with 1 mg adrenaline and 40 ml lidocaine 2% [1–3, 5, 6]. The technique for legs (Figs. 20.3, 20.4, and 20.5) is similar to that for arms (Figs. 20.6, 20.7, and 20.8).

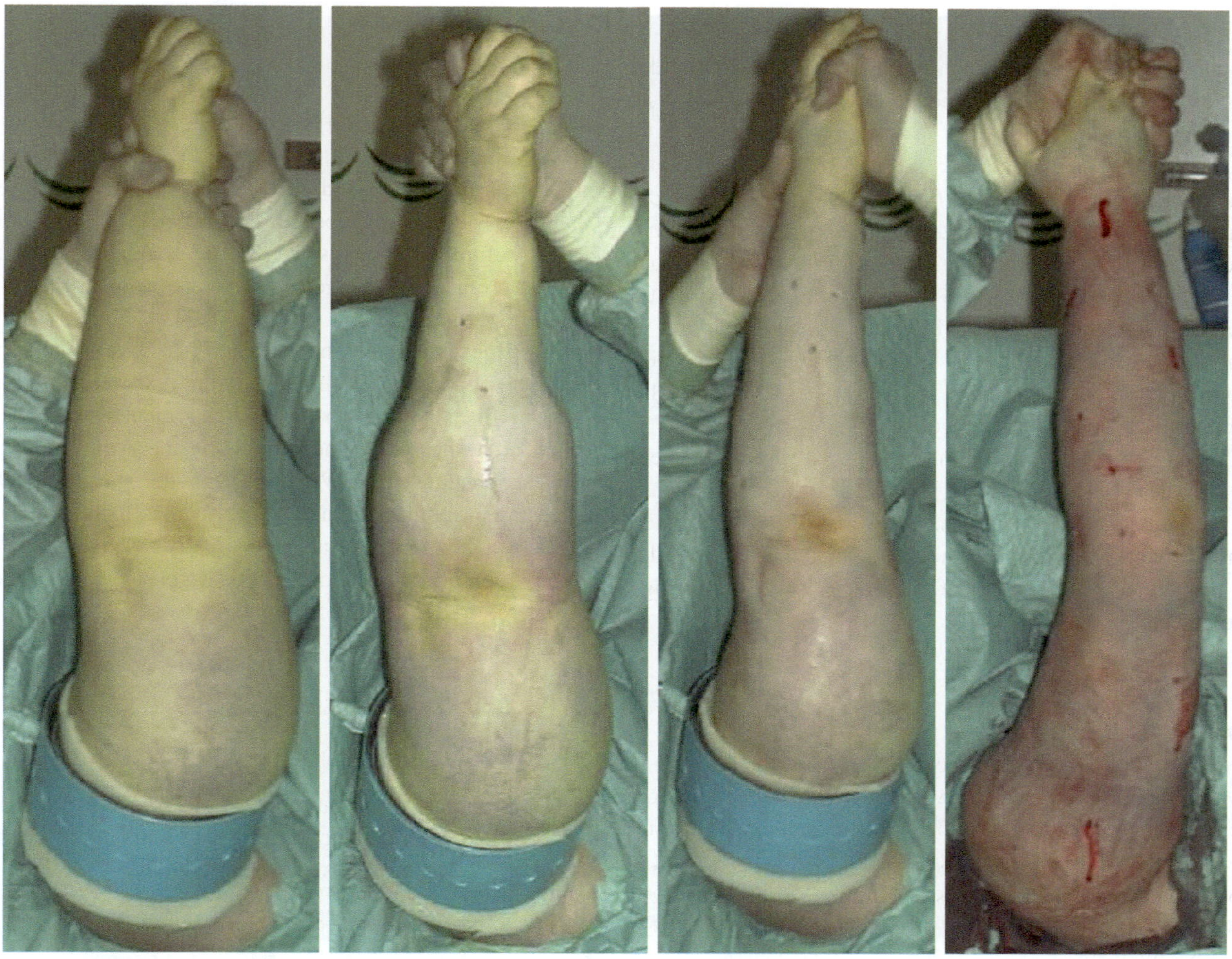

Fig. 20.6 Liposuction of arm lymphedema. The procedure takes about 2 hours. From preoperative to postoperative state (left to right). Note the tourniquet, which has been removed on the right, and the concomitant reactive hyperemia

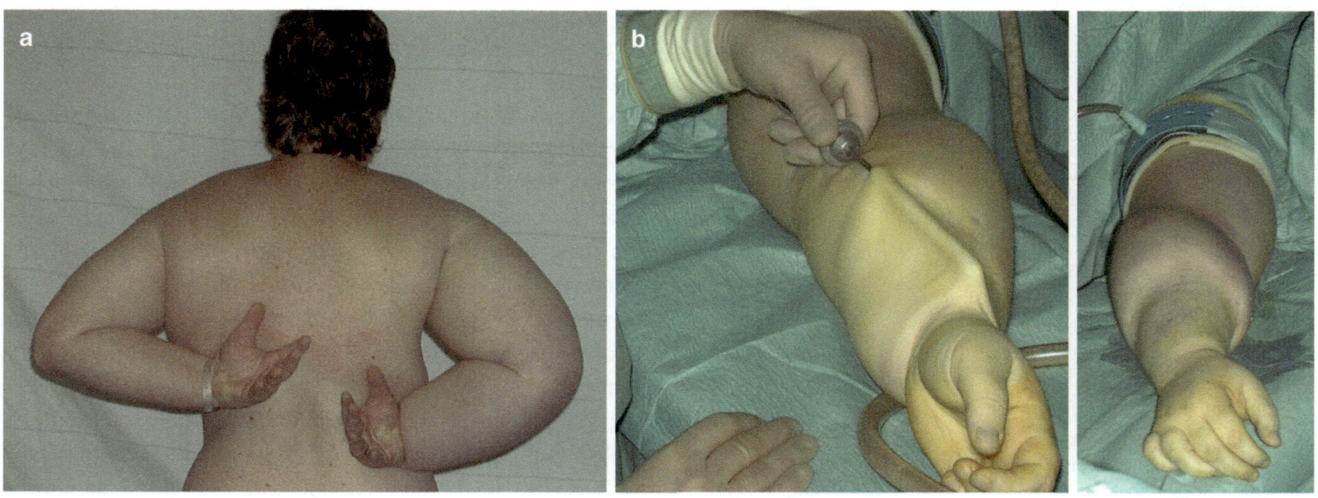

Fig. 20.7 (**a**) Preoperative picture showing a patient with a large right lymphedematous arm (2865 mL excess volume) with decreased mobility; (**b**) the cannula lifts the loose skin of the treated forearm (left); the distal half of the forearm has been treated – note the sharp border between treated (distal forearm) and untreated (proximal arm) areas (right)

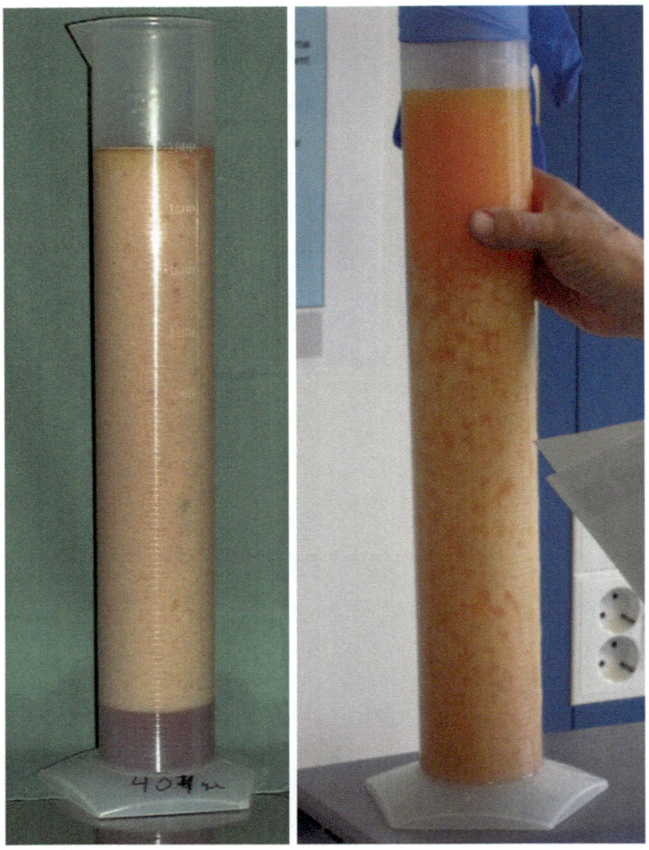

Fig. 20.8 The aspirate contains 90–100% adipose tissue in general. This picture shows typical aspirates collected from a lymphedematous arm before removal of the tourniquet. The aspirate to the left sediments into an upper adipose fraction (90%) and a lower fluid (lymph) fraction (10%). To the right, no fluid fraction is seen

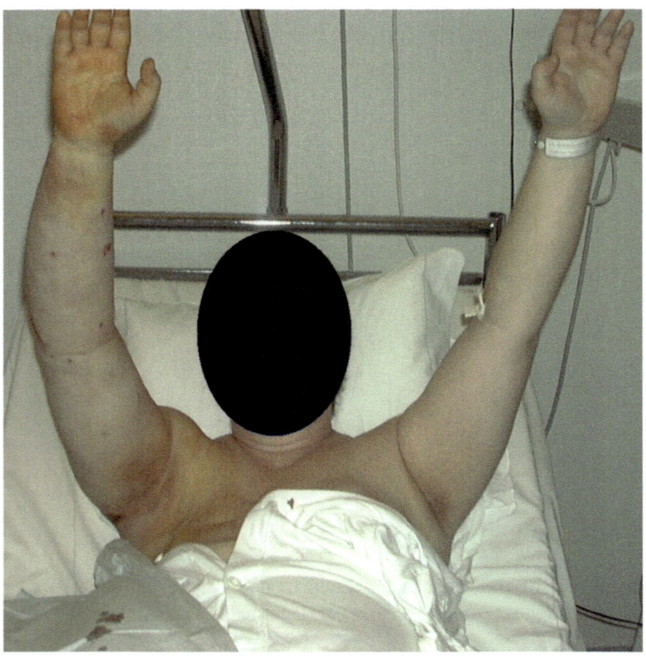

Fig. 20.9 The compression garment is removed 2 days after surgery to take measurements for a custom-made compression garment. A significant reduction of the right arm has been achieved, as compared with the preoperative condition seen in Fig. 20.7a

Postoperative Care

Two days postoperatively, the garments are removed by the patient under supervision so that the patient can take a shower. The arm is lubricated with lotion. Then, the other set of garments are put on, and the used set is washed and dried. Change of garments is repeated by the patient after another 2 days before hospital discharge. The standard glove and gauntlet are usually changed to the made-to-measure glove at the end of the stay.

The patient alternates between the two sets of garments (two sleeves and two gloves) during the first week at home, changing them every other day so that a clean set is always put on after showering and lubricating the arm. Then garments are changed daily. Washing "activates" the garment by increasing the compression due to shrinkage. It also removes products of perspiration that can cause dry and irritated skin. During the subsequent course, this rigorous compression regime, referred to as CCT, is maintained exactly as described in the next section.

Complications

So far, no major complications have occurred. Skin numbness is normal after liposuction and disappears after a couple of weeks. No skin necrosis has occurred.

Controlled Compression Therapy (CCT)

A prerequisite to maintaining the effect of liposuction, and, for that matter, conservative treatment, is the lifelong, continuous (24 h/day) use of a compression garment [1, 2, 5, 6]. If the patient has any doubts about continued CCT, the patient is not accepted for treatment.

After initiating compression therapy, the custom-made garment may be taken in at each visit using a sewing machine to compensate for reduced elasticity and reduced arm volume. This is most important during the first 3 months when the most notable changes in volume occur. At the 1- and 3-month visits, the arm is measured for new custom-made garments. This procedure is repeated at 6, 9, and 12 months. If complete reduction has been achieved at 6 months, the 9-month control may be omitted. If this is the case, it is important to remember to prescribe garments for 6 months.

When the excess volume has decreased as much as possible and a steady state is achieved, new garments can be prescribed using the latest measurements. In this way, the garments (two sets of sleeve and glove garments) are renewed three or four times during the first year. The patient is informed about the importance of hygiene (daily shower with soap and water) and skin care (moisturizing the skin with lotion), as all patients with lymphedema are susceptible to infections [1, 2, 5, 6].

The lifespan of two garments worn alternately is usually 3–6 months. After complete reduction has been achieved, the patient is seen once a year when new garments are prescribed for the coming year, usually four garments and four gloves (or four gauntlets). In active patients, six to eight garments and the same amount of gauntlets/gloves a year are needed.

For legs, it is often necessary to use up to two to three compression garments on top of each other, depending on what is needed to keep pitting away. The larger the diameter of the leg, the more compression is needed according to the law of Laplace. A typical example is Elvarex compression class 3, Elvarex compression class 2, and, when needed, Jobst Bellavar compression class 2. The Elvarex class 2 garment can be a leg-length or a below-the-knee garment. During night only one layer is used. Thus, such a patient needs two sets of two to three garments. It is important to take loose measurements at the ankle since the diameter here is small, giving more compression than needed. An alternative is to order a leg-length garment without the foot part of one of the garments. The follow-up regimen is the same as for arms. CCT can also be used primarily to effectively treat pitting edema as an alternative to CDT, which, in contrast to CCT, comprises daily interventions [1, 2].

Volume Measurements

Volumes are recorded for each patient using the water displacement technique. The displaced water is weighed on a balance to the nearest 5 g, corresponding to 5 mL. Both extremities are always measured at each visit, and the difference in volumes is designated as the edema volume, or more correctly the excess volume. The decrease in the excess volume is calculated in a percentage of the preoperative value [1, 2, 5, 6].

Lymphedema Team

To investigate and treat patients with lymphedema, a team comprising a plastic surgeon, an occupational therapist, and a physiotherapist is needed. An hour is reserved for each scheduled visit to the team when limb volumes are measured, garments are adjusted or renewed, social circumstances are assessed, and other matters of concern are discussed. The patient is also encouraged to contact the team whenever any unexpected problems arise so that these can be tackled without delay. The team also monitors the long-term outcome, and a visit once a year is necessary, in most cases, to maintain a good functional and cosmetic result after complete reduction.

This regimen omits any repeated "maintenance treatment," since if the excess volume increases, it indicates less patient compliance or worn-out garments. Also, one visit a year is economical as compared to conservative treatment, where patients are prescribed massage once a week and repeated maintenance therapies lasting 1–2 weeks.

How Liposuction Helps

For many patients, conservative treatment does not work well or meet their expectations, and no matter what therapy they receive, neither conservative treatment nor microsurgical procedures can remove excess adipose tissue [34–39]. Subcutaneous tissue debulking is the only option to completely reduce the limb excess volume leading to an improvement in the patient's quality of life [13, 14]. In addition, data from a prospective study that evaluated 130 patients with postmastectomy lymphedema treated with liposuction showed that the incidence of erysipelas was reduced by 87% [41]. The mean incidence of pre-liposuction and post-liposuction erysipelas episodes was 0.47 attacks/year (±0.8) and 0.06 attacks/year (±0.3), respectively.

Lymph Transport System and Liposuction

To investigate the effect of liposuction on lymph transport, the author conducted an investigation using indirect lymphoscintigraphy in 20 patients with postmastectomy arm lymphedema. Lymphoscintigraphy was performed before liposuction, with and without wearing a garment. This was repeated after 3 and 12 months. In conclusion, it was found that the already decreased lymph transport was not further reduced after liposuction [42]. Eleven of our patients (6%) with arm lymphedema do not wear any compression. A recent study has shown that liposuction for lymphedema can improve lymph transport [43].

When to Use Liposuction to Treat Lymphedema

A surgical approach, with the intention of removing the hypertrophied adipose tissue, seems logical when conservative treatment has not achieved satisfactory excess volume reduction and the patient has subjective discomfort of a heavy arm.

Initially, lymphedema starts as a swelling that shows pits on pressure. If treated immediately by conservative regimens, the swelling can disappear. If not, or improperly treated, the swelling increases over time and can end up with even more severe pitting edema with concomitant adipose tissue formation. The first and most important goal is to transform a limb with pitting edema into a non-pitting one by conservative regimens like CDT or CCT. "Pitting" means that a depression is formed after pressure exerted on the edematous tissue by the tip of the thumb, resulting in lymph being squeezed into the surroundings (Fig. 20.10a). To standardize the pitting test, the examiner should press as hard as tolerable by the patient with the thumb on the region to be investigated for 1 minute for arms and up to 3 minutes in legs. Following this, the amount of depression is estimated in millimeters. Swelling that is dominated by hypertrophied adipose tissue shows little or no pitting [44] (Fig. 20.10b).

When a patient has been treated conservatively and shows no or minimal pitting, liposuction can be performed. If the patient's quality of life is low, liposuction can be especially effective. The cancer itself is a worry, but the swollen and heavy arm introduces an additional handicap for the patient from a physical, psychosocial, and psychological point of view. Physical problems include pain, limited limb movement and physical mobility, and problems with clothing, thus interfering with everyday activities. Also, the heavy and swollen arm is impractical and cosmetically unappealing, all of which contribute to emotional distress [13, 14].

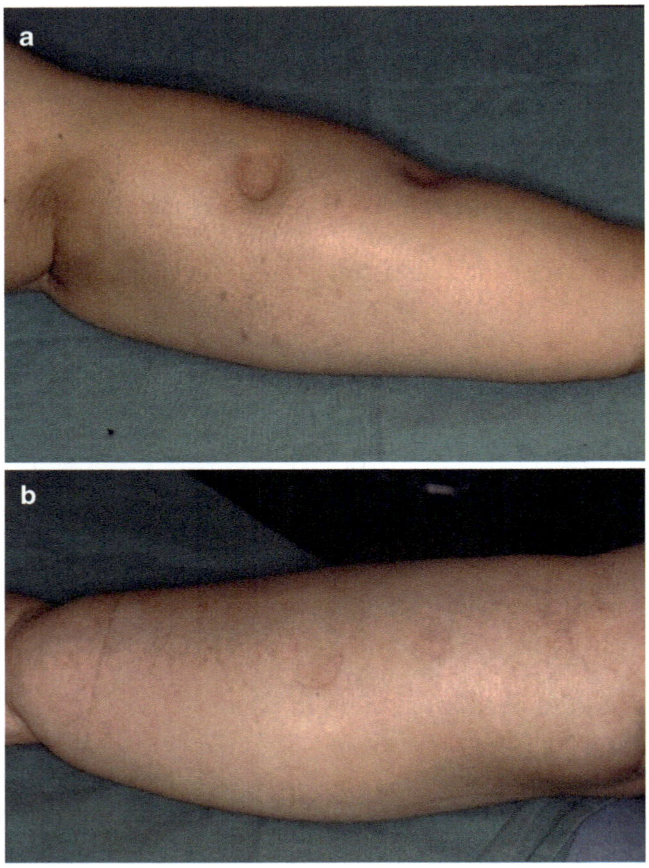

Fig. 20.10 (**a**) Marked lymphedema of the arm after breast cancer treatment, showing pitting several centimeters in depth [International Society of Lymphology (ISL) grade I edema]. The arm swelling is dominated by the presence of fluid, i.e., the accumulation of lymph. (**b**) Pronounced arm lymphedema after breast cancer treatment (ISL grade II edema). There is no pitting in spite of hard pressure by the thumb for 1 minute. A slight reddening is seen at the two spots where pressure has been exerted. The "edema" is completely dominated by adipose tissue. The term *edema* is improper at this stage since the swelling is dominated by hypertrophied adipose tissue and not by lymph. At this stage, the aspirate contains either no or a minimal amount of lymph

When Liposuction Should Never Be Used

Liposuction should not be performed in a patient that has pitting edema (Fig. 20.10a) (see earlier), as it is dominated by accumulated lymph, which can be removed by conservative treatment. In a patient with arm lymphedema, the authors accept around 4–5 mm of pitting, and in leg lymphedema, 5–6 mm. Patients with more pitting than this should be treated conservatively until the pitting has been reduced. Technically, liposuction can be performed in a patient with pronounced pitting, but then you do not know how much adipose tissue comprises the excess volume and how much fat to remove. Also, a patient who never has worn compression garments preoperatively would be less inclined to wear postoperative compression.

Can the Outcome Be Reproduced

Several teams have visited our clinic and published outcomes that parallel ours [43, 45–51].

Pearls and Pitfalls

- Excess arm or leg volume without pitting implies that excess adipose tissue is present.
- Excess adipose tissue can be removed by the use of liposuction. Conservative treatment and microsurgical reconstructions cannot remove adipose tissue.
- As in conservative treatment, the lifelong use (24 hours a day) of compression garments is mandatory for maintaining the effect of surgery.
- Clinically and technically, there is no difference in performing liposuction for primary or secondary lymphedema.
- Any patient with non-pitting swelling that causes a decreased quality of life can be a candidate for surgery.

References

1. Brorson H, Svensson H. Complete reduction of lymphoedema of the arm by liposuction after breast cancer. Scand J Plast Reconstr Surg Hand Surg. 1997;31(2):137–43.
2. Brorson H, Svensson H. Liposuction combined with controlled compression therapy reduces arm lymphedema more effectively than controlled compression therapy alone. Plast Reconstr Surg. 1998;102(4):1058–67; discussion 68.

3. Wojnikow S, Malm J, Brorson H. Use of a tourniquet with and without adrenaline reduces blood loss during liposuction for lymphoedema of the arm. Scand J Plast Reconstr Surg Hand Surg. 2007;41(5):243–9.
4. Brorson H. Liposuction normalizes lymphedema induced adipose tissue hypertrophy in elephantiasis of the leg - a prospective study with a ten-year follow-up. Plast Reconstr Surg. 2015;136(4 Suppl):133–4.
5. Brorson H. Complete reduction of arm lymphedema following breast cancer - a prospective twenty-one years' study. Plast Reconstr Surg. 2015;136(4 Suppl):134–5.
6. Hoffner M, Ohlin K, Svensson B, Manjer J, Hansson E, Troeng T, Brorson H. Liposuction gives complete reduction of arm lymphedema following breast cancer treatment-a 5-year prospective study in 105 patients without recurrence. Plast Reconstr Surg Glob Open. 2018;6(8):e1912.
7. Boccardo F, Casabona F, De Cian F, Friedman D, Murelli F, Puglisi M, Campisi CC, Molinari L, Spinaci S, Dessalvi S, Campisi C. Lymphatic microsurgical preventing healing approach (LYMPHA) for primary surgical prevention of breast cancer-related lymphedema: over 4 years follow-up. Microsurgery. 2014;34(6):421–4.
8. Feldman S, Bansil H, Ascherman J, Grant R, Borden B, Henderson P, Ojo A, Taback B, Chen M, Ananthakrishnan P, Vaz A, Balci F, Divgi CR, Leung D, Rohde C. Single institution experience with Lymphatic Microsurgical Preventive Healing Approach (LYMPHA) for the primary prevention of lymphedema. Ann Surg Oncol. 2015;22(10):3296–301.
9. Gebruers N, Verbelen H, De Vrieze T, Coeck D, Tjalma W. Incidence and time path of lymphedema in sentinel node negative breast cancer patients: a systematic review. Arch Phys Med Rehabil. 2015;96(6):1131–9.
10. Cook JA, Hassanein AH. ASO author reflections: immediate lymphatic reconstruction: a proactive approach to breast cancer-related lymphedema. Ann Surg Oncol. 2021;28:1388–9.
11. Olszewski WL. Lymph stasis: pathophysiology, diagnosis and treatment. 1st ed. Boca Raton, Ann Arbor, Boston, London: CRC Press; 1991. p. 648.
12. Bagheri S, Ohlin K, Olsson G, Brorson H. Tissue tonometry before and after liposuction of arm lymphedema following breast cancer. Lymphat Res Biol. 2005;3(2):66–80.
13. Brorson H, Ohlin K, Olsson G, Långström G, Wiklund I, Svensson H. Quality of life following liposuction and conservative treatment of arm lymphedema. Lymphology. 2006;39(1):8–25.
14. Hoffner M, Bagheri S, Hansson E, Manjer J, Troeng T, Brorson H. SF-36 shows increased quality of life following complete reduction of postmastectomy lymphedema with liposuction. Lymphat Res Biol. 2017;15(1):87–98.
15. Brorson H, Ohlin K, Olsson G, Nilsson M. Adipose tissue dominates chronic arm lymphedema following breast cancer: an analysis using volume rendered CT images. Lymphat Res Biol. 2006;4(4):199–210.
16. Brorson H, Ohlin K, Olsson G, Karlsson MK. Breast cancer-related chronic arm lymphedema is associated with excess adipose and muscle tissue. Lymphat Res Biol. 2009;7(1):3–10.
17. Hoffner M, Peterson P, Mansson S, Brorson H. Lymphedema leads to fat deposition in muscle and decreased muscle/water volume after liposuction: a magnetic resonance imaging study. Lymphat Res Biol. 2018;16(2):174–81.
18. Trinh L, Peterson P, Brorson H, Mansson S. Assessment of subfascial muscle/water and fat accumulation in lymphedema patients using magnetic resonance imaging. Lymphat Res Biol. 2019;17(3):340–6.
19. Trinh L, Peterson P, Leander P, Brorson H, Mansson S. In vivo comparison of MRI-based and MRS-based quantification of adipose tissue fatty acid composition against gas chromatography. Magn Reson Med. 2020;84(5):2484–94.
20. Vague J, Fenasse R. Comparative anatomy of adipose tissue. In: Renold AE, Cahill GF, editors. American handbook of physiology. Section 5. Washington, DC: American Physiology Society; 1965. p. 25–36.
21. Ryan TJ. Lymphatics and adipose tissue. Clin Dermatol. 1995;13(5):493–8.
22. Mattacks CA, Sadler D, Pond CM. The control of lipolysis in perinodal and other adipocytes by lymph node and adipose tissue-derived dendritic cells in rats. Adipocytes. 2005;1(1):43–56.
23. Pond CM. Adipose tissue and the immune system. Prostaglandins Leukot Essent Fatty Acids. 2005;73(1):17–30.
24. Borley NR, Mortensen NJ, Jewell DP, Warren BF. The relationship between inflammatory and serosal connective tissue changes in ileal Crohn's disease: evidence for a possible causative link. J Pathol. 2000;190(2):196–202.
25. Sadler D, Mattacks CA, Pond CM. Changes in adipocytes and dendritic cells in lymph node containing adipose depots during and after many weeks of mild inflammation. J Anat. 2005;207(6):769–81.
26. Harvey NL, Srinivasan RS, Dillard ME, Johnson NC, Witte MH, Boyd K, Sleeman MW, Oliver G. Lymphatic vascular defects promoted by Prox1 haploinsufficiency cause adult-onset obesity. Nat Genet. 2005;37(10):1072–81.
27. Schneider M, Conway EM, Carmeliet P. Lymph makes you fat. Nat Genet. 2005;37(10):1023–4.
28. Jones B, Fishman EK, Hamilton SR, Rubesin SE, Bayless TM, Cameron JC, Siegelman SS. Submucosal accumulation of fat in inflammatory bowel disease: CT/pathologic correlation. J Comput Assist Tomogr. 1986;10(5):759–63.
29. Lantz M, Vondrichova T, Parikh H, Frenander C, Ridderstrale M, Asman P, Aberg M, Groop L, Hallengren B. Overexpression of immediate early genes in active Graves' ophthalmopathy. J Clin Endocrinol Metab. 2005;90(8):4784–91.
30. Zampell JC, Aschen S, Weitman ES, Yan A, Elhadad S, De Brot M, Mehrara BJ. Regulation of adipogenesis by lymphatic fluid stasis: part I. Adipogenesis, fibrosis, and inflammation. Plast Reconstr Surg. 2012;129(4):825–34.
31. Aschen S, Zampell JC, Elhadad S, Weitman E, De Brot M, Mehrara BJ. Regulation of adipogenesis by lymphatic fluid stasis: part II. Expression of adipose differentiation genes. Plast Reconstr Surg. 2012;129(4):838–47.
32. Levi B, Glotzbach JP, Sorkin M, Hyun J, Januszyk M, Wan DC, Li S, Nelson ER, Longaker MT, Gurtner GC. Molecular analysis and differentiation capacity of adipose-derived stem cells from lymphedema tissue. Plast Reconstr Surg. 2013;132(3):580–9.
33. Dayan JH, Wiser I, Verma R, Shen J, Talati N, Goldman D, Mehrara BJ, Smith ML, Dayan E, Coriddi M, Kagan A. Regional patterns of fluid and fat accumulation in patients with lower extremity lymphedema using magnetic resonance angiography. Plast Reconstr Surg. 2020;145(2):555–63.
34. Tambour M, Holt M, Speyer A, Christensen R, Gram B. Manual lymphatic drainage adds no further volume reduction to complete decongestive therapy on breast cancer-related lymphoedema: a multicentre, randomised, single-blind trial. Br J Cancer. 2018;119(10):1215–22.
35. Campisi C, Bellini C, Campisi C, Accogli S, Bonioli E, Boccardo F. Microsurgery for lymphedema: clinical research and long-term results. Microsurgery. 2010;30(4):256–60.
36. Campisi CC, Ryan M, Boccardo F, Campisi C. A single-site technique of multiple lymphatic-venous anastomoses for the treatment of peripheral lymphedema: long-term clinical outcome. J Reconstr Microsurg. 2016;32(1):42–9.
37. Baumeister RG, Siuda S, Bohmert H, Moser E. A microsurgical method for reconstruction of interrupted lymphatic pathways:

autologous lymph-vessel transplantation for treatment of lymphedemas. Scand J Plast Reconstr Surg. 1986;20(1):141–6.
38. Baumeister RG, Mayo W, Notohamiprodjo M, Wallmichrath J, Springer S, Frick A. Microsurgical lymphatic vessel transplantation. J Reconstr Microsurg. 2016;32(1):34–41.
39. Cheng MH, Loh CYY, Lin CY. Outcomes of vascularized lymph node transfer and lymphovenous anastomosis for treatment of primary lymphedema. Plast Reconstr Surg Glob Open. 2018;6(12):e2056.
40. Brorson H, Ohlin K, Olsson G, Svensson B, Svensson H. Controlled compression and liposuction treatment for lower extremity lymphedema. Lymphology. 2008;41(2):52–63.
41. Lee D, Piller N, Hoffner M, Manjer J, Brorson H. Liposuction of Postmastectomy arm lymphedema decreases the incidence of erysipelas. Lymphology. 2016;49(2):85–92.
42. Brorson H, Svensson H, Norrgren K, Thorsson O. Liposuction reduces arm lymphedema without significantly altering the already impaired lymph transport. Lymphology. 1998;31(4):156–72.
43. Greene AK, Voss SD, Maclellan RA. Liposuction for swelling in patients with lymphedema. N Engl J Med. 2017;377(18):1788–9.
44. Brorson H. Liposuction in arm lymphedema treatment. Scand J Surg. 2003;92(4):287–95.
45. Damstra RJ, Voesten HG, Klinkert P, Brorson H. Circumferential suction-assisted lipectomy for lymphoedema after surgery for breast cancer. Br J Surg. 2009;96(8):859–64.
46. Schaverien MV, Munro KJ, Baker PA, Munnoch DA. Liposuction for chronic lymphoedema of the upper limb: 5 years of experience. J Plast Reconstr Aesthet Surg. 2012;65(7):935–42.
47. Boyages J, Kastanias K, Koelmeyer LA, Winch CJ, Lam TC, Sherman KA, Munnoch DA, Brorson H, Ngo QD, Heydon-White A, Magnussen JS, Mackie H. Liposuction for advanced lymphedema: a multidisciplinary approach for complete reduction of arm and leg swelling. Ann Surg Oncol. 2015;22(Suppl 3):S1263–70.
48. Greene AK, Maclellan RA. Operative treatment of lymphedema using suction-assisted lipectomy. Ann Plast Surg. 2016;77(3):337–40.
49. Lamprou DA, Voesten HG, Damstra RJ, Wikkeling OR. Circumferential suction-assisted lipectomy in the treatment of primary and secondary end-stage lymphoedema of the leg. Br J Surg. 2017;104(1):84–9.
50. McGee P, Munnoch DA. Treatment of gynaecological cancer related lower limb lymphoedema with liposuction. Gynecol Oncol. 2018;151(3):460–5.
51. Stewart CJ, Munnoch DA. Liposuction as an effective treatment for lower extremity lymphoedema: a single surgeon's experience over nine years. J Plast Reconstr Aesthet Surg. 2018;71(2):239–45.
52. Brorson H, Ohlin K, Olsson G, Svensson B. Liposuction of postmastectomy arm lymphedema completely removes excess volume: a thirteen year study (Quad erat demonstrandum). Eur J Lymphol. 2007;17:9.

Step-by-Step Instruction: Suction-Assisted Protein Lipectomy Procedure Combined with Vascularized Lymph Node Transfer and/or Lymphaticovenous Anastomosis Surgery as Part of an Integrated Lymphedema Treatment System

21

Jay W. Granzow

Introduction

Lymphedema surgeries, such as suction-assisted protein lipectomy (SAPL), vascularized lymph node transfer (VLNT), and lymphaticovenous anastomosis (LVA) surgeries, for many years clearly have been shown to be safe and effective in the medical literature. When performed properly, lymphedema treatment that includes surgery as a part of a complete treatment process can yield tremendous improvements in a patient's mental and physical condition. The two-phase type approach for the treatment of chronic, solid-predominant lymphedema presented in this chapter is an integral part of this process. This approach is not simply a way of stringing together several operations in a "fire and forget" fashion but rather reflects an overall philosophy that surgery for lymphedema must be part of an ongoing care program for each patient's chronic lymphedema disease condition [1–3].

The most often overlooked and least appreciated part of lymphedema surgery is the appreciation for the overall treatment program and the importance of lymphedema therapy as a key component of this program. Lymphedema is a chronic condition, and lymphedema surgery is not a cure or a "magic bullet" for the treatment for lymphedema. Simply put, to produce consistently successful results, any surgery for lymphedema must be performed in the full context of a complete lymphedema treatment system that includes significant and appropriate lymphedema therapy and utilizes careful patient selection to match the appropriate patient to the correct indication. The nonsurgical details, such as integration of imaging and therapy (Fig. 21.1), are just as important to lymphedema surgery as, for example, they are to hand surgery.

This is in significant contrast to many other types of microsurgery. For example, deep inferior epigastric artery perforator (DIEP) flap breast reconstruction and the subsequent second stage revision are often completed in 3 months after which little to no follow-up may be required if performed properly. Lymphedema surgery, in contrast, is more analogous to metacarpophalangeal (MCP) joint replacement surgery in a patient with chronic rheumatoid arthritis, in which the surgery can provide great improvements in a patient's outcome in the context of a chronic disease process that will continue to require long-term treatment. Lymphedema surgery also does not provide the immediate results and gratification of other types of reconstruction. Swelling after SAPL surgery typically takes months to subside significantly, garments must be downsized and replaced, therapy must be maintained, and patient expectations must be managed appropriately.

Lymphedema surgery and treatment require an ongoing partnership between the patient and the surgeon, lymphedema therapist, and other members of the treatment team. Most lymphedema patients have complex medical histories and presentations. In addition, in my experience, most patients have had significant delays in the diagnosis of their lymphedema and have a limited understanding of their lymphedema or their treatment options. Therefore, the lymphedema surgeon must be prepared to spend significant time with each patient during the initial consultation and in follow-up calls and visits, both before and after surgery. Office staff must be well trained and expect that the time, effort, and care required by lymphedema patients are much higher than most other reconstruction patients.

J. W. Granzow (✉)
Division of Plastic Surgery, Department of Surgery, Harbor-UCLA Medical Center, Torrance, CA, USA
e-mail: info@drgranzow.com

M. V. Schaverien, J. H. Dayan (eds.), *Multimodal Management of Upper and Lower Extremity Lymphedema*,
https://doi.org/10.1007/978-3-030-93039-4_21

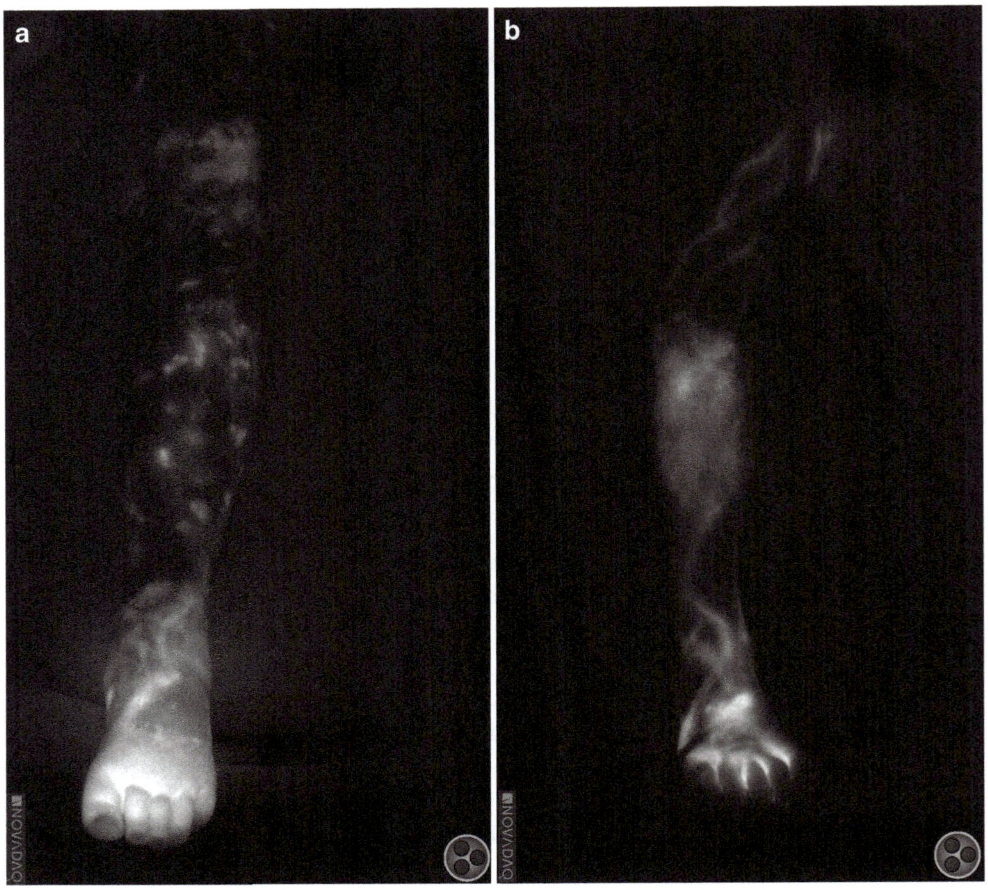

Fig. 21.1 (**a**) Indocyanine green (ICG) imaging of a patient with International Society of Lymphology (ISL) Stage 2 lymphedema of the left leg and (**b**) ISL Stage 0 lymphedema of the right leg

Lymphedema surgeries are arguably more complex and intricate than most other types of microsurgery. Additional training and experience, proper use of lymphedema imaging techniques, integration of lymphedema therapy at all points in the patient's treatment course, and an overall commitment to a significant volume of patients and procedures are essential to produce good outcomes.

Lymphedema surgery should not be undertaken by the casual operator and requires a surgeon who has had proper training and experience with patient selection, surgical techniques, access to and use of appropriate imaging, and integration of high-quality lymphedema therapy at all points of the treatment process. Additional fellowship training and experience specifically in lymphedema surgery are critical to achieve the best results.

Two-Phase Approach Key Points

The two-phase approach was developed based on the significant contributions made by many other talented and dedicated surgeons who described this approach previously, in particular pioneers including Drs. Håkan Brorson, Isao Koshima, Ming-Huei Cheng, and Corinne Becker, among numerous others [4–8]. Many different lymphedema surgery approaches continue to be used elsewhere.

A two-phase approach is used to treat patients with chronic, International Society of Lymphology (ISL) Stage 2 lymphedema whose lymphatic system has suffered severe damage from the lymphedema disease process. These patients first must have undergone and maximized the results of conservative lymphedema therapy administered by an experienced Certified Lymphedema Therapist (CLT). SAPL surgery is used first to remove the inflammatory lymphedema solids that generally consist of fat, protein, and other fibrotic materials. After healing from the SAPL surgery is complete, VLNT and/or LVA is used to decrease the amount of long-term conservative care required.

Specific surgical techniques mentioned below are addressed in great detail elsewhere in this book, and the key points are listed below.

Indications and Patient Selection for Two-Phase Approach

- The two-stage approach is most effective for patients with advanced, chronic, solid-predominant lymphedema.

- These are patients whose arm or leg is characterized by permanent deposits of pathologic excess solids such as fat and lymphedema proteins.
- Patients with pitting lymphedema require high-quality lymphedema therapy before consideration for lymphedema surgery, and the affected limb has minimal or no pitting after this therapy is performed.
- Patients without non-pitting, solid-predominant, solid excess are not candidates.
- Patients must be willing to wear custom, flat-knit compression garments both before surgery and after surgery. Note: In my experience, essentially all patients with chronic, solid-predominant, lymphedema require the ongoing use of current, custom compression garments. The two-phase approach can decrease the need for these garments.
- Poor candidates for lymphedema surgery are patients that have never participated in conservative treatment, have never worn compression garments, are unwilling to participate in complete decongestive therapy (CDT), and/or are looking for a fast "miracle cure."
- Reverse lymphatic mapping is essential when performing VLNT surgery.
- Morbidly obese patients are not candidates [9, 10].
- Lymphatic vesicles that most commonly occur in the toes and genital areas are often best treated once the initial inflammation creating these areas of skin weakness is addressed first.
- Arm lymphedema cases tend to be easier to treat than leg lymphedema cases.
- Family and emotional/mental support for each patient is extremely important and should not be overestimated.

Phase One: Suction-Assisted Protein Lipectomy (SAPL) Surgery

SAPL surgery is based on the technique developed by Dr. Håkan Brorson who first performed his surgery in 1987 [4, 5; see Chap. 20]. Dr. Brorson is a true innovator in the field, and his rigorous, data-driven approach serves as an ideal model for research and training. What is most important to convey is that SAPL surgery is not cosmetic liposuction surgery. Any attempt to treat a lymphedema patient using a cosmetic liposuction or similar protocol will not only fail but may also worsen the patient's condition. The inflamed lymphedema solids present typically are much more adherent and denser than standard fat, and the already impaired lymphatic drainage system present will not allow proper drainage of postoperative inflammation and swelling using a cosmetic-type liposuction protocol.

It has been well known for over 20 years that SAPL does not damage lymphatics [5]. The myth that SAPL surgery somehow causes patients to require compression after surgery that was not required before surgery is also false. In fact, the lymphatic drainage improves, and the inflammation decreases in nearly all patients after SAPL surgery. Even the need for compression and therapy required most often decreases slightly.

SAPL requires the closest cooperation of the lymphedema surgeon and lymphedema therapist preoperatively, perioperatively, and postoperatively. This close involvement of the lymphedema therapist is not optional. The failure of having lymphedema therapy causes persistent swelling, inflammation, prolonged healing, and reaccumulation of the pathologic solids.

Suction-Assisted Protein Lipectomy (SAPL) Surgery Key Points

- Intraoperative indocyanine green (ICG) mapping is usually performed to delineate each patient's individual drainage pattern.
- A surgical tourniquet is used.
- Large, blunt-tip cannulas are used with a power-assisted liposuction machine.

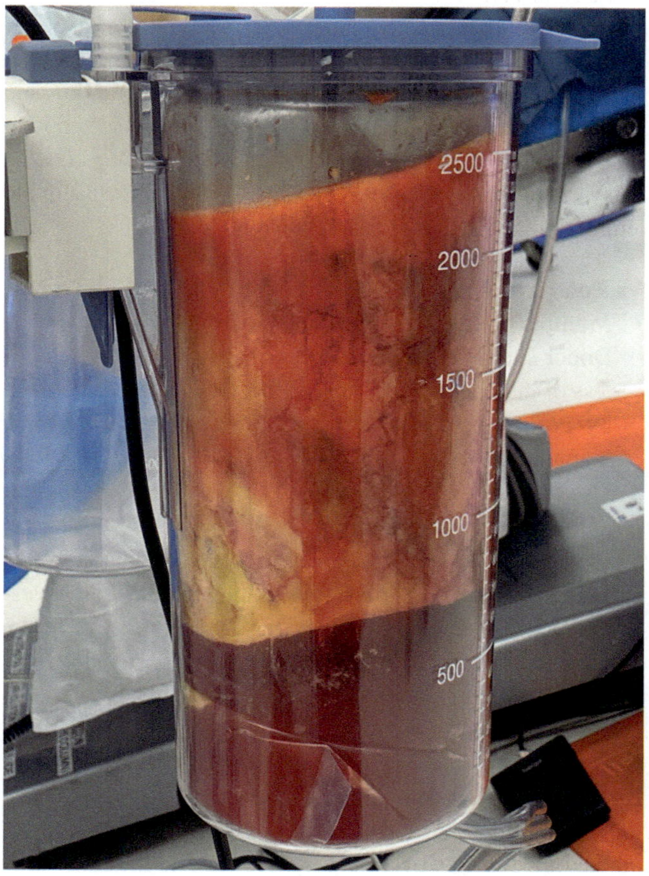

Fig. 21.2 Material removed during suction-assisted protein lipectomy (SAPL) surgery is typically more heterogenous than that removed with cosmetic liposuction. More tumescent fluid is also returned due to the use of the tourniquet

- Use some tumescent fluid but not tumescent technique. The typical volume infused usually is less than overall aspirate volume (Fig. 21.2).
- Aspiration is performed parallel to the direction of the lymphatics whenever possible.
- Intraoperative placement of short-stretch bandages or custom, flat-knit compression garments is optimum.
- Patients require significant postoperative care by the CLT. Bandages especially must be monitored immediately postop after SAPL surgery to ensure that they are not too tight and to avoid issues such as excess recovery room pain and problems with perfusion of finger and toes.
- Surgery time is usually around 4 hours.
- SAPL is an inpatient surgery, and hospital stay is typically 2 nights.
- Long-term lymphedema therapy should be administered by the patient's local lymphedema therapist under the direction of the lymphedema surgeon or surgical lymphedema therapist.

A patient's arm or leg is allowed to heal for an extended period after SAPL surgery, typically 1 year or more, before proceeding to the second-phase VLNT and/or LVA surgery.

Phase Two: Vascularized Lymph Node Transfer (VLNT) and/or Lymphaticovenous Anastomosis (LVA) Surgery

VLNT surgery allows transfer of lymph node containing tissues to areas of deficient lymphatic drainage.

Vascularized Lymph Node Transfer (VLNT) Key Points

- Multiple options exist for donor sites.
- Donor site risk of lymphedema is always present regardless of the donor site, although this risk can be minimized by proper technique and the use of reverse lymphatic mapping.
- Use imaging with Technetium (Tc)-99 and ICG to better define the flap (Fig. 21.3).
- If in doubt, less aggressive harvesting of lymphatic and adjacent tissue is the rule. Divide and repair a pedicle vessel loop rather than dividing crossing lymphatics at the donor site if needed.
- Use a two-team approach whenever possible.

Reverse Lymphatic Mapping During Vascularized Lymph Node Transfer (VLNT) Surgery

Reverse lymphatic mapping is an essential imaging technique used during VLNT surgery. This allows the surgeon to map the lymph nodes most likely to be draining the adjacent structures, such as an arm or leg adjacent to a lymph node donor site, to reduce the possibility of new swelling and lymphedema at or around the donor site. I have used this technique for many years, and it is very well described in Dr. Dayan's excellent manuscript [6]; see Chap. 11. The Tc-99 is injected preoperatively on the morning of surgery or the prior day/evening.

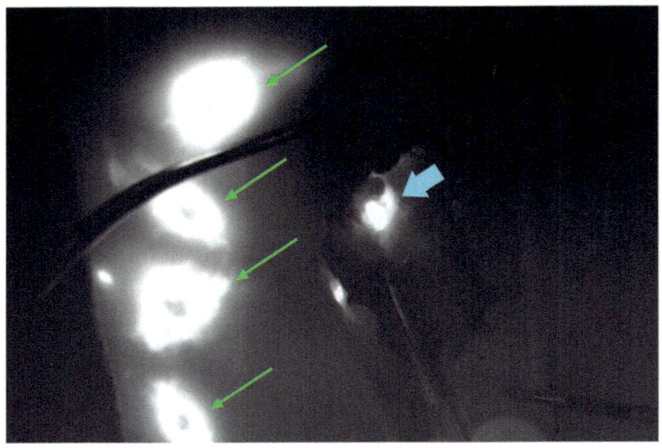

Fig. 21.3 Harvest of lateral thoracic vascularized lymph node transfer (VLNT) flap. Thin green arrows: indocyanine green (ICG) skin injection sites. Thick blue arrow: lymph node seen within flap

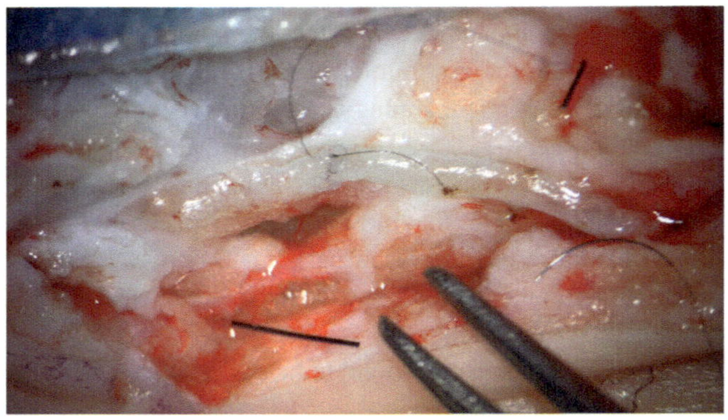

Fig. 21.4 Completed lymphaticovenous anastomosis (LVA) – lymphatic (left) sewn to venule (right) using 11-0 suture

LVA surgery clearly involves some of the smallest vessels and the highest complexity of any type of surgery. The technique involves supermicrosurgery, which is defined by Dr. Koshima as surgery involving vessels less than 0.8 millimeter in diameter [8].

LVA Key Points

- In contrast to most other microsurgery procedures, LVA surgery is performed almost entirely under the operating microscope (Fig. 21.4).
- Specialized, superfine instruments are required as is a very high-power operating microscope as most standard microsurgery microscope configurations and instrument sets are insufficient.
- The operating room/hospital therefore must be willing to invest significant effort and capital to support surgeons performing the LVA surgeries.

- Use ICG imaging to help define optimum incision placements.
- Distally, the protocol tends to lie more along the techniques described by Drs. Koshima and Yamamoto and colleagues [7, 8]; see Chap. 9.
- Proximally, the technique tends to be more similar to that described by Drs. C. Campisi and C.C. Campisi, Boccardo, and colleagues [11]; see Chap. 10.
- A greater number of connections in multiple different sites appear to provide the best long-term results.
- Sew by hand, not with the robot. I have used the robot and found no increase in accuracy but a loss of essential tactile sensation.

Postoperative Care

Proper postoperative care is essential for good outcomes. Compression is applied wherever possible for all surgeries. In my practice, SAPL surgery especially requires a rigorous postoperative compression regimen that includes the use of short-stretch bandaging; flat-knit, custom fitting compression garments; and additional lymphedema therapy and follow-up.

Complications

Patients have standard surgical risks and must have the standard postoperative expectations such as transient postoperative pain, discomfort, and scars at incision sites. True complications from lymphedema surgery are rare and include standard risks such as flap loss, hematoma, seroma, and deep vein thrombosis.

Overall Pearls and Pitfalls

- Lymphedema is, and must be treated as, a chronic disease process that requires ongoing care. Surgery must be performed in the context of an integrated treatment program.
- Complete integration of lymphedema therapy in the preoperative, perioperative, and postoperative treatment timeframes is essential and has often been underappreciated.
- Lymphedema surgery patients typically require significantly more surgeon and staff time and counseling at all phases of the treatment process than other types of surgery.
- Patients will require preoperative and postoperative lifelong use of custom, flat-knit compression garments. The requirement for this compression varies among patients and typically decreases slightly after SAPL surgery and significantly after VLNT/LVA surgeries.
- Solid lymphedema volume excess is addressed with SAPL surgery, while fluid volume excess/reaccumulation is addressed with conservative lymphedema treatment such as manual lymphatic drainage (MLD), bandaging, compression garments, and surgery such as VLNT and LVA.
- SAPL surgery for chronic, solid-predominant lymphedema is not cosmetic liposuction. The use of techniques similar to standard liposuction will provide poor results and may worsen patient outcomes.
- Morbidly obese patients are poor candidates for lymphedema surgery and should pursue weight loss first.

References

1. Granzow JW, Soderberg JM, Kaji AH, Dauphine C. An effective system of surgical treatment of lymphedema. Ann Surg Oncol. 2014;21(4):1189–94.
2. Granzow JW, Soderberg JM, Dauphine C. A novel two-stage surgical approach to treat chronic lymphedema. Breast J. 2014;20:420–2.
3. Granzow JW, Soderberg JM, Kaji AH, Dauphine C. Review of current surgical treatments for lymphedema. Ann Surg Oncol. 2014;21(4):1195–201.
4. Brorson H, Svensson H. Complete reduction of lymphoedema of the arm by liposuction after breast cancer. Scand J Plast Reconstr Surg Hand Surg. 1997;31(2):137–43.
5. Brorson H, Svensson H, Norrgren K, Thorsson O. Liposuction reduces arm lymphedema without significantly altering the already impaired lymph transport. Lymphology. 1998;31:156–72.
6. Dayan JH, Dayan E, Smith ML. Reverse lymphatic mapping: a new technique for maximizing safety in vascularized lymph node transfer. Plast Reconstr Surg. 2015;135(1):277–85.
7. Yamamoto T, Narushima M, Yoshimatsu H, et al. Minimally invasive lymphatic supermicrosurgery (MILS): indocyanine green-guided simultaneous multi-site lymphaticovenular anastomoses via millimeter skin incisions. Ann Plast Surg. 2014;72(1):67–70.
8. Koshima I, Inagawa K, Urushibara K, Moriguchi T. Supermicrosurgical lymphaticovenular anastomosis for the treatment of lymphedema in the upper extremities. J Reconstr Microsurg. 2000;16(6):437–42.
9. Greene AK, Grant FD, Slavin SA, Maclellan RA. Obesity-induced lymphedema: clinical and lymphoscintigraphic features. Plast Reconstr Surg. 2015;135(6):1715–9.
10. Greene AK, Grant FD, Maclellan RA. Obesity-induced lymphedema nonreversible following massive weight loss. Plast Reconstr Surg Glob Open. 2015;3(6):e426.
11. Campisi CC, Ryan M, Boccardo F, Campisi C. A single-site technique of multiple lymphatic-venous anastomoses for the treatment of peripheral lymphedema: long-term clinical outcome. J Reconstr Microsurg. 2016;32(1):42–9.

Step-by-Step Instruction: Direct Excision Combined with Lymphatic Microsurgery

22

Kavan S. Johal and Hung-Chi Chen

Introduction

For the lymphedema population cohort that has failed non-operative management, a number of surgical options are readily available. Decisions on operation choice are based on various factors including disease staging, any previously performed procedures and patient comorbidities. Broadly, we continue to divide available techniques into physiological and excisional. Within the last few years, we have seen an evolution in our own lymphedema practice with modifications to improve existing techniques, including lymphovenous anastomosis (LVA) and vascularized lymph node flap transfer (VLNT), but also an increasing breadth of conditions (both congenital and acquired) that may be suitable for treatment. These include chylous ascites and Klippel-Trenaunay syndrome with lymphedema, to name but a few. Multi-modality treatment represents the cornerstone of success, particularly in advanced disease. Within this chapter, we will discuss the following:

- Donor options for vascularized lymph node flap transfer (VLNT)
- Radical Reduction of lymphedema with Preservation of Perforators (RRPP)
- Hung-Chi Chen (HCC)-modified Charles procedure
- Liposuction
- Algorithm and combination procedures

K. S. Johal
Department of Plastic Surgery, China Medical University Hospital, Taichung, Taiwan

Department of Plastic Surgery, St Thomas' Hospital, London, UK

H.-C. Chen (✉)
Department of Plastic Surgery, China Medical University Hospital, Taichung, Taiwan
e-mail: d19722@mail.cmuh.org.tw

Typical Indications

Numerous factors dictate whether patients are appropriate for surgical treatment:

- Completion of a decongestive therapy program
- Compliance with conservative therapy
- Comorbidities that may exclude candidacy for surgery
- Lymphedema staging

Early staging of lymphedema, as defined by the International Society of Lymphology (ISL) (see Table 22.1) [1, 2], provides easy categorization by patient signs and subjective symptomatology. However, for the clinician, it is more useful to pair these with operative solutions. Correlation of the macroscopic and microscopic disease process with proposed treatments was performed early on by means of a more relevant specifically designed staging system (staging according to Hung-Chi Chen (HCC); Table 22.2) [3]. As per this staging, it becomes easier to categorize patients broadly into likely treatment strategies:

- *Stages 1 and 2*: Conservative treatment including combined decongestive therapy (CDT)
- *Stage 3A*:

Table 22.1 International Society of Lymphology (ISL): lymphedema staging

Stage	Signs and symptoms
0	Latent/sub-clinical stage Impaired lymph transport, possible subjective symptoms
I	Early high protein fluid accumulation, subsides with limb elevation. Pitting may occur
II	Pitting manifests, limb elevation insufficient to reduce swelling, increased fat deposition/fibrosis
III	Lymphostatic elephantiasis, absent pitting, trophic skin changes, progressive fibrosis

M. V. Schaverien, J. H. Dayan (eds.), *Multimodal Management of Upper and Lower Extremity Lymphedema*,
https://doi.org/10.1007/978-3-030-93039-4_22

Table 22.2 Staging according to Hung-Chi Chen (From Chen HC, Liem A, Karonidis A, Karri V, Tang Y-B. Surgical Treatment and Algorithm for Lymphoedema. Elsevier Taiwan LLC; 2011)

Stage	Presentation	Proposed treatment
I	Sentinel decompensation stage, where the lymphatic load exceeds lymphatic transport capacity, intralymphatic pressure builds, flow stagnates, and valvular incompetence occurs	Non-surgical treatment
II	Brief compensation phase where all lymphatic channels are recruited for drainage. This leads to dermal backflow, mild edema and occasional erythema, but the skin remains soft. Patient is unaware	Non-surgical treatment/ combined decongestive therapy (CDT) +/– intermittent positive pressure pumping (IPPP)
III	Fibroblasts, monocytes, adipocytes and keratinocytes Increase in the tissue, along with episodes of infection	
IIIA	Symptoms are obvious, but swelling can be improved after rest	VLNT + LVA + liposuction (day 10)
IIIB	Non-reversible changes are initiated	VLNT + LVA + liposuction (day 10) Or RRPP lower limb + liposuction thigh
IVA	Fibrovascular proliferation is seen: Brawny leather-like skin, crypts and cutaneous ulcers	Radical excision: Charles procedure +/– VLNT
IVB	Stage IVa + severely affected toes; notably swelling with repeated episodes of cellulitis, verrucous hyperkeratosis, deformity or osteomyelitis	Charles procedure and toe Amputation +/– VLNT

VLNT vascularized lymph node transfer, *LVA* lymphovenous anastomosis, *RRPP* Radical Reduction of lymphedema with Preservation of Perforators

- VLNT + LVA (LVA only if patient is not fit for long general anaesthesia) followed by liposuction 10 days later, avoiding the areas of VLNT/LVA.
- Primary option in our unit for VLNT is the gastroepiploic lymph node flap, although in cases of previous abdominal surgery, other options may be utilized (discussed later in this chapter).

- *Stage 3B*:
  - VLNT + LVA + liposuction (as above)
  - Or RRPP (lower limb) + liposuction (thigh)
- *Stage 4:*
  - VLNT (no LVA) + modified Charles procedure +/– toe amputation

Surgical Techniques

Vascularized Lymph Node Flap Transfer (VLNT)

Microsurgical transfer of lymph nodes from a number of sites has been described for the treatment of lymphedema in both the upper and lower extremities. Each institution may have their own preference, but we describe the techniques for a number of flaps we regularly employ and their specific indications.

Donor Site Options

Intra-abdominal Lymph Node Flaps

Gastroepiploic Lymph Node Flap

We first described the use of the right gastroepiploic lymph node flap harvested via an open approach for the successful treatment of both upper and lower limb lymphedema [4]. Harvest is performed via an upper midline laparotomy and proceeds in a stepwise fashion: identifying the left gastroepiploic vessels, dissecting the omentum off the transverse colon, dividing the left gastroepiploic vessels, dissecting away the short segmental gastric branches and thus allowing complete release to visualize the right gastroepiploic vessels. Following harvest, microsurgical transfer is performed, which in our early series was performed as a single flap to the extremity (such as the medial ankle or ulnar side of the wrist) (Fig. 22.1). Success relies on two key principles – improved lymphatic drainage from interstitial fluid into VLNs and then outflow through the flap vein, coupled with omental flap absorption of lymphatic fluid.

Laparoscopic Flap Harvest Modification

Subsequently, our surgical approach was modified to harvest the right gastroepiploic lymph node flap laparoscopically in conjunction with general surgical colleagues, thus reducing abdominal morbidity and facilitating earlier patient mobility/ discharge [5]. Key intra-operative steps include identifying the right gastroepiploic vessels, maintaining omental tissue around the vascular pedicle, separating the omentum from the greater curvature of the stomach (through division of gastric branches) and transverse colon and division of the right gastroepiploic vessels at the mid-gastric area (near the take-off of the middle omental vessels). Adjoining lymph nodes and the local omental tissue must be harvested to maintain intra-flap lymphatics. Flap removal via the umbilical incision is performed, followed by microscopic pedicle dissection ahead of recipient site anastomosis. A small split-skin graft is usually employed to reduce tension over the transferred flap.

Double Gastroepiploic Lymph Node Flaps

Following positive experience with the distally placed gastroepiploic lymph node flap in the extremity, we have further modified our approach to use double flaps placed in the middle and distal limb (popliteal area and ankle, elbow and wrist, respectively) [6]. Harvest is again performed laparoscopically, dissecting towards the origin of the right gastroepiploic artery and then in reverse along the greater curvature before ligation of the left gastroepiploic vessels. Once the right gas-

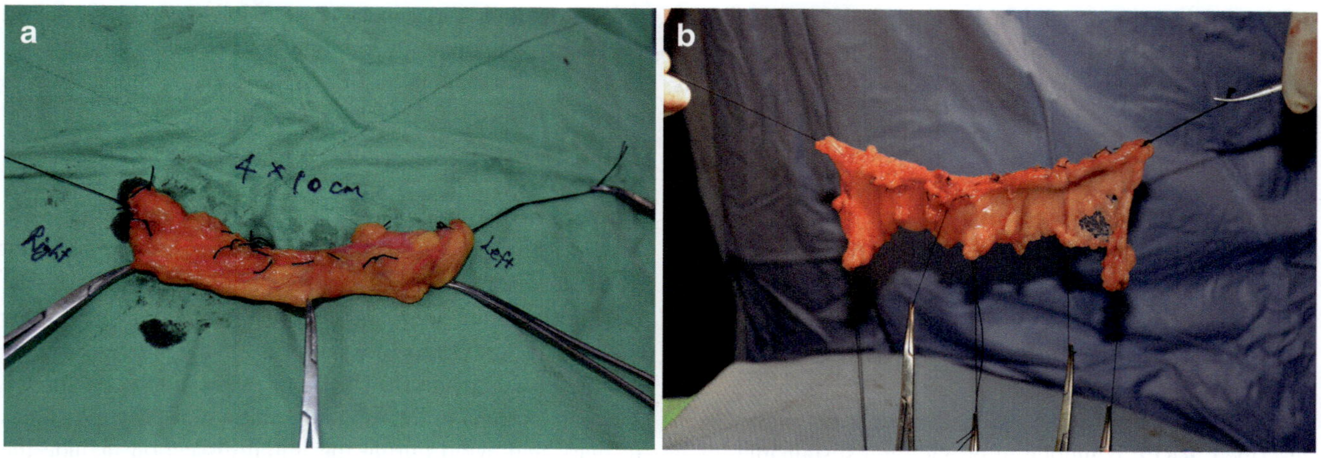

Fig. 22.1 (**a**) Another popular flap source of vascularized lymph nodes was developed in our unit – the gastroepiploic lymph node flap – which can be harvested laparoscopically. If laparoscopy is not available, it can be harvested with a mini-laparotomy technique (another option is robotic harvest; however, this is less frequently used due to higher cost). (**b**) In some circumstances, the lymph node flap can be divided into two or three parts for transfer to different levels

troepiploic vessels have been ligated, the flap is removed, usually being around 15x4cm in dimension. Off-table preparation of the pedicle is performed at two points, distally and approximately at the mid-point of the flap. We normally perform the first set of anastomoses before splitting the flap to reduce ischemia time for the second half. To minimize any potential compression, direct closure over the flap is not advised; however, usually a local flap can be used and the donor defect grafted if required (usually preferred to grafting directly over the gastroepiploic flap).

Combination Flaps and Special Indications

Whilst the gastroepiploic flap provides a valuable option for the treatment of extremity lymphedema, in cases where significant soft tissue coverage is also required, then combining it with a large segment of omentum as a single flap further broadens the possible indications [7]. An excellent example is the treatment of venous ulceration in the lower limb with concurrent lymphedema. Harvest is again performed laparoscopically as previously described, following the right gastroepiploic vessels to their origin and concurrently harvesting the omentum. After anastomosis to the recipient vessels, the omentum may be folded and debulked as required to contour the debrided wound bed, before resurfacing with a meshed split-skin graft. We have used this for progression to rapid wound healing without ulcer recurrence, in combination with marked improvement in lymphedema confirmed by reduction in limb circumference and tonicity.

Peripheral Lymph Node Flaps

Groin Lymph Node Flap

Aside from intra-abdominal harvest, numerous other anatomical sites may be used as VLN flap donors, including the groin. Harvest of a flap from the *contralateral* groin may be based on a number of vascular systems, primarily the superficial circumflex iliac artery (SCIA) but also the superficial inferior epigastric artery (SIEA). Flaps based on the SCIA may be raised either medial to lateral or lateral to medial. For the former, retrograde dissection of the vein and artery from the saphenous vein and femoral artery, respectively, can be performed. Identification of the superficial (medial) and deep (lateral) branches of the artery allows transfer along with the block of lymph nodes usually adjoining the superficial branch. Should no SCIA be present, the flap can be redesigned around the SIEA and adjoining vein. Alternatively, the flap may be raised lateral to medial, initially beginning in the suprafascial plane but switching to subfascial if the SCIA is not initially visualized. By ligating sartorius muscle branches, the SCIA may be followed to its origin, taking care to include the superficial circumflex iliac vein (SCIV) and perivascular nodal tissue.

Supraclavicular Lymph Node Flap and Other Options

Lymph nodes in proximity to the transverse cervical artery (TCA) can be harvested from the posterior triangle (with or without skin) for the treatment of lymphedema [8]. The nodes of interest are usually present deep to the omohyoid muscle and must not be separated from the TCA. Venous outflow is usually via the vena comitans, but the external jugular vein can be harvested for additional drainage.

Other Lymph Node Flaps

Other VLN flap options are numerous. We have published on many donor sites with beneficial results in the extremity, including the use of other intra-abdominal flaps (such as appendicular [9] and ileocaecal [10]) and also flow-through venous flaps incorporating nodal tissue adjacent to the external jugular vein inset into the great saphenous vein in the lower extremity [11]. A case series depicting pre- and post-operative photos with supraclavicular VLN flap harvest is shown (Fig. 22.2a–h).

Post-operative: An inner loose elastic bandage is placed followed by an outer tight compressive bandage with the latter removed at 2 hours post-op in the recovery room. Patients are kept in hospital for 3–5 days to maintain elevation and compression, which is continued on discharge.

Excisional Procedures and Their Combination with Lymphatic Microsurgery

Radical Reduction of Lymphedema with Preservation of Perforators (RRPP)

Whilst a number of excisional procedures have been described, RRPP is unique in providing a sustainable long-term result coupled with acceptable aesthetics [12, 13]. Positive outcomes may be defined by not only the expected reduction in limb circumference but also limb tonicity, episodes of cellulitis/infection and hospital admissions.

Lower Extremity

Pre-operative marking: Mark perforators with handheld Doppler arising from posterior tibial and peroneal arteries above the level of the malleoli. Of particular note in the middle third, a large perforator usually nourishes the medial and lateral flaps, respectively.

Marking: Two anterior and two posterior ellipses are positioned obliquely and parallel to each other. Care must be taken to maintain an adequate skin bridge (at least 4 cm) between the ellipses and both the anterior and posterior aspects. These ellipses represent skin to be excised after the surgical debulking.

Intra-operative: Under tourniquet control, incise down to the fascia. Elevate suprafascially as one unit medially and laterally. Preserve important structures (such as the superficial peroneal and saphenous nerves). Identify and preserve marked perforators. Tangentially excise the skin and the subcutaneous tissue flap to approximately 5 mm thick, preserving a small amount of subdermal fat (and thus the subdermal plexus). Leave a small adipofascial cuff around the two major medial and lateral perforators. Perform haemostasis with the tourniquet deflated, and then close the wound over suction drains.

Upper Extremity

Pre-operative marking: A line from 1 cm below the midpoint of the antecubital fossa to the scaphoid tubercle marks the path of the radial artery. Similarly, a line is drawn from the medial epicondyle to the pisiform; at the junction of the proximal/middle third of this line is the landmark for the ulnar artery that continues along this path distally. Key areas to mark and avoid during the initial dissection include the following: (1) the site of multiple fasciocutaneous perforators arising close to the radial artery origin (adjacent to the takeoff of the radial recurrent artery); (2) fasciocutaneous branches of the ulnar artery found close to the anterior/posterior ulnar recurrent arteries and the common interosseous artery, running between the flexor carpi ulnaris and flexor digitorum superficialis; and (3) superficial palmar branch of the median nerve.

Marking: Volar and dorsal ellipses are marked with a 30° angle. The volar ellipse is drawn between the radial and ulnar marked anatomical lines preserving their main fasciocutaneous branches. The dorsal ellipse is drawn along the central axis.

Intra-operative: Under tourniquet control, incise down to fascia overlying muscle, and elevate medial and lateral flaps. Preserve vascular branches identified and important medial and lateral cutaneous nerves of the forearm. Perform haemostasis with the tourniquet deflated. Excise marked skin ellipse and close over suction drains.

Post-operative: As for the lower extremity.

Hung-Chi Chen (HCC)-Modified Charles Procedure

Following its early description [14], some authors cautioned as to the high morbidity associated with the traditional Charles procedure, and many surgeons remained

Fig. 22.2 (**a**) This 56-year-old woman had cervical cancer 16 years ago, operated on by gynaecology with radical excision followed by chemotherapy. She started to develop progressive swelling of the right lower extremity with repetitive episodes of cellulitis and presented with severe fibrosis of skin and subcutaneous tissue in the right lower limb. Anteroposterior view is shown. (**b**) Posterior view showed bulging of the lateral aspect of the right leg with chronic inflammatory changes of the skin and pigmentation. (**c**) The dorsum of the right foot and toes were swollen with erythema of the great toe and fungal infection in the web spaces. Antibiotics were given for 1 week before surgery. (**d**) In the first stage, a supraclavicular lymph node flap was harvested and transferred to the medial side of the right ankle; EJV, external jugular vein; TCA, transverse cervical artery. (**e**) Ten days later, a modified Charles procedure was performed. She had good care after surgery with regular lubrication over the skin graft every day. At 5 years of follow-up, she did not have any cellulitis since the operation. The two sides were symmetrical in shape, and the surface was smooth. (**f**) Posteroanterior view of the right lower extremity. (**g**) The swelling of the toes had subsided, and there was no residual fungal infection after surgery. (**h**) The donor site was inconspicuous. There was no numbness of skin because the infra-clavicular nerve had been preserved carefully during surgery

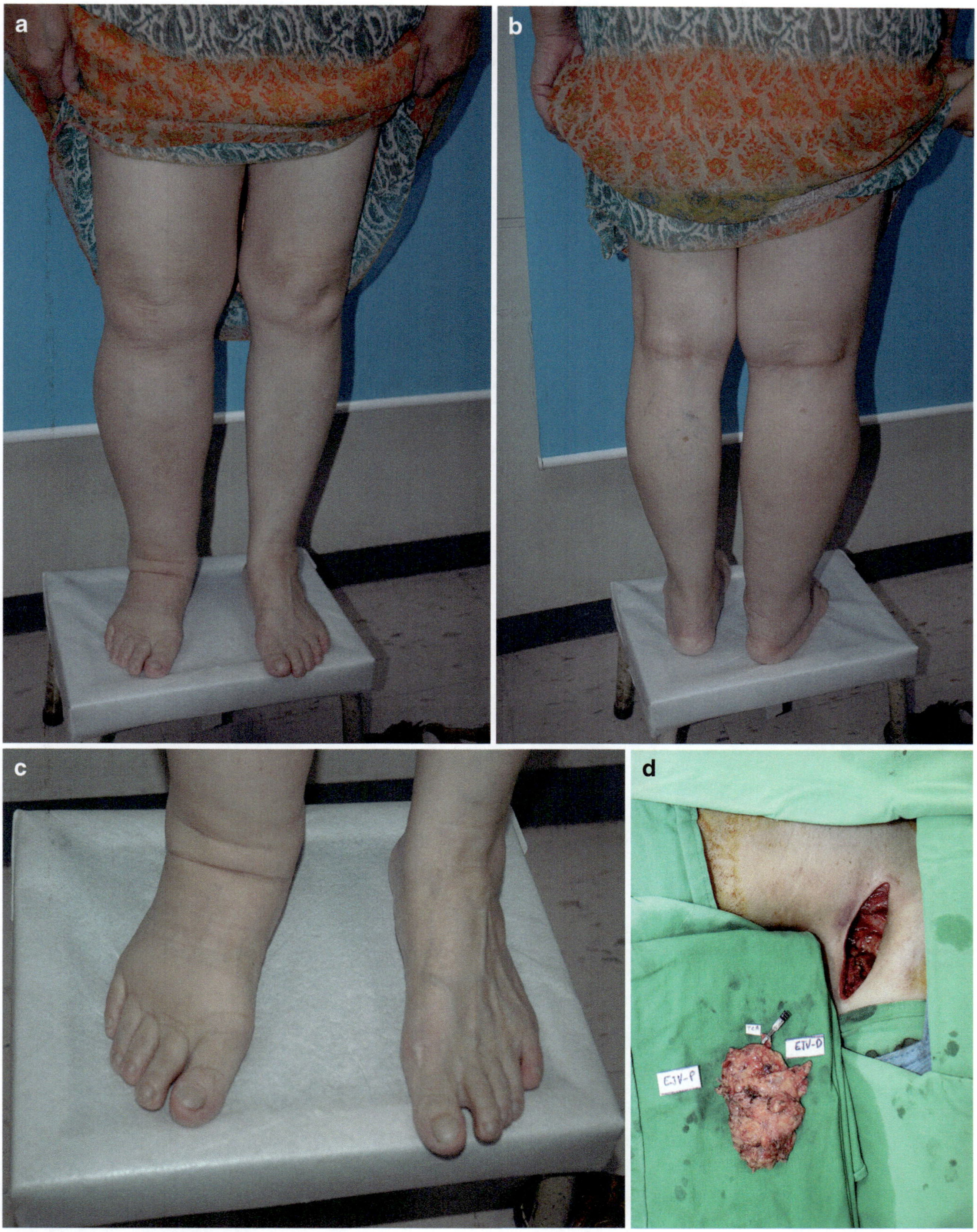
a
b
c
d
TCA
EJV-D
EJV-P

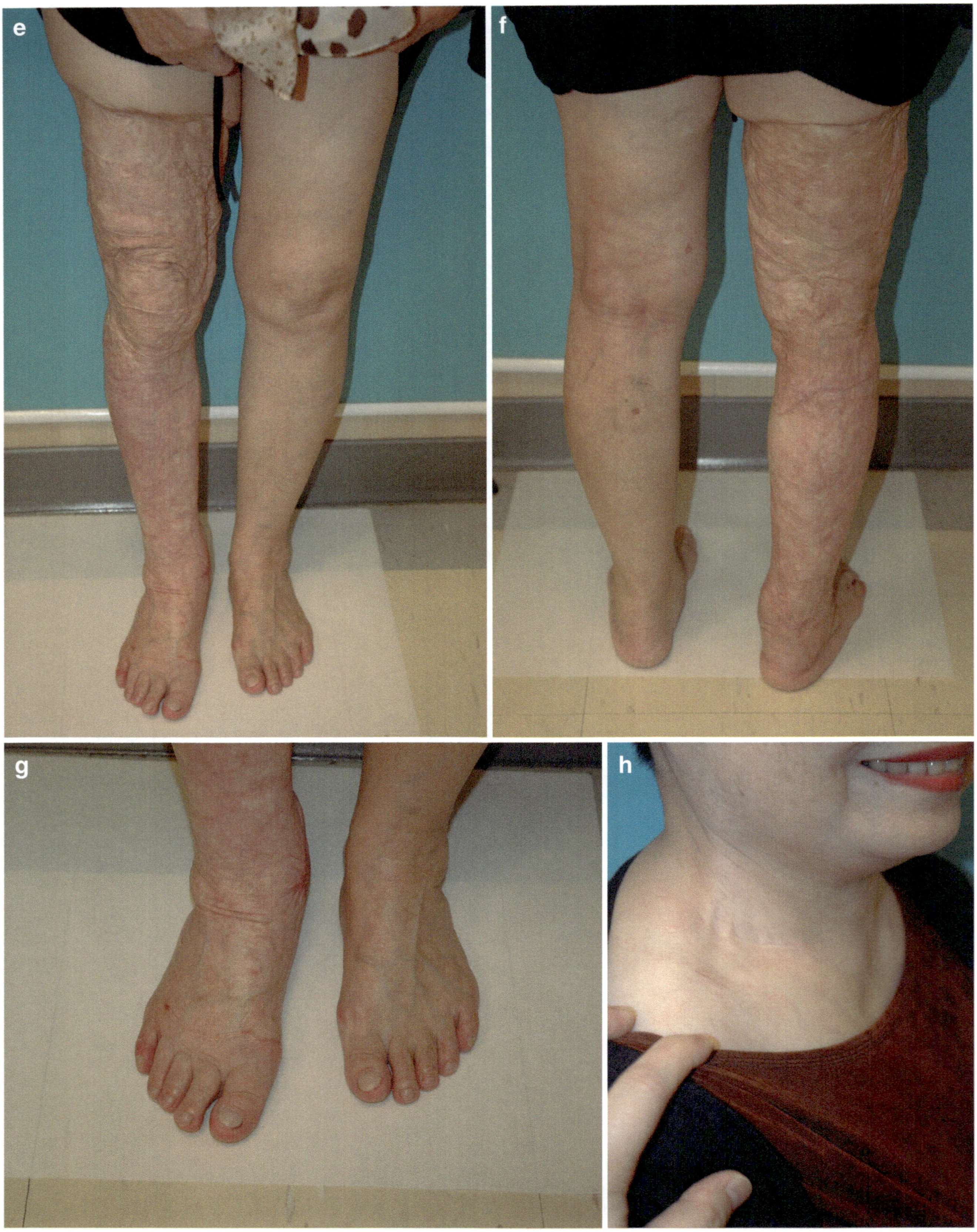

Fig. 22.2 (continued)

reluctant to use it as part of their treatment algorithm [15]. However, in HCC Stage IV disease (Table 22.2), the extent of tissue fibrosis vastly reduces the likelihood of any success with other techniques (including liposuction or any attempt at LVA). In these cases, a modified Charles procedure may be indicated to not only reduce the burden of the tissue for the patient but also to prevent the repeated cycle of cellulitis and infections. For the patient who is prepared to accept the recovery and end-aesthetic result, this procedure can be dramatic in improving the functional use of the limb and quality of life. Case series photographs are shown in Fig. 22.3.

Surgical Technique

- One week prior to surgery, patients are advised to optimize foot hygiene, regular washing and elevation of the affected limb.
- On admission, standard limb measurements are taken.
- A multi-surgeon approach is required to ensure that excision can be safely completed within the tourniquet time.
- Markings are dictated by extent of involved tissue and discussions with the patient on the proximal limit of excision.
- In general:
  - One limb is operated on at a time.
  - The surgery is performed as a single stage.
  - Pre-operative antibiotics are given as standard.
  - Medial and lateral wedge excisions are marked vertically at the proximal thigh terminating in a transverse circumferential incision. These will allow subcutaneous debulking and smooth the transition from normal tissue to the excised and grafted area. Distal to this point, the tissue is planned for circumferential excision down to the foot, but preserving the heel, plantar foot and web spaces between the toes. Should there be less disease above-knee, or as per the patient wishes, excision can be limited to below-knee.
  - The first step is to harvest long split-thickness grafts from the entire affected limb using an air/electric-powered dermatome (taken at 12/1000th inch).
  - The limb is exsanguinated and excision is begun under tourniquet control (350–375 mmHg).

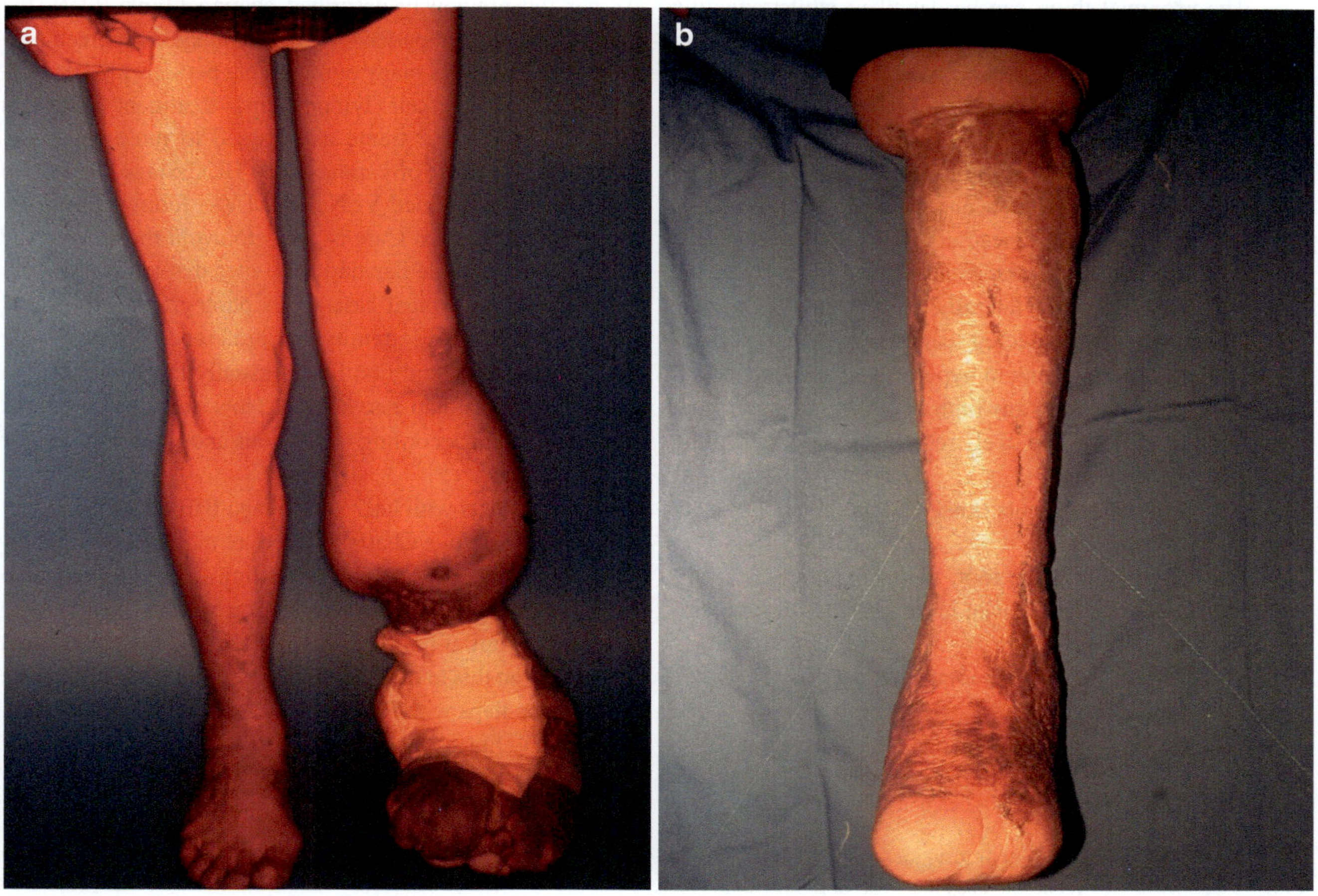

Fig. 22.3 (**a**) This is a case of advanced lymphedema presenting with repetitive infective episodes and destruction of toes in a 41-year-old male. The lymphedema was due to trauma accompanied by prolonged infection. (**b**) A modified Charles procedure was done with amputation of all toes. This is the ultimate solution for the most severe lymphedema. The patient had no more infections after the radical surgery

- Excision proceeds full thickness down to the deep fascia, from the circumferential thigh incision to the toes.
- Care should be taken to preserve the great saphenous vein and its major branches – this forms an important part of the modified technique [16].
- The deep fascia is often thickened and abnormal, so it should be thinned to normal limits.
- Once the anterior excision is complete, a 3-mm pin can be inserted into the tibia to allow elevation of the limb for posterior excision and also elevation of the grafted limb in the ward. Removal of the pin can be done at the bedside after ensuring grafts are well taken.
- For the foot, the toes may require amputation if prone to recurrent and severe infections, proven osteomyelitis, or verrucous hyperkeratosis (as per HCC Stage IVB). Otherwise, removal of nail plate and nail beds with coverage by C-V rotation-advancement flaps is appropriate to preserve length. Minimal trimming of the distal phalanx can be undertaken to allow tension-free soft tissue closure. The algorithm for toe management is presented in Table 22.3 [17–19].
- Adrenaline soaks and compressive bandaging are applied.
- The proximal thigh can be debulked whilst awaiting haemostasis. The mid-axial wedge excisions are undermined circumferentially and going proximally around 10 cm. The resulting anterior/posterior thigh flaps are thinned tangentially to around 2 cm and sutured together, down to the deep fascia.
- Once haemostasis has been achieved, the limb is resurfaced with the fenestrated split-thickness grafts, ensuring horizontal placement of the grafts with the free edges meeting laterally with 1 cm of overlap. Avoiding medial/inner leg seams is important, particularly in patients prone to hypertrophic scarring. Small overlap accounts for any limb swelling and gap formation that would more likely result in secondary healing and poor scarring.
- All grafts around joints (knee and ankle) should meet laterally.
- For the dorsum of the foot, in our experience, a full-thickness graft has proven more resistant to problematic scarring and hyperkeratosis (due to friction with compression garments or footwear).
- Non-adherent dressings, gauze, compression wrapping and a posterior Plaster-of-Paris splint are subsequently applied.
- Elevation of the limb (aided by the tibial pin) is important to avoid shearing and graft loss.

Table 22.3 Management of toes in advanced lymphedema

Stage	Infection	Treatment
HCC-stage IVA	No	Nail plate removal
HCC-stage IVA	Yes	Nail plate + bed removal
HCC-stage IVB	Yes	Removal of 2–4 toes (or all toes if no request to keep the great toe)

HCC Hung-Chi Chen Staging

Therapeutic Liposuction

Liposuction plays an integral adjunctive role in the surgical treatment of lymphedema patients, particularly in HCC Stage II and III disease (Fig. 22.4). It may be used alone but more commonly is used in combination with other surgical procedures. It has an important role in potentially reducing the lymphatic loading of the affected limb, allowing improved functioning of the residual lymphatics and/or reconstructive drainage procedures such as LVA and VLNT.

Combined Procedures

As per the previously described staging (Table 22.2), the majority of surgical patients we treat undergo combined procedures. This serves many purposes but perhaps most importantly completes their lymphedema treatment within a relatively short time frame as opposed to multiple procedures. The majority of patients with HCC Stage III disease will undergo combined VLNT and LVA, followed by liposuction 10 days later. Care is taken to avoid the sites of the previous lymph node flap and LVA sites that are marked out pre-operatively. Typical case-series photographs are shown in Fig. 22.4. For the extremity, our preference is now double lymph node flaps, and first line is usually laparoscopic gastroepiploic VLN flap harvest [6]. However, donor options can be modified according to previous abdominal surgery or patient preference.

Some patients with later HCC Stage IIIB disease that will likely culminate in a Charles procedure may be better candidates for initial RRPP to the lower limb with liposuction to the thigh. A decision can be made on whether to combine this with an initial lymph node flap, and we have published previously on this to include the use of double gastroepiploic lymph node flaps with RRPP in advanced lymphedema [20].

For HCC Stage IV disease, we generally find that a radical excision (modified Charles procedure), with treatment of toes, is indicated. However, we would still consider primary VLNT in these cases followed by later excision. Clearly, with the extent of tissue fibrosis and occlusion of lymphatic ducts, there is little scope for LVA.

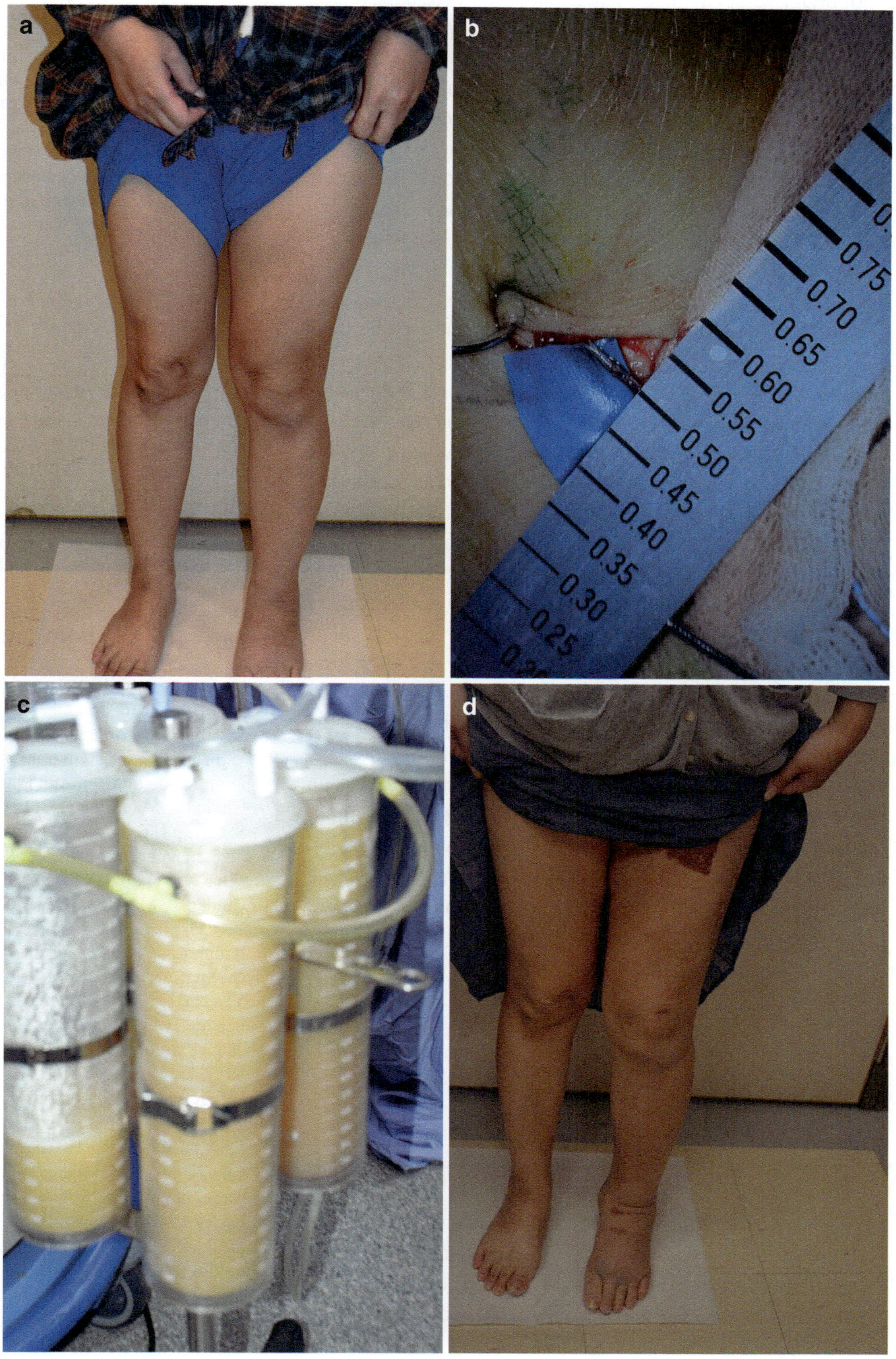

Fig. 22.4 (**a**) For moderate lymphedema (without fibrotic change of soft tissue as measured by tonometry), the patient does not need a modified Charles procedure. This is a 43-year-old female patient with previous cervical cancer. The left lower limb developed progressive swelling, but she did not have a history of cellulitis. Pre-operative picture is shown. (**b**) She was treated with lymphaticovenular anastomosis (LVA) at the dorsum of the left foot and lymph node flap transfer to the medial side of the left ankle. This was the LVA performed at the dorsum of the left foot. The gastroepiploic lymph node flap was harvested laparoscopically in this patient. (**c**) Ten days later, extensive therapeutic liposuction lipectomy was done to decrease the lymphatic loading of the left lower limb. For this patient, a modified Charles procedure was not necessary. (**d**) The swelling gradually subsided. This was the picture taken at 6 months after surgery

Complications

The majority of cases are uncomplicated, and to date, we have not experienced any donor extremity lymphedema, intra-abdominal harvest complications or microvascular lymph node flap loss. However, we did have rare cases of lymphorrhea or seroma from donor sites or at sites where lymph node flaps had been placed; this can be reduced by careful dissection and direct microscopic visualization and ligation of lymph channels. Also of note is that when using the gastroepiploic lymph node flap (particularly when taken as an omental flap), it may be a less suitable bed for skin graft take and may rarely need re-grafting for partial take.

Special Indications

The majority of lymphedema cases that clinicians encounter will be secondary to prior oncological treatment; however, an important subset may be due to other acquired or congenital pathology. Worldwide, the commonest adult cause of lymphedema remains filariasis, and, where facilities allow, many of these patients can successfully be treated by combinations of VLNT and excisional procedures [21].

The presentation of congenital lymphedema may be mild and go unnoticed for some time; conversely, it may be detected in utero due to gross limb abnormalities and associated systemic manifestations. In a lymphedema practice, one should expect to encounter such patients and be able to offer solutions. Milroy disease, classically described as presenting with unilateral lymphedema (but often also bilateral), may be successfully treated with lymph node flaps followed by therapeutic liposuction [22]. Treatment can occur in childhood/adolescence depending on severity. Klippel-Trenaunay syndrome may have a vast array of clinical features other than the cutaneous manifestations, including not only limb hypertrophy but also significant intra-abdominal pathology with potential bleeding tendencies. For the extremity, hypertrophy with lymphedema may be aided by lymph node flaps but will almost certainly require excisional procedures such as the modified Charles procedure when severe. Other more unusual cases include the treatment of abdominal distension due to chylous ascites with vascularized lymphatic cable flaps (based on the deep inferior epigastric vascular system) [23]; however, one can safely adopt treatment algorithms for any cause of lymphedema, whether it be congenital or acquired [24].

Pearls and Pitfalls

- For most surgical patients, combination surgery is required.
- When excising lymphedematous tissue to place extremity lymph node flaps, meticulous dissection and lymph channel ligation are needed to avoid lymphorrhea.
- In all cases of VLN flap transfer, the pocket should be slightly over-sized.
- For intra-abdominal flap harvest, it is important to have a good working relationship with general surgical teams to ensure refinement of techniques and atraumatic vascular pedicle dissection.
- The modified Charles procedure, if carried out carefully, can achieve good results. Re-grafting is sometimes required for the foot and distal leg if verrucous hyperkeratosis occurs years later.

References

1. International Society of Lymphology Executive Committee. The diagnosis and treatment of peripheral lymphedema. Lymphology. 1995;28:113–7.
2. International Society of Lymphology. The diagnosis and treatment of peripheral lymphedema: 2013 Consensus Document of the International Society of Lymphology. Lymphology. 2013;46(1)
3. Chen HC, Liem A, Karonidis A, Karri V, Tang Y-B. Surgical Treatment and Algorithm for Lymphoedema. Elsevier Taiwan LLC; 2011.
4. Ciudad P, Kiranantawat K, Sapountzis S, Yeo MS, Nicoli FA, Maruccia MI, Sirimahachaiyakul P, Chen HC. Right gastroepiploic lymph node flap. Microsurgery. 2015;35(06):496–7.
5. Ciudad P, Maruccia M, Socas J, Lee MH, Chung KP, Constantinescu T, Kiranantawat K, Nicoli F, Sapountzis S, Yeo MS, Chen HC. The laparoscopic right gastroepiploic lymph node flap transfer for upper and lower limb lymphedema: technique and outcomes. Microsurgery. 2017;37(3):197–205.
6. Ciudad P, Manrique OJ, Date S, Agko M, Perez Coca JJ, Chang WL, Lo Torto F, Nicoli F, Maruccia M, López Mendoza J, Chen HC. Double gastroepiploic vascularized lymph node tranfers to middle and distal limb for the treatment of lymphedema. Microsurgery. 2017;37(7):771–9.
7. Di Taranto G, Chen SH, Elia R, Bolletta A, Amorosi V, Sitpahul N, Chan JC, Ribuffo D, Chen HC. Free gastroepiploic lymph nodes and omentum flap for treatment of lower limb ulcers in severe lymphedema: killing two birds with one stone. J Surg Oncol. 2020;121(1):168–74.
8. Sapountzis S, Singhal D, Rashid A, Meo D, Chen HC. Lymph node flap based on the right transverse cervical artery as a donor site for lymph node transfer. Ann Plast Surg. 2014;73(4):398–401.
9. Ciudad P, Manrique OJ, Date S, Chang WL, Nicoli F, Sapountzis S, Cheng HT, Agko M, Chen HC. Vascularized appendicular lymph node transfer for treatment of extremity lymphedema: a case report. Microsurgery. 2018;38(5):553–7.
10. Ciudad P, Manrique OJ, Agko M, Liu EW, Chang WL, Sze-Wei Yeo M, Huang TC, Chilgar RM, Chen HC. Ileocecal vascularized lymph node transfer for the treatment of extremity lymphedema: a case report. Microsurgery. 2019;39(1):81–4.
11. Visconti G, Constantinescu T, Araki J, Salgarello M, Chen HC. The venous lymph node flap for the treatment of peripheral lymphedema: preliminary evidence. Microsurgery. 2017;37(1):86–7.
12. Salgado CJ, Mardini S, Spanio S, Tang WR, Sassu P, Chen HC. Radical reduction of lymphedema with preservation of perforators. Ann Plast Surg. 2007;59(2):173–9.
13. Salgado CJ, Sassu P, Gharb BB, Di Spilimbergo SS, Mardini S, Chen HC. Radical reduction of upper extremity lymphedema with preservation of perforators. Ann Plast Surg. 2009;63(3):302–6.
14. Charles RH. The surgical technique and operative treatment of elephantiasis of the generative organs based on a series of 140 consecutive successful cases. Ind Med Gaz. 1901;36:84.
15. Miller TA. Charles procedure for lymphedema: a warning. Am J Surg. 1980;139(2):290–2.
16. Sapountzis S, Ciudad P, Lim SY, Chilgar RM, Kiranantawat K, Nicoli F, Constantinides J, Wei MY, Sönmez TT, Singhal D, Chen HC. Modified Charles procedure and lymph node flap transfer for advanced lower extremity lymphedema. Microsurgery. 2014;34(6):439–47.
17. Ciudad P, Agko M, Huang TC, Manrique OJ, Chang WL, Nicoli F, Maruccia M, Lo Torto F, Chen HC. Comprehensive multimodal surgical treatment of end-stage lower extremity lymphedema with toe management: the combined Charles', Homan's, and vascularized lymph node transfer (CHAHOVA) procedures. J Surg Oncol. 2019;119(4):430–8.

18. Karonidis A, Chen HC. Preservation of toes in advanced lymphedema: an important step in the control of infection. Ann Plast Surg. 2010;64(4):446–50.
19. Chen HC, Gharb BB, Salgado CJ, Rampazzo A, Xu E, Di Spilimbergo SS, Su S. Elective amputation of the toes in severe lymphedema of the lower leg: rationale and indications. Ann Plast Surg. 2009;63(2):193–7.
20. Ciudad P, Manrique OJ, Adabi K, Huang TC, Agko M, Trignano E, Chang WL, Chen TW, Salgado CJ, Chen HC. Combined double vascularized lymph node transfers and modified radical reduction with preservation of perforators for advanced stages of lymphedema. J Surg Oncol. 2019;119(4):439–48.
21. Chilgar RM, Khade S, Chen HC, Ciudad P, Yeo MS, Kiranantawat K, Maruccia M, Li K, Zhang YX, Nicoli F. Surgical treatment of advanced lymphatic filariasis of lower extremity combining vascularized lymph node transfer and excisional procedures. Lymphat Res Biol. 2019;17(6):637–46.
22. Bolletta A, Di Taranto G, Chen SH, Elia R, Amorosi V, Chan JC, Chen HC. Surgical treatment of Milroy disease. J Surg Oncol. 2020 Jan;121(1):175–81.
23. Chen SH, Yeh LF, Chen HC. Successful surgical treatment of intractable chylous ascites using the lymphatic cable flap: a retrospective review study. World J Surg. 2017;41(12):3100–4.
24. Sabbagh MD, Agko M, Huang TC, Manrique OJ, Román C, Reynaga C, Delgado R, Maruccia M, Chen HC. Surgical management of lower extremity lymphedema: a comprehensive review. Indian J Plast Surg. 2019;52(01):081–92.

Step-by-Step Instruction: Immediate Lymphatic Reconstruction for Lymphedema Risk Reduction in Breast Cancer Management

23

Melisa D. Granoff, Ryoko Hamaguchi, and Dhruv Singhal

Introduction

Breast cancer-related lymphedema (BCRL) will affect one in five of the over 3.5 million breast cancer survivors in the United States [1]. Patients are at increased risk for the development of this disease if they have undergone axillary lymph node dissection (ALND) and regional lymph node radiation (RLNR), although many other risk factors have been described [1, 2]. The standard of care for BCRL is palliative in nature, focusing mostly on compression, manual lymphatic drainage (MLD), and other physical therapy techniques. In recent years, microsurgical techniques to reconstruct lymphatic function, often called physiologic procedures, have become more popular, including vascularized lymph node transplant (VLNT) and lymphovenous bypass (LVB) [3]. Similarly, liposuction has been demonstrated to be effective in reducing the fat hypertrophy often present with BCRL [4, 5]. However, while good results have been reported from all of these procedures, none are curative [6]. Therefore, the focus on preventive approaches to lymphedema remain critical. Immediate lymphatic reconstruction (ILR), originally described as the LYmphatic Microsurgical Preventive Healing Approach (LYMPHA), is one technique that has demonstrated potential to reduce the risk of developing BCRL [7–10].

Supplementary Information The online version of this chapter (https://doi.org/10.1007/978-3-030-93039-4_23) contains supplementary material, which is available to authorized users.

M. D. Granoff · D. Singhal (✉)
Boston Lymphatic Center, Division of Plastic and Reconstructive Surgery, Beth Israel Deaconess Medical Center, Harvard Medical School, Boston, MA, USA
e-mail: dsinghal@bidmc.harvard.edu

R. Hamaguchi
Harvard Medical School, Boston, MA, USA

Typical Indications

- Breast cancer patients undergoing ALND.
- Although we do not have a minimum body mass index (BMI) requirement, Boccardo et al. requires a BMI >30 to be considered a surgical candidate [11]. If a patient has a BMI <30, they are still eligible for ILR if their transport index on lymphoscintigraphy is ≥10.

Anatomy

Familiarity with the nerves and veins of the axilla is important when performing ILR (Fig. 23.1). Veins that can be identified in the axilla include the accessory vein, which is most often used for the lymphovenous anastomosis (LVA) in our experience, as well as the medial pectoral, lateral thoracic, thoracodorsal, and serratus branch of the thoracodorsal vein. The accessory vein is most often found 2 cm anterior to the thoracodorsal nerve. In some patients, the accessory vein has been sacrificed during the ALND or is otherwise not available. This vein has been found suitable for use 59% of the time according to our internal data.

Nerves in the axilla include the intercostobrachial, long thoracic, and thoracodorsal nerves. Regarding ILR, the intercostobrachial nerve most often crosses anteriorly across the accessory vein and thus is most at risk for injury during isolation of this vein.

Patient Selection

Surgical Candidacy

Patients are candidates for ILR if they are undergoing ALND as part of their breast cancer surgical therapy. Due to the nature of a breast cancer cohort with nodal disease, these patients have also often undergone neoadjuvant chemotherapy

M. V. Schaverien, J. H. Dayan (eds.), *Multimodal Management of Upper and Lower Extremity Lymphedema*,
https://doi.org/10.1007/978-3-030-93039-4_23

Fig. 23.1 Axillary anatomy

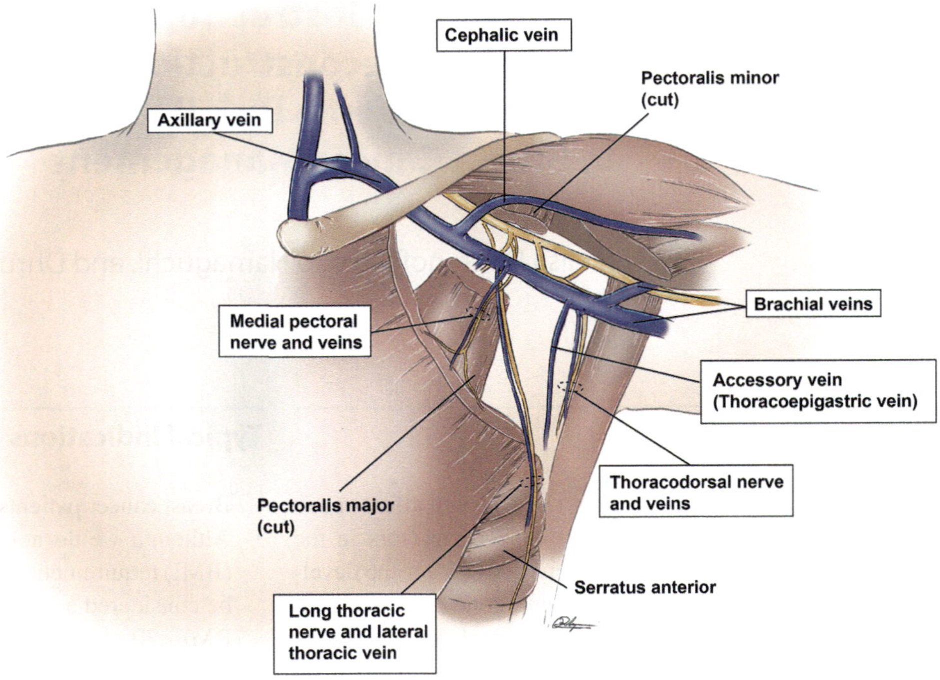

and are likely to require adjuvant RLNR. Aside from the patient's ability to safely undergo an ALND, there are no other specific exclusion criteria used at our institution.

Preoperative Measurements

All patients must undergo baseline lymphedema measurements with a Certified Lymphedema Therapist (CLT) preoperatively [12]. Baseline measurements include L-Dex (ImpediMed, California, USA), perometry, and limb circumferential measurements. These three measurement modalities are taken to establish a baseline with which to compare postoperative measurements. Patients also complete subjective metrics of disease preoperatively, specifically the Lymphoedema Quality of Life Questionnaire (LYMQOL) and the Short-Form (SF-36) Health Survey. The LYMQOL is validated for use in patients with chronic lymphedema and evaluates domains including function, appearance, symptoms, and mood [13]. The instrument includes a self-reported measure where patients are asked to rate their quality of life from 0 (poor) to 10 (excellent). Patients complete this survey preoperatively to establish a baseline should they develop lymphedema in the future. The SF-36 assesses health-related limitations or exacerbations in eight domains: physical activities, social activities, usual roles (physical and emotional), bodily pain, mental health, vitality, and general health [14].

Preoperative Indocyanine Green (ICG) Lymphography

Preoperative indocyanine green (ICG) lymphography is performed to establish a baseline of each patient's lymphatic anatomy prior to surgical intervention. In the case that the patient develops lymphedema postoperatively, the preoperative lymphogram can be referenced by CLTs for optimal planning of MLD along the patient's known lymphatic pathways. Lymphography is performed by intradermal injection of 0.1 cc stock ICG (Akorn Inc., Illinois, USA) with albumin in the first and fourth web spaces, the distal third of the volar forearm, and over the cephalic vein 4 cm proximal to the antecubital crease. A near-infrared (NIR) imaging device, the PDE-Neo II (Hamamatsu Photonics KK, Hamamatsu, Japan), is used for visualization.

Operative Technique (see supplementary material)

- Position the patient supine with the operative extremity abducted at a 90-degree angle.
- Palpate the brachial artery to identify its location.
- Immediately prior to the start of the ALND, inject 0.25 cc 2% fluorescein isothiocyanate (FITC) solution with albumin into the medial upper arm at two sites 4 cm apart, as well as 0.25 cc at the level of the muscle fascia at each site (total 1 cc injection) [15]. Take care to avoid the brachial artery.

- Use ultrasound localization to identify the cephalic vein [16]. Inject 1 cc isosulfan blue into the skin and deep soft tissues 4 cm proximal to the elbow crease over the vein [17]. Take care to avoid an intra-vascular injection of the dye.
- Incisions for the ALND include the mastectomy incision versus a counter-incision in the axilla. The choice of access is most often dictated by the breast surgeon. If the counter-incision is made in the axilla, the breast surgeon often places this incision at the inferior aspect of the axillary hairline.
- Following completion of the ALND, note the length and location of available veins (e.g., accessory, thoracodorsal, lateral thoracic, medial pectoral) including the presence or absence of valves. Note the location of the intercostobrachial nerve, thoracodorsal nerve, and long thoracic nerve (Fig. 23.1).
- Confirm that an adequate vein is available. Confirm the absence of venous back bleeding. If an adequate vein is not available anywhere in the field, the ILR will need to be aborted.
- Visualize the axilla through a MM51 Mitaka Microscope (Colorado, USA) with a 560-nm filter activated to confirm dye flow through the lymphatic channels.
- Mobilize the targeted vein and position it adjacent to the target lymphatic channel(s).
- Given that there is often a lymphatic to vein size mismatch, we most commonly perform an anastomosis between the vein and one or more lymphatics utilizing the intussusception technique.
- Pexy the target vein adjacent to the lymphatic channel utilizing backwall sutures (Fig. 23.2).
- Place a U-stitch through the anterior wall of the vein and the lymphatic channel. Guide the lymphatic channel into the vein as tension is placed on the sutures exiting the anterior wall of the vein (Fig. 23.3).
- Sutures are placed from the front wall of the vein to the soft tissues above the lymphatic channel (Fig. 23.4).
- Remove the U-stitch.
- Visualize patency by looking for FITC in the vein via the 560-nm filter.
- Wrap a fat graft around the anastomosis. Secure with a triple stitch (Fig. 23.5).
- Place a #15 Blake drain into the axilla (avoiding the anastomosis) and secure with a 2–0 silk suture.

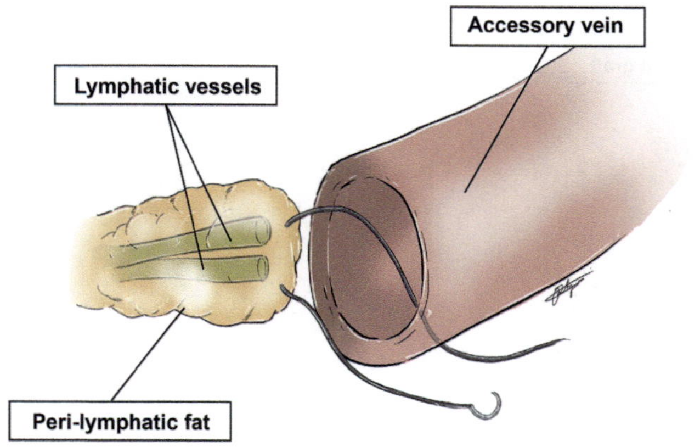

Fig. 23.2 Accessory vein with backwall sutures

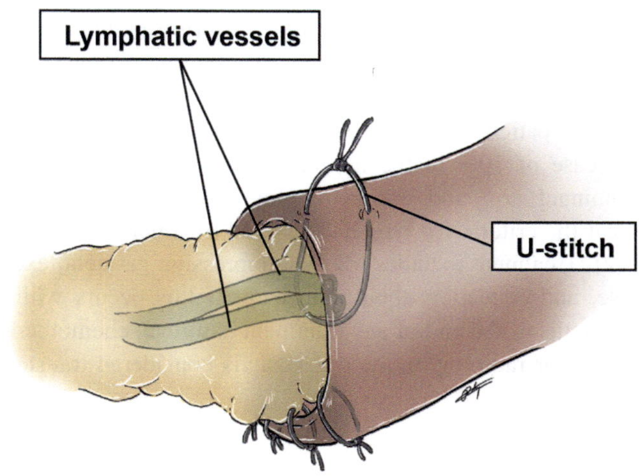

Fig. 23.3 U-stitch

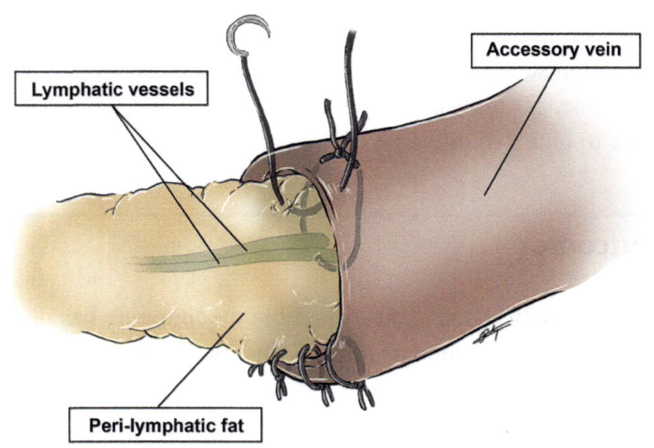

Fig. 23.4 Front wall stitch

Postoperative Care

Patients are seen in the surgical clinic 2 weeks postoperatively. The drain can be removed after the output is less than 20 cc/day for two consecutive days. This can be done in postoperative follow-up with the breast or lymphatic surgery service. Patients are then seen for postoperative surveillance visits with CLTs at 4 weeks and then every 3 months for

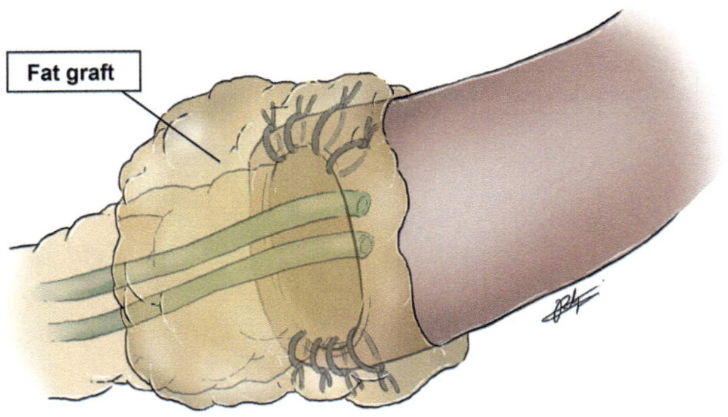

Fig. 23.5 Fat graft

2 years. At each surveillance visit, perometry, L-Dex, and circumferential measurements are taken. The patients also complete the LYMQOL and SF-36 at 3 months, 6 months, and then annually. After 2 years without the development of lymphedema, patients are surveilled every 6 months for an additional 2 years, for a total of 4 years postoperative surveillance.

If a patient develops either an L-Dex >10 or volume increase of 10% in the dominant arm or 7% in the non-dominant arm and has symptoms of lymphedema, they meet the criteria for lymphedema and treatment is initiated [12]. Treatment includes MLD, compression garment, exercise, and education about skin care. If this occurs within 6 months of the end of any treatment (surgical, chemotherapeutic, or radiologic), the diagnosis is considered transient lymphedema.

Complications

Complications are rare and include local skin reactions and anaphylaxis to isosulfan blue dye. To prevent anaphylaxis, we administer prophylaxis to all patients with 100 mg hydrocortisone, 50 mg diphenhydramine, and 20 mg famotidine prior to blue dye injection [18].

Outcomes

As previously stated, data reported in the literature has demonstrated good outcomes from this procedure. A recent meta-analysis reports that in patients who have undergone ALND, incidence of BCRL went from 14.1% without ILR to 2.1% with ILR, and in those who underwent ALND and RLNR, 33.4% to 10.3% [1]. At our institution, the incidence of BCRL diagnosed in all patients who have undergone ILR is 5.6% [12].

ILR is not only effective but also cost-effective. In a recent cost-utility analysis, the cost utility of ILR in patients undergoing ALND and in patients undergoing ALND with RLNR was evaluated. In both the patients who underwent ALND and those who underwent ALND with RLNR, the addition of ILR was more cost-effective, with incremental cost-utility ratios (ICURs) of $1587.73/quality of life year (QALY) and $699.84/QALY, respectively [19].

Pearls and Pitfalls

- Collaboration with the Breast Surgery Service is critical to overall success.
  - Preoperatively, identify appropriate surgical candidates in collaboration with the Breast Surgery Service.
  - Intraoperatively, work with the breast surgeons to preserve suitable veins.
- ILR requires multidisciplinary planning and execution. Before offering this procedure, be sure that a surveillance team and protocol are in place, with clear instructions to patients and appropriate personnel for long-term follow-up.

References

1. Johnson AR, Kimball S, Epstein S, Recht A, Lin SJ, Lee BT, et al. Lymphedema Incidence After Axillary Lymph Node Dissection: Quantifying the Impact of Radiation and the Lymphatic Microsurgical Preventive Healing Approach. Ann Plast Surg. 2019;82(4S Suppl 3):S234–41.
2. Johnson AR, Singhal D. Immediate lymphatic reconstruction. J Surg Oncol. 2018;
3. Basta MN, Gao LL, Wu LC. Operative treatment of peripheral lymphedema: a systematic meta-analysis of the efficacy and safety of lymphovenous microsurgery and tissue transplantation. Plast Reconstr Surg. 2014;133(4):905–13.
4. Brorson H, Svensson H. Complete reduction of lymphoedema of the arm by liposuction after breast cancer. Scand J Plast Reconstr Surg Hand Surg. 1997;31(2):137–43.
5. Brorson H, Svensson H. Liposuction combined with controlled compression therapy reduces arm lymphedema more effectively than controlled compression therapy alone. Plast Reconstr Surg. 1998;102(4):1058–67; discussion 1068.
6. Johnson AR, Bravo MG, Granoff MD, Kang CO, Critchlow JF, Tsai LL, et al. Flow-through omental flap for vascularized lymph node transfer: a novel surgical approach for delayed lymphatic reconstruction. Plast Reconstr Surg Glob Open. 2019;7(9):e2436.
7. Boccardo F, Casabona F, De Cian F, Friedman D, Villa G, Bogliolo S, et al. Lymphedema microsurgical preventive healing approach: a new technique for primary prevention of arm lymphedema after mastectomy. Ann Surg Oncol. 2009;16(3):703–8.
8. Feldman S, Bansil H, Ascherman J, Grant R, Borden B, Henderson P, et al. Single institution experience with Lymphatic Microsurgical Preventive Healing Approach (LYMPHA) for the primary prevention of lymphedema. Ann Surg Oncol. 2015;22(10):3296–301.
9. Hahamoff M, Gupta N, Munoz D, Lee BT, Clevenger P, Shaw C, et al. A lymphedema surveillance program for breast cancer patients reveals the promise of surgical prevention. J Surg Res. 2018;
10. Johnson AR, Fleishman A, Granoff MD, Shillue K, Houlihan MJ, Sharma R, et al. Evaluating the impact of immediate lymphatic

reconstruction for the surgical prevention of lymphedema. Plast Reconstr Surg. 2020;
11. Boccardo F, Casabona F, De Cian F, DeCian F, Friedman D, Murelli F, et al. Lymphatic microsurgical preventing healing approach (LYMPHA) for primary surgical prevention of breast cancer-related lymphedema: over 4 years follow-up. Microsurgery. 2014;34(6):421–4.
12. Johnson A, Fleishman A, Tran BN, Shillue K, Carroll B, Tsai L, et al. Developing a lymphatic surgery program: a first-year review. Plast Reconstr Surg [Internet]. 2019[cited 2020 Apr 24];144(6). Available from: insights.ovid.com
13. Keeley V, Crooks S, Locke J, Veigas D, Riches K, Hilliam R. A quality of life measure for limb lymphoedema (LYMQOL). J Lymphoedema. 2010;5(1):26–37.
14. McHorney CA, Ware JE, Raczek AE. The MOS 36-Item Short-Form Health Survey (SF-36): II. Psychometric and clinical tests of validity in measuring physical and mental health constructs. Med Care. 1993;31(3):247–63.
15. Spiguel L, Shaw C, Katz A, Guo L, Chen H-C, Lee BT, et al. Fluorescein isothiocyanate: a novel application for lymphatic surgery. Ann Plast Surg. 2017;78(6S Suppl 5):S296–8.
16. Johnson AR, Granoff MD, Suami H, Lee BT, Singhal D. Real-time visualization of the Mascagni-Sappey pathway utilizing ICG lymphography. Cancers. 2020;12(5):1195.
17. Johnson AR, Bravo MG, James TA, Suami H, Lee BT, Singhal D. The all but forgotten Mascagni-Sappey pathway: learning from immediate lymphatic reconstruction. J Reconstr Microsurg. 2020;36(1):28–31.
18. Raut CP, Hunt KK, Akins JS, Daley MD, Ross MI, Singletary SE, et al. Incidence of anaphylactoid reactions to isosulfan blue dye during breast carcinoma lymphatic mapping in patients treated with preoperative prophylaxis. Cancer. 2005;104(4):692–9.
19. Johnson AR, Asban A, Granoff MD, Kang CO, Lee BT, Chatterjee A, et al. Is immediate lymphatic reconstruction cost-effective? Ann Surg. 2019;

Key Topic: Evidence-Based Outcomes of Lymphedema Microsurgery

24

Mark V. Schaverien and Joseph H. Dayan

Background

Surgical options for the treatment of lymphedema include lymphovenous bypass (LVB), vascularized lymph node transplant (VLNT), suction-assisted lipectomy (SAL), direct excision, as well as combinations of these physiological and debulking procedures [1–3]. The evidence base supporting the effectiveness of surgery at treating lymphedema is informed by systematic reviews and meta-analyses, a randomized-controlled trial (RCT), and prospective and retrospective cohort and comparative studies. Primary outcomes for these surgical procedures included change in limb circumference or volume excess, lymphedema symptom reduction, patient-reported outcomes (PROs) and health-related quality of life (HRQoL), lymphedema-related cellulitis, and complications. There is also growing evidence supporting the efficacy of immediate lymphatic reconstruction (ILR) at the time of axillary lymphadenectomy for breast cancer treatment at reducing the risk of lymphedema. Three systematic reviews compared outcomes of different surgical treatments for chronic lymphedema:

- A systematic review evaluated outcomes of LVB, VLNT, SAL debulking, excisional procedures, and combined surgical procedures [4]. A search of PubMed-MEDLINE, Cochrane Library databases, Embase, Scopus, and Web of Science from January 2000 to May 2016 was conducted. Two reviewers independently reviewed 4144 abstracts, and 69 studies were included. Studies were scored using the Methodological Index for NOnRandomized Studies (MINORS) scoring system, and 39 studies were found to be high quality through these criteria (12 LVB, ten VLNT, four liposuction debulking, five excisional procedures, and eight combined surgical procedures), scoring >12/16 or >19/24, with loss to follow-up the most common cause of low scores. Overall, the mean volume reduction was 33.1% [95% confidence interval (CI): 14.4–51.9%] for LVB, 26.4% (95% CI: – 7.98–60.8%) for VLNT, and 96.6% (95% CI: 86.2–107%) for liposuction debulking
- A systematic review and meta-analysis of the efficacy and safety of LVB and VLNT was performed, searching Ovid MEDLINE and then rating studies on methodological quality based on the American Society of Plastic Surgeons (ASPS) Evidence Rating Scale for Therapeutic Studies [5]. In total, 27 studies were included, three with level III and 24 with level IV evidence; ten concerned upper extremity outcomes, 11 lower extremity, and five examined both. LVB procedures were the subject of 22 studies and five concerned VLNT – of these, 20 studies were suitable for meta-analysis. Overall, the study population consisted of 1619 patients with a mean follow-up among all studies of 3.3 years. Studies reporting change in volume demonstrated reduction in excess volume by 56.6% (±9.1), and absolute volume reduction was 23.6% (±2.1). Overall limb excess circumference was reduced by 48.8% (±6.0), and absolute circumference was reduced by 3.3 cm (±0.73). Overall, 11.8% had no improvement in their lymphedema postoperatively. Subjective improvement was reported by 91.2% of patients, and 64.8% of patients discontinued compression garments at follow-up. Patients that underwent VLNT reported a greater subjective improvement than those that received LVB (100% versus 89.2%, respectively) and were more likely to discontinue compression garments (78% versus 56.3%, respectively; $p = 0.04$). Overall complications included surgical site infection in 4.7%, lymphorrhea in 7.7%, and reexploration for flap congestion in 2.7%. The authors

M. V. Schaverien (✉)
Department of Plastic Surgery, The University of Texas MD Anderson Cancer Center, Houston, TX, USA
e-mail: mvschaverien@mdanderson.org

J. H. Dayan (✉)
Division of Plastic and Reconstructive Surgery, Memorial Sloan Kettering Cancer Center, New York, NY, USA
e-mail: dayanj@mskcc.org

M. V. Schaverien, J. H. Dayan (eds.), *Multimodal Management of Upper and Lower Extremity Lymphedema*, https://doi.org/10.1007/978-3-030-93039-4_24

noted that although complication rates were higher for VLNT, a reporting bias likely contributed to this finding as these studies reported complications whereas several LVB studies did not.

- A systematic review of cellulitis outcomes following lymphedema surgery, including LVB, VLNT, or SAL debulking, was performed by searching the Embase, MEDLINE, and Cochrane databases to January 2016 [6]. In total, 25 studies were included: two case-control studies, 17 case series, and six case reports. Studies ranged between four and five on the Oxford Centre for Evidence-Based Medicine (CEBM) quality rating scale. All studies (LVB, $n = 9$; VLNT, $n = 5$; SAL, $n = 2$) reported a decrease in the incidence of cellulitis. One study compared outcomes of VLNT with a control group and found a reduction in lymphedema incidence. Limitations of the studies reviewed included retrospective study design in some of the included studies and low follow-up rates.

Lymphovenous Bypass (LVB) Procedure

Available literature evaluating LVB as a surgical intervention for the treatment of lymphedema includes systematic reviews and prospective studies. Studies reporting outcomes of both upper and lower extremity lymphedema consistently demonstrated a reduction in limb volume and circumferential measurements, with greater mean limb volume excess reductions reported in earlier compared with later stage lymphedema. There is heterogeneity in the measurement modalities used between different studies but consistency within individual studies, most often using limb circumferential measurements or water-displacement plethysmography. In all studies assessing these outcomes, reductions were found in mean limb volume, lymphedema-specific symptoms, and cellulitis incidence, with all studies reporting a decrease in the mean number of infections postoperatively. Improvement in functional assessment and patient-reported QoL measures were reported. The rate of discontinuation or decrease in the compression class of compression garments postoperatively, where reported, ranged from approximately 56% to 85% of patients. The complication rate was low across the studies.

Systematic Reviews

- The systematic review by Carl et al. evaluated outcomes of LVB [4]. Studies were scored using the MINORS scoring system, and of these, 39 studies were found to be high quality using MINORS scoring system criteria – 12 high-quality studies (mean MINORS score of 13.9 ± 1.2) included 3074 patients that received LVB. Overall, the mean limb volume reduction was 33.1% (weighted average; 95% CI: 14.4–51.9%), mean reduction in limb excess circumference was 16.1%, and mean reduction in absolute circumference was 5.8%. Five studies reported QoL outcomes: specifically, one study reported a 91.7% symptom improvement, two studies reported an average satisfaction rate of 94.5%, and two other studies reported improved QoL in 90% of patients and subjective improvement in 50%. Lymphedema stage ranged from Stages I to III on the International Society of Lymphology (ISL) staging system and from Stages Ib to V on the Campisi scale. Two patient complications were reported (partial skin ulceration, $n = 1$, and wound dehiscence, $n = 1$).
- In the systematic review and meta-analysis by Basta et al., the efficacy and safety of LVB were evaluated [5]. Ovid MEDLINE was searched and then the studies were rated on methodological quality based on the ASPS Evidence Rating Scale for Therapeutic Studies, of which 22 studies concerned LVB procedures. Overall limb excess circumference was reduced by 48.9% (CI, 40.7–57.2), and 87.8% of patients reported a quantitative improvement. Subjective improvement was reported by 89.2% of patients, and 56.3% of patients discontinued compression garment use at follow-up. Complications included surgical site infection (3.9%) and lymphorrhea (4.1%).
- A systematic review focusing on LVB surgery queried the PubMed database up to September 2016, and data extraction was performed by two independent reviewers [7]. In total, 293 titles were identified, of which 18 studies, including 939 patients, were included, comprising eight prospective studies and ten retrospective observational cohort studies; there were no RCTs. The majority of studies reported outcomes of secondary lymphedema only ($n = 9$), and eight studies included both primary and secondary lymphedema. The review found that all studies reported objective reductions in limb circumference measurements (83% of patients showing improvement) and in limb volume (2–44% of patients showing improvement), subjective symptom relief was found in 50–100% of patients, and there was a reduction in the number of cellulitis episodes in all investigated cases. The authors concluded that LVB surgery resulted in both objective and subjective improvements in most patients and found that limitations of the current evidence included heterogeneity in surgical techniques, number of anastomoses performed, and supplementary interventions, and only one study that reported subjective symptom improvement used a validated tool, the 36-item short-form health survey (SF-36).
- A systematic literature search using MEDLINE, Embase, and the Cochrane Library to July 2017 was conducted to identify all studies of the use of LVB for the treatment of breast cancer-related lymphedema (BCRL) [8]. The primary outcome was limb volume or circumference reduc-

tion, and the secondary outcome was improvement in QoL. The search yielded 686 results, of which 15 articles were included. Of these, 13 reported a positive surgical effect on reduction in limb volume or circumference, and 12 studies reported symptom improvement and improvement in QoL, with 50–100% of patients reporting improvement in symptoms. The authors concluded that although the outcomes were variable, LVB was effective in early-stage BCRL.

Prospective Cohort or Comparative Studies

- A prospective evaluation of HRQoL following LVB was conducted for 74 patients with upper or lower limb lymphedema [9]. Evaluations were made using the Lymphoedema Quality of Life (LyMQoL) tool, a validated lymphedema disease-specific PRO instrument. All patients were evaluated preoperatively, 1 month after surgery, and every 3 months up to 1 year. The study found significant improvements in LyMQoL scores postoperatively ($p < 0.001$) for both upper (2.3 points) and lower (2.6 points) extremities at a mean follow-up of 8.5 months (range, 2–21 months), with significant improvements in all four LyMQoL domains (function, body image, symptoms, and mood; $p < 0.01$).
- Cornelissen et al. conducted a prospective study of QoL outcomes of LVB for upper extremity BCRL including 20 consecutive women with ISL Stage 1 or 2A lymphedema that had undergone complete decongestive therapy (CDT) for at least 3 months [10]. Mean follow-up was 7.8 (±1.5) months. Significant improvements in QoL using the Lymphoedema Functioning, Disability and Health (Lymph-ICF) were found for the total score and for all QoL domains ($p < 0.05$) after 1 year of follow-up. Using the Upper Extremity Lymphedema (UEL) index, there was a reduction in the mean relative volume difference from 14.92 (±8.01) preoperatively to 12.99 (±7.47) postoperatively ($p = 0.582$). The use of compressive garments was discontinued in 85% of patients ($n = 17$).
- A prospective study of outcomes of 100 consecutive LVB cases for treatment of extremity lymphedema (89 upper extremity and 11 lower extremity) by Chang et al. was conducted with a mean follow-up of 30.4 months (range, 3–84 months) [11]. Symptom improvement was reported in 96% of patients overall. In patients with upper extremity lymphedema, quantitative improvement was noted in 74%; mean overall differential volume reduction was 42% at 12 months postop using perometer (33% at 3 months and 36% at 6 months). Of the seven patients that underwent lower extremity LVB, only four (57%) noted symptom improvement, and volumetric measurements were incomplete. The mean volume differential reductions were significantly better in patients with MD Anderson Cancer Center (MDACC) indocyanine green (ICG) Stage 1 or 2 lymphedema (58%, 52%, and 61%, respectively, at 3, 6, and 12 months; $n = 16$) than for Stage 3 or 4 lymphedema (12%, 16%, and 17%, respectively, at 3, 6, and 12 months; $n = 14$). There were no postoperative complications, and no patient experienced worsening of lymphedema during the study period.
- A prospective cohort study by Akita et al. was performed to assess lymphatic function at standardized intervals by ICG lymphography in 192 lower limbs of 96 consecutive patients that underwent pelvic and/or para-aortic lymph node dissection for gynecological cancer [12]. Of patients that developed lower extremity lymphedema with stardust pattern dermal backflow that did not improve with a trial of compression therapy, 29 underwent LVB surgery and 24 underwent conservative therapy alone [mean follow-up 12.5 (±7.7) and 12.0 (±4.9) months, respectively]. In the LVB group, the Lower Extremity Lymphedema (LEL) index of limb circumference significantly improved: the ICG imaging improved in 17 patients; compression therapy was discontinued in 13 patients (44.8%) and was decreased in four patients. In the conservative treatment group, the LEL index was unchanged: 15 had stable ICG imaging and nine had worsening, four of which increased their compression therapy requirements. The authors therefore concluded that CDT alone did not slow the progression of lower extremity lymphedema and that when patients become symptomatic or stardust pattern is observed, then LVB can prevent worsening or improve lymphatic function.

Retrospective Cohort or Comparative Studies

- A study by Koshima and colleagues evaluated outcomes of 52 patients that underwent LVB for lower extremity lymphedema followed by postoperative compression garments [13]. Surgery was effective in 82.5% of patients even with Campisi Stage III and IV lymphedema at a mean follow-up of 14.5 (±10.2) months; however, the others had no improvement. The mean decrease in limb circumference in unilateral cases was 41.8% (±31.2), and 17 patients had a reduction in limb circumference of over 4 cm. The authors concluded that LVB surgery was effective for lower extremity lymphedema even in early acute Campisi Stage III and fibrotic Stage IV.
- The largest published series of lymphatic microsurgery by Campisi et al. reported outcomes of more than 2600 patients affected by upper and/or lower limb lymphedema, between 1973 and 2013 [14]. Techniques used included multiple lymphatic-venous anastomoses (MLVA) or lymphatic pathway reconstruction using inter-

positioned vein-grafted shunt multiple lymphatic venous lymphatic anastomoses (MLVLA) performed at a single surgical site – either the axillary or inguinal-crural region. Patients were followed for a minimum of 5 years to over 20 years. The authors reported a significant reduction in limb excess volume postoperatively of over 84%, with an average follow-up of 10 years or more. Over 86% of patients with earlier stages of disease (Campisi Stage IB or IIA) progressively stopped using conservative therapies, and 42% of patients with later stage disease (Campisi Stage IIB and III) decreased the frequency of use of physical therapies. The frequency of cellulitis episodes was reduced by over 91%.

- Mihrara et al. performed a retrospective study of 95 patients with lymphedema (84 patients with lower extremity and 11 with upper extremity lymphedema) that underwent LVB to evaluate the change in incidence of cellulitis using predefined criteria extracted from medical records and telephone interviews [15]. Mean follow-up was 27.3 months (range, 12–57). The mean number of episodes of cellulitis was significantly reduced in the year after surgery (0.18; range, 0–3) compared with in the year preceding surgery (1.46; range, 0–12; $p < 0{\cdot}001$).
- A retrospective study of 37 patients that underwent LVB (ten patients with upper extremity and 27 with lower extremity lymphedema) and were followed for 1 year was conducted to evaluate the change in incidence of cellulitis using predefined criteria and collected with telephone interviews [16]. The incidence of cellulitis significantly decreased in all patients, from a mean of 1.7 episodes/year preoperatively to 0.1 episodes/year postoperatively ($p = 0.0012$). Specifically, the incidence of upper extremity cellulitis decreased from an average of 1.4 episodes/year to 0.07 after surgery; in the lower extremity, cellulitis incidence decreased from an average of 2.8 episodes/year to 0.2 postoperatively.

Vascularized Lymph Node Transplant (VLNT) Procedure

Available literature for VLNT includes systematic reviews and meta-analyses, an RCT, and prospective and retrospective cohort and comparative studies. Studies included patients with both upper and lower extremity lymphedema. Varying types of flaps were included, and there was heterogeneity in the measurement modalities between different studies but consistency within individual studies. In all studies assessing these outcomes, a mean overall reduction in limb volume was reported, as well as a reduction in infection incidence, functional improvement, and improved QoL measures, and 53 to 78% of patients were able to discontinue compression therapy postoperatively; subjective improvement was reported in 84 to 100% of patients. The RCT concluded that surgical intervention was superior to conservative management alone.

Systematic Reviews

- The systematic literature review by Carl et al. evaluated outcomes of VLNT procedures [4]. Using the MINORS scoring system, ten studies of VLNT that included 185 patients with lower extremity ($n = 74$) and upper extremity ($n = 111$) lymphedema were found to be high quality [MINORS score of 14.1 (±0.9)]. The lymphedema stage of patients included ranged from ISL Stage IIa to III. Overall, the mean excess volume reduction was 26.4% (weighted average; 95% CI: −7.98–60.8%), and the excess circumference reduction was 39.5%. Four studies reported quality of life outcomes, including improved function, appearance, and mood along with decreased pain. The most common complications were cellulitis, lymphocele, and donor site pain, seroma, and lymphedema.
- A systematic review of the outcomes of free VLNT for the treatment of lymphedema was conducted by Ozturk et al. by searching the PubMed, Embase, and Cochrane Central Register of Controlled Trials (CENTRAL) electronic databases for English language articles published between 1980 and 2015 [17]. Of these, 18 studies including 305 patients (309 limbs; 195 upper extremity and 114 lower extremity lymphedema) were reviewed independently by four coauthors and rated using ASPS guidelines for therapeutic studies and assigned a level of evidence. The mean quality score was 5.3 (3–7), and the levels of evidence were Level II-3, Level III-13, and Level IV-2. The patient age ranged from 13 to 80 years, and the length of follow-up ranged from 2 to 132 months. Among 182 patients that underwent limb circumference assessment, 165 (91%) showed postoperative improvement, and reduction in limb volume was reported in 98 of 114 (86%) patients. In those evaluated for this outcome, 53% were able to reduce their daily use of garments and were able to reduce or discontinue compression therapy. Postoperative lymphoscintigraphy or lymphangiography was performed in 92 patients, of which 55 (60%) demonstrated moderate or significant improvement of flow. Patient satisfaction was evaluated in 105 patients, and with exception of seven patients, all reported a high satisfaction level with significant relief in symptoms and improved QoL. A reduction in infectious episodes was reported in all studies that reported this outcome. The most common donor site complication reported was delayed wound healing ($n = 8$, 4.1%), and persistent donor extremity lymphedema was

not reported in any of the cases. The authors found that the limitations of the studies included heterogeneity of the patient populations, inconsistent reporting of staging of lymphedema, and lack of standardized methods for reporting outcomes.

- In the systematic review and meta-analysis by Basta et al., the efficacy and safety of VLNT were evaluated, rating studies on methodologic quality using the ASPS Evidence Rating Scale for Therapeutic Studies, and five studies were evaluated [5]. Quantitative improvement was found in 90.7% patients; overall, the limb excess circumference was reduced by 48.5% (CI, 35.3–61.6). Subjective improvement was reported in 100% of patients, and 78% discontinued the use of compression garments. Complications included surgical site infection (7.8%), lymphorrhea (14.7%), and reexploration for flap congestion (2.7%).

Randomized Controlled Trials

- Dionyssiou et al. conducted a prospective RCT of women with a diagnosis of ISL Stage II unilateral BCRL and at least one infectious episode in the last year [18]. Using random allocation, 36 patients were divided into two equal groups: in group A, patients underwent microsurgical groin VLNT followed by 6 months of standardized physiotherapy and compression; in group B, patients were managed by standardized physiotherapy and compression alone for 6 months. Using the truncated cone formula based on 4 cm intervals, limb volume reduction was significantly greater in group A (57%) than in group B (18%; $p = 0$). In group A, the mean number of episodes of cellulitis per year was significantly reduced compared with group B (1.94 to 0.27 and 1.61 to 1.16, respectively; $p = 0.001$). All group A patients reported significant reduction of pain and feeling of heaviness of the affected extremity with significant overall functional improvement, compared with no significant improvement in these parameters in group B, with significantly better outcomes in group A for all three parameters ($p = 0$). At 1 year postoperatively, patients in group A had a significantly lower recurrence rate of lymphedema, as compared to group B where almost 80% of patients returned to their previous lymphedema state. Group A patients underwent postoperative lymphoscintigraphy, 6 months after the microsurgical procedure, which showed functional activity of the implanted lymph nodes in 13 out of 18 patients (72%). A lifetime cost advantage was estimated for group A (€6465 versus €26,175), not including treatment of infectious episodes (€119,944). Limitations of the study include the small group sizes, medium-term follow-up (18 months), and use of subjective visual analogue scaling systems to assess pain, heaviness, and functional disturbances.

Prospective Cohort or Comparative Studies

- Beederman et al. prospectively evaluated outcomes of 274 patients with secondary lymphedema affecting the upper ($n = 197$) or lower extremities ($n = 77$) treated by physiological microsurgery with a mean follow-up time of 15.0 (±13.8) months [19]. The majority of patients with upper extremity lymphedema underwent a combination of both VLNT and LVB ($n = 104$, 52.8%); VLNT donor sites included the supraclavicular VLN flap ($n = 78$, 43.8%), groin VLNT combined with autologous breast reconstruction ($n = 57$, 32.0%), and lateral thoracic VLNT ($n = 43$, 24.2%). The majority of patients with lower extremity lymphedema also underwent a combination of both VLNT and LVB ($n = 64$, 83.1%); VLNT donor sites included supraclavicular ($n = 64$, 85.3%), lateral thoracic ($n = 10$, 13.3%), and pedicled groin VLNT ($n = 1$, 1.3%). Postoperatively, all patients underwent immediate compression wrapping performed by physical therapists until 4 weeks after surgery. After 4 weeks, patients resumed their regular lymphedema therapies (including lymphatic massage, compression garments, compression pump). Overall, greater than 87% of upper extremity patients and 60% of lower extremity patients had a reduction in excess limb volume during at least one time point postoperatively. At 12 months postoperatively, patients with upper extremity lymphedema had a 25.7% reduction in volume difference between limbs, 47.4% at 24 months and 47.7% at 4 years. There was no statistically significant difference in volume differential reduction when the three donor site groups were compared. When comparing percent reduction in volume differential between upper extremity and lower extremity patients, upper extremity patients had a greater reduction at each time point; however, results were only statistically significant at 3 months and 12 months. For the lower extremity, at 24 months postoperatively, the average reduction in volume differential was 34.8% among the patients who showed improvement. Overall, greater than 86% of upper extremity and 75% of lower extremity patients also had improvement in Lymphedema Life Impact Scale (LLIS) scores during at least one time point postoperatively. In total, 59 experienced at least one postoperative complication, for an overall complication rate of 12.9% (upper extremity, 10.7%; lower extremity, 17.7%). There were 17 donor site complications, including seroma ($n = 8$), hematoma ($n = 2$), abscess ($n = 1$), cellulitis ($n = 3$), superficial wound dehiscence ($n = 1$), and deep vein thrombosis requiring anticoagulation ($n = 1$). No patient who underwent VLNT harvest reported subsequent donor site lymphedema; however, two patients had a significant chyle leak following supraclavicular VLN harvest, requiring operative management. Thirty-one patients had recipient site complications, including cellulitis ($n = 9$), wound dehiscence/partial flap loss ($n = 8$), and microvascular complications ($n = 9$). There was one delayed lower extremity flap loss (<1.0%).

- Schaverien et al. performed a prospective study of consecutive patients undergoing VLNT to treat primary and secondary lymphedema affecting the upper or lower extremities with all patients optimized preoperatively to achieve maximal reductions by conservative therapy [20]. There were 134 patients (115 upper extremity; 19 lower extremity) included, and VLN flaps included jejunal mesenteric ($n = 25$), groin ($n = 43$), lateral thoracic ($n = 31$), omental/right gastroepiploic ($n = 21$), and submental ($n = 14$). Synchronous LVB procedures were performed in 76 patients. Patients prominently had MDACC Lymphedema Stage III [$n = 55$ (41%)] and IV [$n = 39$ (29.1%)] lymphedema, and the mean length of postoperative follow-up was 20.1 months (±9.7). At 12 months postoperatively, there were significant reductions in mean limb volume change [34.7% (±4.1), $p < 0.001$], mean L-Dex score [49.4% (±4.7), $p < 0.001$], and mean LLIS score [53.8% (±3.9), $p < 0.001$], compared with preoperatively. At 24 months postoperatively, these had all improved further: there were significant reductions in mean limb volume change [45.7% (±8.7), $p = 0.002$], mean L-Dex score [59.8% (±8.7), $p < 0.001$], and mean LLIS score [61.6% (±5.9), $p < 0.001$]. At 3 and 6 months postoperatively, limb volume change was significantly greater for the upper than the lower extremity ($p = 0.014$ and $p < 0.001$, respectively); otherwise, outcomes were similar. There were no flap losses, and there was a low flap-related complication rate; no patient developed clinical donor extremity lymphedema during follow-up. Overall outcomes in limb volume change, L-Dex score, and LLIS score were similar between the different VLN flaps at 6 and 12 months postoperatively. Postoperatively, 97.1% of patients had a decrease in L-Dex score, and 90.2% had a reduction in limb volume excess; 98.9% of patients had an improvement in at least one of these measures. In 96.2% of patients, there was an improvement in the LLIS score postoperatively. All patients with lower extremity lymphedema had an improvement in LVC, L-Dex, and LLIS score. There were minimal clinically important differences (MIDs) for limb volume change in 89.6% patients, for L-Dex score in 91.1%, and for LLIS score in 94.8% of patients. In 35.2% of patients, there was a history of cellulitis, 56.7% of which reported multiple cellulitis episodes, and 86.7% had at least one episode of cellulitis in the 12 months before surgery; at up to 24 months follow-up postoperatively, there was only one episode of cellulitis reported (97.9%, $p < 0.001$). Overall, in patients eligible to reduce their compression therapy postoperatively, 63.1% had either discontinued (42.1%) or significantly reduced (21.1%) their use of compression garments at a mean of 12.1 months (±8) postoperatively; however, for the lower extremity, compression stocking use was typically continued.
- Chang et al. reported outcomes of a prospective study of patients that underwent DIEP flap breast reconstruction with groin VLNT; thirty-three underwent adjunctive LVB (combined group) and 21 did not [21]. Subjective symptomatic improvement was reported in 100% of patients in the combined group compared to 81% of patients that received VLNT only ($p = 0.019$). There were significant differences in postoperative limb volume reduction (measured using perometer) between the two groups at 3 months (40.7% vs. 20.0%, $p = 0.037$) and 6 months (57.0% vs. 44.5%, $p = 0.043$), but this was not statistically significant at 12 months (60.4% vs. 57.8%, $p = 0.43$). A decrease in regular compression garment use was reported in 81.8% of patients ($n = 27$) in the combined group and 76.2% ($n = 16$) in the VLNT-only group. In each group, five patients developed complications, and no patient developed donor site lower extremity lymphedema. Limitations included the small study size and non-randomized approach.
- A prospective study by Patel et al. of 25 patients that underwent VLNT for upper or lower extremity lymphedema evaluated QoL parameters at multiple time points during the 12-month perioperative period using the LyMQoL questionnaire [22]. The mean limb circumference reduction was 24.4% (±14.7) at 12 months in the upper extremity ($n = 15$; 13 groin VLN flaps and two submental VLNTs) and 35.2% (±23.9) at 12 months in the lower extremity ($n = 10$; all submental VLNTs). These improvements were mirrored by improvements in all HRQoL domains and overall quality of life (upper limb, 2.1–5.8; $p < 0.01$; lower limb, 3.0–7.1; $p < 0.01$). The function, body appearance, symptom, and mood domains were all found to be significantly improved during the postoperative evaluation, with continued improvement being reported throughout the study period ($p < 0.01$ within each domain). The occurrence of cellulitis was also significantly decreased in both cohorts (upper limb: $p = 0.05$; lower limb: $p < 0.01$). There were no partial or complete flap losses.
- Akita et al. [23] evaluated outcomes in patients ($n = 27$) with secondary upper extremity lymphedema that underwent groin VLNT combined with DIEP flap surgery [$n = 13$; mean follow-up 13.9 (±6.5) months] compared with those that underwent groin VLNT only [$n = 14$; mean follow-up 13.2 (±4.4) months]. Mean follow-up

was 18.8 (± 1.7) months. Mean circumference reduction rate using the Upper Extremity Lymphedema (UEL) index was similar at 6 months postop [13.9 (±4.1) in the combined group, compared with the groin flap-only group [13.2 (±1.5); $p = 0.75$). In the combined group, there was a significant improvement using ICG lymphography in 6/13 patients, compared with 4/14 patients in the groin flap-only group. In the combined group, compression therapy was discontinued in six patients and reduced in a further four patients; in the groin LN flap-only group, compression therapy was discontinued in only three patients; the proportion of patients that reduced their compression garment use was significantly higher in the groin LNT + DIEP flap group (ten of 13 patients) than in the groin flap alone group (three of 14 patients; $p = 0.04$).

- Akita et al. [24] evaluated outcomes in patients with ISL late stage II or more severe lower extremity lymphedema treated with LVB (43 limbs treated in 33 patients) compared with supraclavicular VLNT (performed in 13 patients to the distal thigh or lower leg). No significant complications occurred in the LVA group, whereas three patients in the supraclavicular VLNT group required reoperation for complications without flap loss ($p < 0.01$). Improvement in circumference reduction rate using Lower Extremity Lymphedema (LEL) index was significantly greater in the VLNT group than in the LVB group [mean 21.2 (±2.0) compared with 26.5 (±4.4), respectively; $p = 0.032$]. No patient discontinued compression stocking use.

Retrospective Comparative Studies

- Cheng et al. evaluated outcomes in ten patients with postmastectomy upper limb ISL Stage 2 lymphedema with repeated episodes of cellulitis that underwent groin VLNT to either the wrist or elbow compared with ten control patients who chose to undergo physical therapy only [25]. Mean follow-up was 39.1 months (± 15.7). Mean circumferential measurement reduction rate was significantly greater in the VLNT group [40.4% (±16.1)] than in the physical therapy group [8.3% (±34.7); $p = 0.02$], as was the mean improvement of circumferential difference measured at 10 cm above the elbow and 10 cm below the elbow [7.3% (± 2.7) compared with 1.7% (±4.6); $p < 0.01$]. There was a greater reduction rate of episodes of cellulitis in the surgery group [1.3 (±1) versus 0.9 (±0.4)] although this difference was not significant.
- Engel et al. evaluated outcomes of lymphedema microsurgery in 124 patients with BCRL, 37 of whom underwent microvascular breast reconstruction (MBR) [mean follow-up, 12.7 (±1.8) months] and 87 that did not [mean follow-up, 25.5 (±8.9) months], comparing CDT alone, with LVB alone, and VLNT alone (submental VLNT, $n = 27$; or groin VLNT, $n = 18$; 42 flaps transferred to the wrist and three to the elbow) [26] (Table 24.1). The study found that in both groups, mean improvement in circumferential difference, reduction rate, and episodes of cellulitis was significantly greater with VLNT than with LVB or CDT ($p = 0.04$, 0.04, and 0.06, respectively) at a mean follow-up of 19.1 (±5.3) months (range, 5.7–62.8 months). Improvement in circumferential difference, reduction rate, and episodes of cellulitis was significantly greater in the LVB and VLNT groups than in those that underwent CDT alone ($p = 0.04$, 0.04, and 0.03, respectively). The mean episodes of cellulitis were improved from 6.2% (±1.9) to 1.9% (±1.8) ($p = 0.03$), but this improvement did not differ by treatment modality in either group. Improvements in the circumferential difference, circumferential reduction rate, and episodes of cellulitis did not significantly differ between patients that received MBR and those that did not ($p = 0.06$, 0.07, and 0.06, respectively). The overall complication rate was 8.1% ($n = 10$), and no flap losses occurred. One of 18 patients that underwent groin VLNT developed lower limb lymphedema that was successfully treated by LVB.

Retrospective Cohort Studies

- This study retrospectively reported outcomes in 38 patients (41 legs) with secondary leg lymphedema that underwent VLNT [27]. There was a history of limb cellulitis in 15 patients, and all patients were compliant with continuous compression garment use. The study included 23 legs; in 15 patients with unilateral lymphedema there was an average 46.3% (±34.7) reduction in limb excess volume (measured using the truncated cone volume formula) at a mean follow-up of 12.8 months (±10.7); of these, two patients recovered completely. Outcomes were significantly better (defined as >30% limb excess volume reduction) in patients with smaller preoperative excess volume ($p = 0.045$). Minor complications occurred in 11 patients (28.9%); none required operative intervention. The authors noted limitations of the study including retrospective data collection and uncontrolled data acquisition.
- Gratzon and colleagues evaluated clinical outcomes and PROs in 50 patients with ISL Stage 1 or 2 BCRL resistant to conservative therapy treated with VLNT (including groin, lateral thoracic, or supraclavicular) to the axilla [28] (Fig. 24.1). The median follow-up time for the cohort was 12 months, with a total study period of 24 months. Patients underwent a 2-week CDT protocol before surgery and were evaluated preoperatively and postopera-

Table 24.1 Outcomes in patients with upper extremity breast cancer-related lymphedema (BCRL) that underwent complete decongestive therapy (CDT), lymphovenous bypass (LVB), or vascularized lymph node transplant (VLNT), with or without microsurgical breast reconstruction (MBR). Adapted from Engel et al. [26]

	Mean circumference difference reduction (%) (mean ± SD)			Mean reduction rate (%) (mean ± SD)			Cellulitis episode reduction (per year) (mean ± SD)			Mean follow-up (months) (mean ± SD)		
	Lymphedema intervention only ($n = 87$)	MBR and lymphedema intervention ($n = 37$)	*P*-value	Lymphedema intervention only ($n = 87$)	MBR and lymphedema intervention ($n = 37$)	*P*-value	Lymphedema intervention only ($n = 87$)	MBR and lymphedema intervention ($n = 37$)	*P*-value	Lymphedema intervention only ($n = 87$)	MBR and lymphedema intervention ($n = 37$)	*P*-value
CDT ($n = 52$)	4.1 (±1.6)	1.8 (±0.8)	0.07	9.8 (±2.5)	7.6 (±2.3)	0.07	2.3 (±2.1) vs 1.2 (±0.9)	6.3 (±1.0) vs 2.4 (±4.7)	0.06	8.5 (±3.4)	16.3 (±1.0)	0.04*
LVB ($n = 27$)	9.3 (±2.7)	11.1 (±4.9)	0.06	17.3 (±6.0)	11.6 (±5.7)	0.06	4.4 (±1.5) vs 1.4 (±0.2)	8.4 (±2.5) vs 1.2 (±0.7)	0.06	9.7 (±4.2)	6.4 (±2.5)	0.06
VLNT ($n = 45$)	25 (±8.2)	19.7 (±10.2)	0.04	34.0 (±6.9)	24.9 (±10.0)	0.04*	7.4 (±2.3) vs 2.6 (±2.3)	8.0 (±1.8) vs 2.8 (±1.8)	1	58.3 (±19.1)	15.4 (±1.8)	0.04*
Mean	12.8 (±4.2)	11.5 (±5.3)	0.06	20.4 (±5.1)	14.7 (±6)	0.04*	1.7 (±1.1)	2.1 (±2.4)	0.06	25.5 (±8.9)	12.7 (±1.8)	0.04*

MBR microvascular breast reconstruction, *SD* standard deviation, *CDT* complete decongestive therapy, *LVB* lymphovenous bypass, *VLNT* vascularized lymph node transplant. *$p < 0.05$

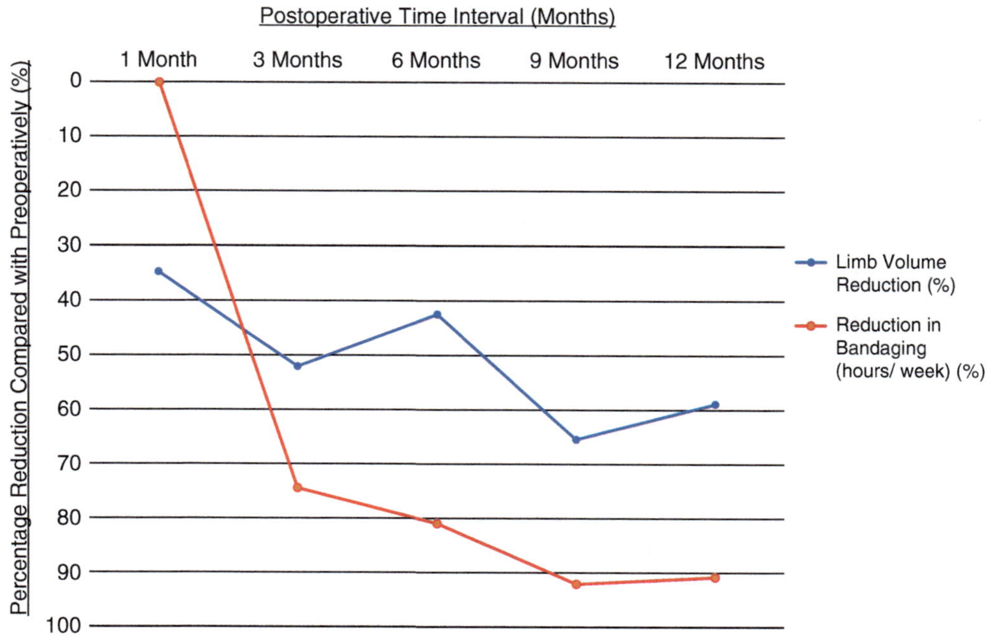

Fig. 24.1 Change in arm volume and need for bandaging following vascularized lymph node transplantation (VLNT). (Adapted from Gratzon et al. [28])

tively at standardized intervals using circumferential measurements (truncated cone formula), pain/heaviness scales, and the LyMQoL questionnaire. The study found a mean decrease in arm volume of 58.7% at 12 months postoperatively ($n = 24$ patients), with significant patient-reported reductions in mean arm pain and heaviness (both $p < 0.01$), as well as significant improvements in mean overall LyMQoL scores (from 5.72 preop to 7.79 at 12 months, $p < 0.01$) and for all domains. Preoperatively, 10/50 patients (20%) reported a preoperative cellulitis episode; postoperatively, there was a reduction in episodes of infection in nine patients (90%), with seven having no further lymphedema-associated cellulitis episodes during follow-up. The need for bandaging decreased from an average of 76.8 hours per week to an average of 7.3 hours per week at 12 months postoperatively, with seven patients (14%) discontinuing all forms of CDT. Complications occurred in 17 patients, with three requiring reoperative intervention.

- De Brucker et al. evaluated QoL outcomes in 25 female patients with BCRL that underwent groin VLNT, 22 of which underwent simultaneous DIEP flap MBR with groin VLNT [29]. Postoperatively, 21 patients (84%) had an improvement in QoL evaluated using the Upper Limb Lymphedema-27 (ULL-27) questionnaire, with significant improvements in mean physical, psychological, and social scores ($p < 0.001$). There were no postoperative cellulitis episodes in 50% of cases. In 11 patients (44%), compression therapy was discontinued at a mean postoperative time interval of 29 months; in the other patients, the average frequency of compression therapy decreased from three sessions to one session per week. Complications included seroma ($n = 3$), donor-site wound breakdown ($n = 4$), and one flap loss; no patient developed donor site lymphedema during follow-up. Limitations of the study included that the questionnaire was completed at the time of the final postoperative visit which may have introduced recall bias.
- This study evaluated outcomes in 29 consecutive patients with refractory BCRL that underwent MBR with simultaneous groin VLNT [30]. Mean follow-up was 11 months. The mean differential volume reduction measured using perometer was 48% at 12 months (decreasing from 21% preoperatively to 20%, 19%, 14%, and 10% at 1, 3, 6, and 12 months postoperatively, respectively). Sustained symptomatic improvement was reported postoperatively in 23 patients (79%). Donor site wound complications occurred in six patients (21%) all resolving with conservative measures, and no patients developed donor site lymphedema.
- Nguyen et al. evaluated outcomes in 42 patients who underwent free omental lymphatic flap transplant to treat lymphedema of the upper ($n = 19$) or lower ($n = 24$) extremities, 39 of which were harvested laparoscopically, with an average follow-up of 14 months [31]. The mean duration of lymphedema symptoms was 5.8 years. Overall, 83% of patients reported a subjective improvement, with a mean volumetric improvement (perometer) of 22%. There was a history of cellulitis in 74% ($n = 31$) of patients, whereas cellulitis occurred postoperatively in only 5% ($n = 2$) of patients. Complications occurred in 16% ($n = 7$) of patients; major complications included one episode of pancreatitis and one flap loss. The study findings were limited by incomplete collection of QoL outcomes measures.

- Ciudad and colleagues evaluated long-term outcomes in 83 patients with upper or lower extremity lymphedema that underwent VLNT, including groin, supraclavicular, and gastroepiploic (open and laparoscopic flap harvest) [32]. Of these, 30 patients had upper extremity and 53 patients had lower extremity lymphedema, with 47 diagnosed with ISL Stage II and 36 with Stage III lymphedema. The mean follow-up was 32.8 months (range, 24–49). The mean circumference reduction rate was significant in both Stage II and III lymphedema ($p < 0.0001$), with a significantly greater reduction in Stage II [29.1% (±8)] than Stage III [17.9% (±7.6)] lymphedema. At 1 year postoperatively, lymphoscintigraphy showed an improvement in lymphatic drainage in 96.4% of patients, with only three patients having no improvement in symptoms or on lymphoscintigraphy. There was a history of recurrent infections in 77 patients preoperatively, and 51 patients did not experience any cellulitis episodes postoperatively ($p < 0.05$), with a significant decrease in the number of infectious episodes in the remaining patients.

Suction-Assisted Lipectomy (SAL) Debulking

Available literature includes systematic reviews and meta-analyses, and prospective cohort and comparative studies. All patients adhered to a postoperative compression regimen, and the overall incidence of complications was low.

Systematic Reviews

- The systematic review of outcomes of SAL debulking by Carl et al. identified four high-quality studies (MINORS score of 14.25 ± 0.5) that included 105 patients with upper extremity ($n = 99$) or lower extremity ($n = 6$) lymphedema [4]. All four studies reported an excess volume reduction, with a weighted average reduction of 96.6% (95% CI: 86.2–107%, I2: 0.0%). Of the two studies that reported the ISL stage, all patients were stage II or III. QoL outcomes were reported in three studies, finding improved overall well-being and decreased depression and anxiety postoperatively. All patients continued to wear compression garments postoperatively. No operative or postoperative complications were reported.
- A systematic review of all studies evaluating the efficacy of the use of SAL debulking for upper extremity lymphedema was conducted following the Preferred Reporting Items for Systematic Reviews and Meta-Analyses (PRISMA) guidelines for article identification and final selection [33]. A PubMed database search screened 129 articles, of which 13 met inclusion criteria – ten studies reported outcomes of liposuction followed by controlled compression therapy (CCT), and the three other studies compared outcomes in patients following liposuction with CCT with those treated with CCT alone. Overall, there was a greater than 100% relative limb volume reduction in all patients that underwent SAL followed by CCT, and in two studies, there was also a decrease in L-Dex scores. Across these studies, there was an increase in QoL, a decrease in incidence of infection, and an improvement in range of motion in the surgery group.

Prospective Cohort or Comparative Studies

- Hoffner et al. reported results of a prospective study of 105 patients that underwent SAL with CCT to treat arm lymphedema with 5 years of postoperative follow-up [34] (Fig. 24.2). The preoperative mean excess volume was 1573 (±645) ml (range, 570–3520). At 5 years, the mean limb volume reduction was 117% (±26) (range, 25–191) with an excess volume of −188 (±300) ml (range, −920 to 1010); ninety-six patients (91.4%) achieved at least a 90% reduction. No complications were reported.
- Brorson et al. reported outcomes of a long-term prospective study of the use of SAL to treat upper extremity BCRL [35]. The study included 146 women with a mean duration of lymphedema of 9 years (range, 1–38). The preoperative mean excess volume was 1568 ml (range, 545–4235), and the postoperative mean reduction was 103% (range, 50–194) at 3 months and greater than 100% at up to 21 years of follow-up. The preoperative mean volume ratio between affected and unaffected arms was 1.5 and was 1.0 at 3 months postoperatively, and less than 1.0 after 1 year.
- A prospective cohort study of 130 patients on the effect of SAL debulking on the incidence of cellulitis in postmastectomy arm lymphedema was conducted [36]. The total number of pre-liposuction observation years was 1147, and total post-liposuction observation years was 983. Following liposuction debulking, there was a reduction in mean excess volume of 109% (range, 61–198; SD 27; $p < 0.001$) at 6 months. The incidence of cellulitis decreased significantly by 87% ($p < 0.001$) from 0.47 attacks/year (range, 0–5.0; SD 0.8 attacks/year) to 0.06 attacks/year (range, 0–3.0; SD 0.3 attacks/year) after liposuction. The total number of cellulitis episodes decreased from 534 to 60 after liposuction, and of 76 patients that experienced at least one cellulitis episode preoperatively, only 13 (17%) patients experienced cellulitis postoperatively.
- Stewart and Munnoch conducted a prospective study of 69 patients with leg lymphedema (72 legs; 42 primary and 30 secondary lymphedema) who were consecutively treated with liposuction with CCT by a single surgeon over a 9-year period [37]. The mean preoperative limb volume measured using circumferential measurement and truncated cone calculation was 4372 mL (range, 229–15,166),

and the mean reduction in limb volume was 88% at 1 year (n = 60), 94% at 2 years (n = 41), and 90% at 5 years (n = 15). The mean limb volume reduction at 1 year postoperatively was 84.3% (31.3–169.9; n = 38) in patients with primary and 95.6% (50–163.8; n = 22) in those with secondary lymphedema. There were no major surgical complications. Limitations of the study included loss of 17 patients from follow-up over time (five due to cancer recurrence) and ten patients who were noncompliant with the postoperative compression garment regimen.

Retrospective Cohort or Comparative Studies

- Outcomes of 88 patients with lower extremity lymphedema treated with SAL, comparing outcomes in primary (n = 47 patients) with secondary lymphedema (n = 41 patients), were evaluated by Lamprou et al. [38]. The mean volume reduction was 89% at 2 years postop: 101% in the secondary lymphedema group and 79% in the primary group. The incidence of cellulitis was significantly reduced ($p < 0.001$): in the secondary group, from 6 episodes/year to 0.3 episodes/year ($p < 0.001$) and in the primary group, from 8 episodes/year to 0.2 episodes/year ($p < 0.001$).
- Hoffner et al. evaluated HRQoL outcomes following SAL debulking in 60 female patients with arm lymphedema (of 90; non-responders demographically similar) that were followed for a 1-year period after surgery; the SF-36 was used and compared with normative data for Swedish women [39]. The preoperative excess arm volume measured using the water displacement technique was 1365 (±73) mL. Starting at 1 month postoperatively, scores for mental health were significantly improved. Commencing at 3 months, there were significant improvements in physical functioning, bodily pain, and vitality, and at 1 year, there was a significant improvement in social functioning. Compared with the SF-36 normative data, there were significant improvements in general health, bodily pain, vitality, mental health, and social functioning postoperatively. Limitations to the study included the relatively small number of patients and use of a generic rather than disease-specific outcomes questionnaire.
- Brorson et al. patients evaluated outcomes in female BCRL patients with arm lymphedema that underwent liposuction with postoperative CCT (n = 35) compared with CCT with custom compression garments only (n = 14) [40]. There were significant reductions in edema volumes in both groups at 6 months and at 1 year postoperatively; however, the reductions were significantly greater in the SAL group, compared with compression therapy only, at both 6 months ($p < 0.0001$) and at 1 year (103% compared with 50%; p = 0.0001). There was a decrease in pain, swelling of the hand, and difficulties with activities of daily living at 1 year postoperatively in the liposuction group, whereas in the compression-only group, there was no change. There were greater improvements in the surgery group on the Nottingham Health Profile, the Psychological General Well-Being Index, and the Hospital Anxiety Depression Test. The authors concluded that liposuction results in greater arm volume reduction and improvement in patient QoL, particularly qualities associated with everyday activities, compared with conservative therapy alone.

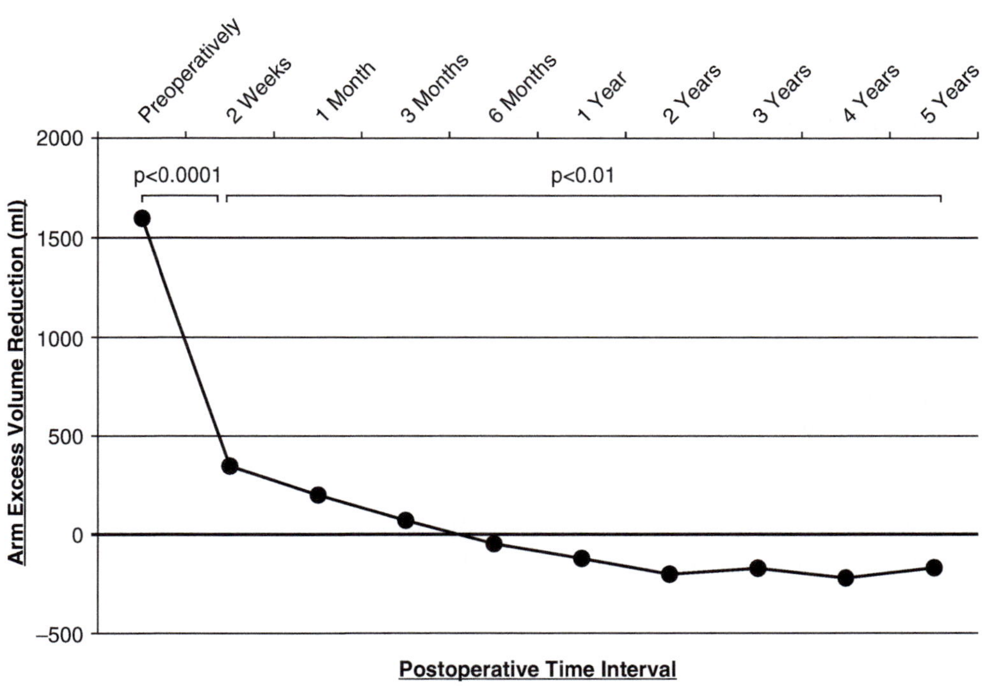

Fig. 24.2 Pre- and postoperative arm excess volume reduction (mean) in patients that underwent suction-assisted lipectomy (SAL) with controlled compression therapy (CCT). (Adapted from Hoffner et al. [34])

Combined Procedures

In their meta-analysis, Carl et al. evaluated the outcomes of combined procedures to treat lymphedema [4]. There were eight high-quality studies [MINORS score of 14.3 (±1.3)] identified that included 135 patients with lower extremity ($n = 50$) or upper extremity ($n = 59$) lymphedema. In two studies combining SAL debulking and VLNT, there was a weighted average reduction of excess circumference of 70.8%; one study that reported QoL outcomes found an improvement in the two case studies presented. Complications were reported in five studies, the most frequently occurring of which were partial skin graft/skin flap loss, delayed healing, and donor-site lymphedema.

Excisional Procedures

In the meta-analysis by Carl et al., outcomes of excisional procedures to treat lymphedema in patients with the most advanced stages of disease who were experiencing persistent swelling and fibrosis were evaluated [4]. In total, five high-quality studies [MINORS score of 14.0 (±0.7)] were evaluated including 76 patients (lower extremity, $n = 65$; upper extremity, $n = 11$). QoL outcomes were reported in two studies, both showing improvements in well-being and function postoperatively. Complications were reported in four studies, most commonly prolonged numbness, cellulitis, wound breakdown, and the need for additional skin grafting.

Immediate Lymphatic Reconstruction (ILR)

The available evidence for ILR includes two systematic reviews and meta-analyses, and an RCT.

Systematic Reviews

- A review of lymphedema incidence after ILR was conducted by Johnson et al. following a search of PubMed, Embase, Web of Science, and Cochrane databases through 2018 [41]. In total, 19 studies were included, and data were extracted from 3035 patients, 711 with lymphedema. The pooled cumulative incidence of lymphedema was 14.1% in the axillary lymphadenectomy (ALND) group versus 2.1% in the ALND with ILR [Lymphatic Microsurgical Preventive Healing Approach (LYMPHA) technique] group, a difference of 12.0% ($p = 0.029$). In the group that underwent ALND with regional lymph node radiation (RLNR) therapy, the pooled cumulative incidence of lymphedema was 33.4% versus 10.3% in the ALND with RLNR group that underwent ILR, a difference of 23.1% ($p = 0.004$).
- Jorgensen et al. performed a systematic meta-analysis of studies treating patients with a cancer diagnosis receiving lymphadenectomy of either the axillary or groin area with prophylactic lymphovenous anastomosis (LVA) for the prevention of secondary lymphedema following lymphadenectomy [42]. A systematic search was conducted in MEDLINE and Embase to August 2016; of 1453 articles, 86 full-text studies were assessed for eligibility and yielded 12 articles included in the qualitative analysis, and four of these were further eligible to be included in the quantitative analysis. The qualitative analysis comprised a total of 270 cases treated with prophylactic LVA, of which 17 developed lymphedema during the follow-up period. In the quantitative analysis, four studies with a control group were included. A total of 12 out of 82 patients treated with prophylactic LVA developed lymphedema, and 94 patients acted as controls, of which 53 went on to develop lymphedema. Clinical lymphedema occurred only in six of the included studies using prophylactic LVA. All included studies but one revealed a lower lymphedema incidence than expected from the literature, with a pooled lymphedema rate of 0% for iliac, 12% for ilioinguinal, 5% for axillary, and 7% for para-aortic lymph node dissection. Patients treated with prophylactic LVA had a significant reduction in lymphedema incidence (relative risk, 0.33; 95% CI: 0.19–0.56) when compared to patients that received no prophylactic treatment ($p < 0.0001$). Postoperative complications from the procedure were only reported in one patient (lymphorrhea). The authors conclude that prophylactic LVA can reduce the lymphedema incidence to 1/3 compared with no intervention. Limitations include the low number of eligible studies and method heterogeneity between these studies.

Randomized Controlled Trials

- Boccardo et al. randomly allocated 46 women undergoing ALND for breast cancer treatment into two groups: 23 underwent LYMPHA at the time of ALND and 23 did not (control group) [43]. Patients were followed up at standardized intervals up to 18 months postoperatively with arm volume measurements (truncated cone formula). The lymphedema incidence in the LYMPHA group was 4.3% compared with 30.4% in the control group. No statistically significant differences in the arm volume were observed in the treatment group during follow-up compared with preoperatively, while the arm volume in the control group showed a significant increase after 1, 3, and 6 months postoperatively (all $p < 0.001$). Arm volumes compared with preoperatively were significantly higher in the control group compared to the treatment group at all postoperative timepoints (all $p < 0.01$). Lymphoscintigraphy was performed after 18 months postoperatively in 41 patients, demonstrating anastomotic patency in all 21 patients in the LYMPHA group.

Retrospective Comparative Studies

- In a study by Feldman and colleagues, female patients with breast cancer undergoing planned ALND were offered ILR using the LYMPHA technique at a single institution [44]. Of these, 37 women underwent attempted LYMPHA at the time of ALND, with successful completion in 27, 17 (63%) of which received axillary radiotherapy; LYMPHA was not completed in ten either because of extensive axillary disease or lack of suitable vessels. Of 24 patients that underwent LYMPHA (patients excluded if preoperative lymphedema or less than 3 months follow-up), the lymphedema rate as measured using circumferential measurements and L-Dex was three patients (12.5%), compared with four (50%) of eight in unsuccessfully treated patients ($p = 0.05$) at a mean follow-up of 6 months (range, 3–24 months). Lymphoscintigraphy was performed postoperatively at 3 months (n = 16) and at 18 months (n = 5) in the LYMPHA group; only one had abnormal ipsilateral lymphatic drainage visualized. Limitations of the study included the non-randomized study design and limitations in the measurement of preclinical lymphedema.

Retrospective Cohort Studies

- Boccardo et al. evaluated lower limb lymphedema outcomes in 27 patients that underwent LYMPHA at the time of inguinofemoral lymphadenectomy using circumferential measurements [45]. Persistent lower extremity lymphedema occurred in one patient (9%) and transient lymphedema in one patient (6.25%). Lymphoscintigraphy was performed in all patients postoperatively and was abnormal in six patients, only one of which had clinical lymphedema. No lymphocele or infectious complication occurred in the cohort.

Conclusions

The current available evidence demonstrates improved clinical outcomes for lymphedema surgery including LVB, VLNT, SAL debulking, and combinations of these surgeries, including in limb circumference/volume measurements, lymphedema-specific symptoms, patient-reported HRQoL, and episodes of lymphedema-related cellulitis, in patients who are appropriately diagnosed with lymphatic disease and who do not respond to conservative treatments (Table 24.2). In studies where surgery with compression therapy was compared to compression therapy only, more pronounced objective and subjective improvements were seen in the surgery group. Although there was heterogeneity in assessment modalities used between different studies, modes of assessment were consistent within all studies for pre- and postoperative measurements. Complications were infrequent across studies. The available evidence supports the efficacy of surgery to treat chronic lymphedema and in risk reduction following ALND in the treatment of breast cancer.

Table 24.2 Data from key observational case-control studies of outcomes of surgical interventions for lymphedema

Comparator groups	Study	Extremity	Primary or secondary	Study design	Study groups	Outcomes
Comparison of CDT with LVB and/or VLNT	Dionyssiou et al., *Breast Cancer Res Treat. 2016* [18]	UE	Secondary	Randomized controlled trial	18 pts. treated with groin VNLT (to axilla) followed by 6 mo of standardized CDT 18 pts. received 6 mo of standardized CDT alone	Limb volume reduction (measured using truncated cone formula based on 4 cm intervals) greater in VLNT (57%) group than in CDT (18%; $p = 0$) group. Mean number of episodes of cellulitis per year significantly reduced in VLNT compared with CDT group (1.94 to 0.27, and 1.61 to 1.16, respectively; $p = 0.001$). All patients that received VLNT reported significant symptomatic and functional improvement, compared with no significant improvement in the CDT only group ($p = 0$). At 1-year postoperatively patients in the VLNT group had a significantly lower recurrence rate of their lymphedema. At 6 months postoperatively, lymphoscintigraphy showed functional activity of the implanted lymph nodes in 13 out of 18 patients (72%). A lifetime cost advantage was estimated for the VLNT group (€6465 versus €26,175 respectively, not including treatment of infectious episodes of €119,944).

(continued)

Table 24.2 (continued)

Comparator groups	Study	Extremity	Primary or secondary	Study design	Study groups	Outcomes
	Cheng et al., *Plast Reconstr Surg. 2013* [25]	UE	Secondary	Retrospective comparative study	10 pts. underwent groin VLNT (to wrist or elbow) [mean f/u 39.1 (±15.7) mo] 10 patients underwent CDT only	Mean circumferential measurement reduction rate significantly greater [40.4% (±16.1)] in VLNT compared with CDT group [8.3% (±34.7); $p = 0.02$]. Mean improvement of circumferential difference measured at 10 cm above the elbow and 10 cm below the elbow also significantly greater [7.3% (± 2.7)] in VLNT compared with CDT group [1.7% (±4.6); $p < 0.01$]. Greater reduction rate of episodes of cellulitis in the VLNT group [1.3 (±1) versus 0.9 (±0.4)] although this difference was not significant.
	Akita et al., *J Plast Reconstr Aesthet Surg. 2014* [12]	LE	Secondary	Prospective cohort study	29 pts. underwent LVB surgery [mean f/u 12.0 (±4.9) mo] 24 pts. underwent CDT alone [mean f/u 12.5 (±7.7) mo]	Patients that underwent pelvic and/or para-aortic LN dissection for gynecological cancer and developed stardust pattern dermal backflow on ICG imaging that did not improve with a trial of compression therapy included. In LVB group, LEL index of limb circumference significantly improved; ICG imaging improved in 17 pts.; CDT discontinued in 13 (44.8%) and decreased in 4. In CDT group, LEL index was similar; 15 had stable ICG imaging and 9 had deterioration, 4 of which increased compression therapy requirements.
	Engel et al., *Ann Surg. 2018* [26]	UE	Secondary	Retrospective comparative study	37 pts. underwent MBR [mean f/u 12.7 (±1.8) mo] 87 pts. did not undergo MBR [mean f/u 25.5 (±8.9) mo]	Outcomes of CDT alone, LVB, and VLNT compared [submental VLNT ($n = 27$) or groin VLNT ($n = 18$); all transferred to wrist or elbow] with and without MBR. In both groups (with and without MBR), mean improvement in circumferential difference, reduction rate, and episodes of cellulitis significantly greater with VLNT than with LVB or CDT ($p = 0.04$, 0.04, and 0.06, respectively) at a mean follow-up of 19.1(±5.3) months. Mean episodes of cellulitis improved from 6.2% (±1.9) to 1.9% (±1.8) ($p = 0.03$), but this improvement not significantly different by treatment modality. One of 18 patients that underwent groin VLNT developed lower limb lymphedema that was successfully treated by LVB.

Table 24.2 (continued)

Comparator groups	Study	Extremity	Primary or secondary	Study design	Study groups	Outcomes
Comparison of CDT with SAL	Brorson et al., *Lymphology. 2006* [40]	UE	Secondary	Retrospective comparative study	35 pts. underwent SAL with postoperative CCT 14 pts underwent CCT with custom compression garments only	Significant reductions in edema volumes in both groups at 6 months and at 1 year postoperatively, however the reductions were significantly greater in the SAL group compared with compression therapy only at both 6 months ($p < 0.0001$) and at 1 year (103% compared with 50%; $p = 0.0001$). Decrease in pain, swelling of the hand, and difficulties with activities of daily living at 1 year postoperatively in the liposuction group, whereas in the compression only group there was no change. Greater improvements in the liposuction group on the Nottingham Health Profile, the Psychological General Well-Being Index, and the Hospital Anxiety Depression Test.
Comparison of LVB with VLNT	Akita et al., *Ann Plast Surg. 2015* [24]	LE	Secondary	Prospective comparative study	13 pts. underwent supraclavicular VLNT (to distal thigh or lower leg) 43 limbs underwent LVB in 33 pts	Improvement in circumference reduction rate using LEL index was significantly greater in the VLNT group than in the LVB group [mean 21.2 (±2.0) compared with 26.5 (±4.4), respectively; $p = 0.032$]. ICG lymphography or lymphoscintigraphy improved in significantly more pts. following VLNT ($n = 7$) than LVB ($n = 10$). No significant complications occurred in the LVB group, whereas 3 patients in the supraclavicular VLNT group required reoperation for complications without flap loss ($p < 0.01$).
Comparison of different VLNTs	Ciudad et al., *J Surg Oncol. 2017* [32]	UE/LE	Primary and secondary	Retrospective cohort study	Comparative outcomes in 83 patients (UE, 30 pts.; LE, 53 pts) that underwent groin, supraclavicular, and gastroepiploic (open and laparoscopic flap harvest) VLNT [mean follow-up was 32.8 mo (range, 24–49)]	Mean circumference reduction rate was significant in both ISL stage II and III lymphedema ($p < 0.0001$), with a significantly greater reduction in stage II [29.1% (±8)] than stage III [17.9% (±7.6)] lymphedema. Similar good outcomes for patients with ISL stage II lymphedema [groin VLNT 28.5% (±7.8; $n = 10$); supraclavicular VLNT 26.2% (±9.8; $n = 10$); and gastroepiploic VLNT 30.4% (±7.3; $n = 25$)]. Similar modest outcomes for ISL stage III disease [groin VLNT 11.7% (±10.2; $n = 3$); supraclavicular VLNT 18.9% (±8.90; $n = 15$); and gastroepiploic VLNT 18.2% (±11; $n = 17$)]. Complication rate: groin VLNT 30.8%; supraclavicular VLNT 28%; gastroepiploic VLNT 24%; no donor site lymphedema. In pts. with prior cellulitis, there were no further episodes in 61.4% ($p < 0.05$), and a significant reduction in 27.7%. At 1 year postoperatively lymphoscintigraphy showed an improvement in lymphatic drainage in 96.4% patients.

(continued)

Table 24.2 (continued)

Comparator groups	Study	Extremity	Primary or secondary	Study design	Study groups	Outcomes
	Akita et al., *J Reconstr Microsurg. 2017* [23]	UE	Secondary	Prospective comparative study	13 pts. underwent chimeric DIEP-groin VLNT [mean f/u 13.9 (±6.5) mo] 14 pts. underwent groin LN flap alone [to axilla; mean f/u 13.2 (±4.4) mo]	Mean circumference reduction rate using UEL index similar at 6 mo post-op: DIEP-groin VLNT group 13.9 (±4.1); groin VLNT group 13.2 (±1.5). In DIEP-groin VLNT group, significant improvement using ICG lymphography in 6 pts.; in groin VLNT only group, significant improvement in 4 pts. In DIEP-groin VLNT group, significantly more patients reduced their compression garment use than in the VLNT only group (10 of 13 patients, compared with 3 of 14 patients; $p = 0.04$).
	Schaverien et al., *J Am Coll Surg. 2021* [20]	UE/LE	Primary/ secondary	Prospective comparative study	134 pts. (115 UE; 19 LE) underwent VLNT following maximal CDT; VLNTs included jejunal mesenteric ($n = 25$), groin ($n = 43$), lateral thoracic ($n = 31$), omental/right gastroepiploic ($n = 21$), and submental ($n = 14$). Synchronous LVB performed in 76 pts	Significant reductions in mean limb volume change [12 mo: 34.7% (±4.1), $p < 0.001$; 24 mo: 45.7% (±8.7), $p = 0.002$], mean LDex score [12 mo: 49.4% (±4.7), $p < 0.001$; 24 mo: 59.8% (±8.7), $p < 0.001$], and mean Lymphedema Life Impact Scale (LLIS) score [12 mo: 53.8% (±3.9), $p < 0.001$; 24 mo: 61.6% (±5.9), $p < 0.001$], compared with preoperatively. Outcomes similar between the different VLN flaps. Postoperatively 97.1% of patients had a decrease in LDex score and 90.2% had a reduction in limb volume excess; 98.9% of patients had an improvement in at least one of these measures. In 96.2% of patients there was an improvement in the LLIS score postoperatively. There were minimal clinically important differences (MIDs) for limb volume change in 89.6% patients, for LDex score in 91.1%, and for LLIS score in 94.8% of patients. In 35.2% of patients there was a history of cellulitis, and at up to 24 months follow-up postoperatively there was only one episode of cellulitis reported (97.9%, $p < 0.001$). In patients eligible to reduce their compression garments postoperatively, 63.1% had either discontinued (42.1%) or significantly reduced (21.1%) their use. There were no flap losses and there was a low flap-related complication rate; no patient developed clinical donor extremity lymphedema during 20.1 mo (±9.7) f/u.

UE upper extremity, *LE* lower extremity, *BCRL* breast cancer-related lymphedema, *ICG* indocyanine green, *LVB* lymphovenous bypass, *VLNT* vascularized lymph node transplant, *CDT* complete decongestive therapy, *CCT* controlled compression therapy, *LEL* lower extremity lymphedema, *UEL* upper extremity lymphedema, *MBR* microvascular breast reconstruction, *ISL* International Society of Lymphology, *DIEP* deep inferior epigastric artery perforator flap, *SAL* suction-assisted lipectomy, *pts* patients, *mo* months, *f/u* follow-up

References

1. Chang DW, Masia J, Garza R 3rd, Skoracki R, Neligan PC. Lymphedema: surgical and medical therapy. Plast Reconstr Surg. 2016;138:209–18.
2. Schaverien MV, Coroneos CJ. Surgical treatment of lymphedema. Plast Reconstr Surg. 2019;144(3):738–58.
3. Silva AK, Chang DW. Vascularized lymph node transfer and lymphovenous bypass: novel treatment strategies for symptomatic lymphedema. J Surg Oncol. 2016;113:932–9.
4. Carl H, Walia G, Bello R, et al. Systematic review of the surgical treatment of extremity lymphedema. J Reconstr Microsurg. 2017;33:412–25.
5. Basta MN, Gao LL, Wu LC. Operative treatment of peripheral lymphedema: a systematic meta-analysis of the efficacy and safety of lymphovenous microsurgery and tissue transplantation. Plast Reconstr Surg. 2014;133:905–13.
6. Sharkey AR, King SW, Ramsden AJ, Furniss D. Do surgical interventions for limb lymphoedema reduce cellulitis attack frequency? Microsurgery. 2017;37(4):348–53.
7. Scaglioni MF, Fontein DBY, Arvanitakis M, et al. Systematic review of lymphovenous anastomosis (LVA) for the treatment of lymphedema. Microsurgery. 2017;37:947–53.
8. Cornelissen AJM, Beugels J, Ewalds L, et al. Effect of lymphaticovenous anastomosis in breast cancer-related lymphedema: a review of the literature. Lymphat Res Biol. 2018;16:426–34.
9. Salgarello M, Mangialardi ML, Pino V, et al. A prospective evaluation of health-related quality of life following lymphaticovenular anastomosis for upper and lower extremities lymphedema. J Reconstr Microsurg. 2018;34:701–7.
10. Cornelissen AJM, Kool M, Lopez Penha TR, et al. Lymphaticovenous anastomosis as treatment for breast cancer-related lymphedema: a prospective study on quality of life. Breast Cancer Res Treat. 2017;163(2):281–6.
11. Chang DW. Lymphaticovenular bypass for lymphedema management in breast cancer patients: a prospective study. Plast Reconstr Surg. 2010;126:752–8.
12. Akita S, Mitsukawa N, Kuriyama M, et al. Suitable therapy options for sub-clinical and early-stage lymphoedema patients. J Plast Reconstr Aesthet Surg. 2014;67:520–5.
13. Koshima I, Nanba Y, Tsutsui T, et al. Minimal invasive lymphaticovenular anastomosis under local anesthesia for leg lymphedema: is it effective for stage III and IV? Ann Plast Surg. 2004;53(3):261–6.
14. Campisi CC, Ryan M, Boccardo F, Campisi C. A single-site technique of multiple lymphatic-venous anastomoses for the treatment of peripheral lymphedema: long-term clinical outcome. J Reconstr Microsurg. 2016;32(1):42–9.
15. Mihara M, Hara H, Furniss D, et al. Lymphaticovenular anastomosis to prevent cellulitis associated with lymphoedema. Br J Surg. 2014;101(11):1391–6.
16. Gennaro P, Gabriele G, Salini C, et al. Our supramicrosurgical experience of lymphaticovenular anastomosis in lymphoedema patients to prevent cellulitis. Eur Rev Med Pharmacol Sci. 2017;21(4):674–9.
17. Ozturk CN, Ozturk C, Glasgow M, et al. Free vascularized lymph node transfer for treatment of lymphedema: a systematic evidence based review. J Plast Reconstr Aesthet Surg. 2016;69:1234–47.
18. Dionyssiou D, Demiri E, Tsimponis A, et al. A randomized control study of treating secondary stage II breast cancer-related lymphoedema with free lymph node transfer. Breast Cancer Res Treat. 2016;156:73–9.
19. Beederman M, Garza RM, Agarwal S, Chang DW. Outcomes for physiologic microsurgical treatment of secondary lymphedema involving the extremity. Ann Surg. 2020;
20. Schaverien MV, Asaad M, Selber JC, et al. Outcomes of vascularized lymph node transplantation for the treatment of lymphedema. J Am Coll Surg. 2021;
21. Chang EI, Ibrahim A, Liu J, Robe C, Suami H, Hanasono MM, Nguyen AT. Optimizing quality of life for patients with breast cancer-related lymphedema: a prospective study combining DIEP flap breast reconstruction and lymphedema surgery. Plast Reconstr Surg. 2020;145(4):676–85.
22. Patel KM, Lin CY, Cheng MH. A prospective evaluation of lymphedema-specific quality-of-life outcomes following vascularized lymph node transfer. Ann Surg Oncol. 2015;22:2424–30.
23. Akita S, Tokumoto H, Yamaji Y, et al. Contribution of simultaneous breast reconstruction by deep inferior epigastric artery perforator flap to the efficacy of vascularized lymph node transfer in patients with breast cancer-related lymphedema. J Reconstr Microsurg. 2017;33(8):571–8.
24. Akita S, Mitsukawa N, Kuriyama M, et al. Comparison of vascularized supraclavicular lymph node transfer and lymphaticovenular anastomosis for advanced stage lower extremity lymphedema. Ann Plast Surg. 2015;74(5):573–9.
25. Cheng MH, Chen SC, Henry SL, et al. Vascularized groin lymph node flap transfer for postmastectomy upper limb lymphedema: flap anatomy, recipient sites, and outcomes. Plast Reconstr Surg. 2013;131(6):1286–98.
26. Engel H, Lin CY, Huang JJ, Cheng MH. Outcomes of lymphedema microsurgery for breast cancer-related lymphedema with or without microvascular breast reconstruction. Ann Surg. 2018;268(6):1076–83.
27. Batista BN, Germain M, Faria JC, Becker C. Lymph node flap transfer for patients with secondary lower limb lymphedema. Microsurgery. 2017;37(1):29–33.
28. Gratzon A, Schultz J, Secrest K, Lee K, Feiner J, Klein RD. Clinical and psychosocial outcomes of vascularized lymph node transfer for the treatment of upper extremity lymphedema after breast cancer therapy. Ann Surg Oncol. 2017;24:1475–81.
29. De Brucker B, Zeltzer A, Seidenstuecker K, et al. Breast cancer-related lymphedema: quality of life after lymph node transfer. Plast Reconstr Surg. 2016;137:1673–80.
30. Nguyen AT, Chang EI, Suami H, Chang DW. An algorithmic approach to simultaneous vascularized lymph node transfer with microvascular breast reconstruction. Ann Surg Oncol. 2015;22(9):2919–24.
31. Nguyen AT, Suami H, Hanasono MM, Womack VA, Wong FC, Chang EI. Long-term outcomes of the minimally invasive free vascularized omental lymphatic flap for the treatment of lymphedema. J Surg Oncol. 2017;115(1):84–9.
32. Ciudad P, Agko M, Perez Coca JJ, et al. Comparison of long-term clinical outcomes among different vascularized lymph node transfers: 6-year experience of a single center's approach to the treatment of lymphedema. J Surg Oncol. 2017;116:671–82.
33. Forte AJ, Huayllani MT, Boczar D, et al. Lipoaspiration and controlled compressive therapy in lymphedema of the upper extremity: a comprehensive systematic review. Cureus. 2019;11(9):e5787.
34. Hoffner M, Ohlin K, Svensson B, et al. Liposuction gives complete reduction of arm lymphedema following breast cancer treatment-a 5-year prospective study in 105 patients without recurrence. Plast Reconstr Surg Glob Open. 2018;6:1912.
35. Brorson H. Complete reduction of arm lymphedema following breast cancer: a prospective twenty-one years' study. Plast Reconstr Surg. 2015;136:134–5.
36. Lee D, Piller N, Hoffner M, et al. Liposuction of postmastectomy arm lymphedema decreases the incidence of erysipelas. Lymphology. 2016;49:85–92.
37. Stewart CJ, Munnoch DA. Liposuction as an effective treatment for lower extremity lymphoedema: a single surgeon's experience over nine years. J Plast Reconstr Aesthet Surg. 2018;71:239–45.
38. Lamprou DA, Voesten HG, Damstra RJ, Wikkeling OR. Circumferential suction-assisted lipectomy in the treatment of primary and secondary end-stage lymphoedema of the leg. Br J Surg. 2017;104:84–9.

39. Hoffner M, Bagheri S, Hansson E, et al. SF-36 shows increased quality of life following complete reduction of postmastectomy lymphedema with liposuction. Lymphat Res Biol. 2017;15:87–98.
40. Brorson H, Ohlin K, Olsson G, et al. Quality of life following liposuction and conservative treatment of arm lymphedema. Lymphology. 2006;39:8–25.
41. Johnson AR, Kimball S, Epstein S, et al. Lymphedema incidence after axillary lymph node dissection: quantifying the impact of radiation and the lymphatic microsurgical preventive healing approach. Ann Plast Surg. 2019;82:S234–41.
42. Jorgensen MG, Toyserkani NM, Sorensen JA. The effect of prophylactic lymphovenous anastomosis and shunts for preventing cancer-related lymphedema: a systematic review and meta-analysis. Microsurgery. 2018;38(5):576–85.
43. Boccardo FM, Casabona F, Friedman D, Puglisi M, De Cian F, Ansaldi F, Campisi C. Surgical prevention of arm lymphedema after breast cancer treatment. Ann Surg Oncol. 2011;18(9):2500–5.
44. Feldman S, Bansil H, Ascherman J, et al. Single institution experience with lymphatic microsurgical preventive healing approach (LYMPHA) for the primary prevention of lymphedema. Ann Surg Oncol. 2015;22(10):3296–301.
45. Boccardo F, Valenzano M, Costantini S, et al. LYMPHA technique to prevent secondary lower limb lymphedema. Ann Surg Oncol. 2016;23(11):3558–63.

Key Topic: Evaluating Outcomes of Lymphedema Surgery

25

Mark V. Schaverien and Joseph H. Dayan

Introduction

There is a large and robust body of evidence, including systematic reviews and meta-analyses, randomized controlled trials (RCTs), and prospective comparative and cohort studies, demonstrating the effectiveness of surgery to treat lymphedema (Chap. 24). These surgical treatments include lymphovenous bypass (LVB), vascularized lymph node transplant (VLNT), suction-assisted lipectomy (SAL) debulking with controlled compression therapy (CCT), and direct excisional procedures, as well as combined physiological and debulking procedures. A limitation of the current evidence base is that although there is consistency within individual studies regarding objective measurement modalities used pre- and postoperatively, there is heterogeneity in those used between different studies. For example, most commonly studies report limb volume measurements calculated using limb circumferential measurements; however, the utility of these remains limited by significant inter- and intrarater variability [1, 2]. Other studies have used water-displacement plethysmography, which, although it is the most accurate tool available for measuring limb volume, is not commonly utilized in the clinical setting due to practical limitations. The ability to allow comparison between different studies to enable pooling of data and meta-analysis is therefore limited, and there remains a pressing need for consistency in longitudinal outcomes data including objective measurements and patient-reported outcomes (PROs).

Similar to the multimodal evaluation of the lymphedema patient preoperatively as detailed in Chap. 5, during postoperative follow-up of surgery to treat their lymphedema, a standardized approach involving measurement of multiple objective metrics and PROs should be instituted at fixed interval periods [1, 3]. These include the change in excess limb volume, extracellular fluid measurement using bioimpedance spectroscopy (BIS), conservative care requirements, episodes of cellulitis, as well as PROs, at each postoperative time interval compared with preoperatively and between each successive time interval [1, 4]. It is important that patient evaluation incorporates multiple assessment methods to increase the reliability of the lymphedema assessments [5]. Other metrics may include restaging, typically at yearly intervals postoperatively, using indocyanine green (ICG) fluorescent lymphography [6, 7] or radioisotope lymphoscintigraphy [8]. Lymphoscintigraphy or magnetic resonance lymphangiography (MRL) may also be used to evaluate the physiological functioning of the VLNT [9, 10].

Many of these metrics have been shown to correlate, which increases their reliability: one study of upper and lower extremity lymphedema found a correlation between limb circumference change in response to VLNT and all domains using the validated condition-specific Lymphedema Quality-of-Life (LYMQOL) questionnaire [4]. Multiple studies have demonstrated that L-Dex score correlates with limb volume excess, and one study found that both of these were responsive to surgical intervention including LVB and VLNT [1, 11, 12].

Here, we present a framework for evaluation of evidence-based postoperative outcomes for patients undergoing surgical treatment of their lymphedema (Table 24.1).

Lymphedema-Specific Symptoms

Evaluation should include self-reports of lymphedema-specific symptoms of swelling and heaviness in the affected limb, currently and previously, as well as change in frequency and relation to provoking activities. Lymphedema-

M. V. Schaverien (✉)
Department of Plastic Surgery, The University of Texas MD Anderson Cancer Center, Houston, TX, USA
e-mail: mvschaverien@mdanderson.org

J. H. Dayan (✉)
Division of Plastic and Reconstructive Surgery, Memorial Sloan Kettering Cancer Center, New York, NY, USA
e-mail: dayanj@mskcc.org

M. V. Schaverien, J. H. Dayan (eds.), *Multimodal Management of Upper and Lower Extremity Lymphedema*,
https://doi.org/10.1007/978-3-030-93039-4_25

Table 24.1 Recommended minimal clinical postoperative measurements/investigations for patients that have undergone surgery for lymphedema

Measurement/investigation	6 months	12 months	24 months
Lymphedema-specific symptoms including swelling and heaviness currently and in the past 12 months, and change in frequency/relation to activities	X	X	X
Episodes of lymphedema-related cellulitis in the past 12 months and treatment required (oral/intravenous antibiotics)	X	X	X
Detailed treatment history including number of hours using bandaging or compression garment, and compression type/class; frequency of use of an intermittent pneumatic compression device/week; frequency of use of night compression/week and type	X	X	X
Degree of pitting edema measured using the pitting edema scale	X	X	X
Limb volume measurement using perometer or limb circumferential measurements with truncated cone formula	X	X	X
Extracellular fluid measurement using L-Dex score	X	X	X
Patient-reported outcomes using LLIS (v2), LYMQOL, or ULL27	X	X	X
Physiological restaging imaging using ICG fluorescent lymphography (MRL or lymphoscintigraphy alternatives), either scheduled or as indicated by disease response		X	X

LLIS Lymphedema Life Impact Scale, *LYMQOL* Lymphedema Quality-of-Life, *ULL*-27 Upper Limb Lymphedema 27, *ICG* Indocyanine green, *MRL* Magnetic resonance lymphangiography

specific symptoms are sensitive for diagnosis and longitudinal evaluation and include impaired limb mobility, limb swelling, truncal swelling, heaviness, tightness, numbness, tenderness, pain, aching, and tingling (paresthesia) [13]; evaluation of multiple symptoms improves the sensitivity and specificity of assessment [5]. The Lymphedema Breast Cancer Questionnaire (LBCQ) is a structured, self-report tool that assesses 19 symptoms and the frequency of their occurrence that has demonstrated reliability when used in prospective lymphedema surveillance [14]. Within this tool, a self-report of limb swelling or heaviness is most closely associated with a lymphedema diagnosis [15]; this is supported by the findings of a study of patients with upper extremity secondary lymphedema that the most common symptoms reported were swelling (97.5%) and heaviness (71%) [1].

Recommendation: *At each interval, self-report of swelling and heaviness in the affected extremity should be recorded.*

Episodes of Lymphedema-Related Cellulitis

The number of episodes of lymphedema-related cellulitis in the affected limb annually and the treatment required (oral/intravenous antibiotics) should be sought and documented, together with the cause (i.e., spontaneous or following trauma), frequency, and timing. The frequency of episodes of cellulitis is typically reduced following physiological and debulking surgeries for lymphedema [16, 17].

Recommendation: *At each interval, the number of episodes of cellulitis in the affected extremity annually and treatment required should be recorded.*

Detailed Treatment History

A detailed treatment history should be documented at each interval to determine the longitudinal changes in these requirements in response to surgery. This history should include the number of hours using bandaging or compression garments, as well as the compression type and compression class, the frequency of use of their intermittent pneumatic compression device (PCD) per week and treatment duration if applicable, as well as the frequency of use of night compression per week and type of garment (including bandaging), if applicable. The use of these in the last week can be documented by the patient in a diary to improve accuracy.

Recommendation: *At each interval, a detailed treatment history in the past week should be recorded.*

Degree of Pitting Edema

The degree of pitting edema at each time interval can be measured using the pitting edema scale. The presence of pitting edema is a sensitive sign of lymphedema, occurring in 71% of patients in one study of upper extremity secondary lymphedema [1]. The presence of pitting edema is assessed by pressing the examiner's thumb into consistent locations for 60 seconds; the severity of pitting edema can be measured approximately and expressed using the pitting edema scale [18]. Its presence and distribution correspond to the dermal backflow visualized on lymphatic imaging (i.e., ICG lymphography, lymphoscintigraphy, MRL) [19], and the degree of pitting edema correlates with the L-Dex score but not limb volume difference, likely due to the associated fibrosis that characterizes the advanced lymphedema phenotype [12].

Recommendation: *At each time interval, the degree of pitting edema and distribution should be recorded.*

Limb Volume Measurement

Limb volume measurements using a perometer should be conducted at each time interval. Alternatively, limb circumferential measurements using a tape measure at 4 cm intervals can be used to calculate limb volume using the truncated cone formula; there is significant inter- and intra-rater variability due to difficulty replicating both the exact reference points and the tension applied to the tape, and standardization is essential [1, 2].

The perometer is very accurate due to its availability and ease of use – it is fast, valid, and reliable [12, 20, 21]. The differences between the affected and unaffected limbs are expressed as relative and absolute limb volume excess ratios; in bilateral lymphedema, the excess volume cannot be determined, and so the percentage change in volume for each limb from baseline is calculated. A minimal clinically important difference (MCID) in limb volume has been estimated at 10% [22]. To achieve accuracy and low variance, measurements are taken from defined and reproducible points with the same limb length used for each measurement and for each limb by consistent trained investigators; a variance of less than 1% between successive measurements should be achieved, with the variance in measurements of the unaffected limb a useful benchmark between successive measurement intervals. It is important in the clinical setting that the perometer is regularly recalibrated to maintain accuracy.

Recommendation: *At each interval, limb volume measurements of the affected and unaffected extremities using a perometer or limb circumference measurements (using truncated cone volume calculation) should be recorded.*

Bioimpedance Spectroscopy (L-Dex Score)

Bioimpedance spectroscopy (BIS) measurement enables rapid and reliable noninvasive measurement of extracellular water in an extremity. The L-Dex® U400 (ImpediMed, Carlsbad, CA), a portable adhesive electrode and lead-based system, has been the most studied BIS device for lymphedema; however, a significant amount of training and standardization are required for consistent results; the SOZO® (ImpediMed, Carlsbad, CA) uses contact electrode pads at the palm and sole to reduce user error and improve reliability. Measurement of the L-Dex score is reliable for the diagnosis of secondary upper extremity breast cancer-related lymphedema (BRCL) [1, 20, 21, 23–25] and significantly correlates with lymphedema severity stage and limb volume excess [12, 26]; it is also highly responsive to nonsurgical and surgical interventions [1, 12].

The L-Dex score is derived from the ratio of the impedance values between the affected and unaffected limbs calculated after adjusting for sex, upper/lower limb, and right/left dominance [27], and a limitation of BIS remains the ability to independently and reliably measure bilateral extremity lymphedema. Although no MCID has been established as a threshold for the L-Dex score, an estimate for a given population can be made utilizing the distribution-based method using half a standard deviation [28].

Recommendation: *At each interval, the L-Dex score should be recorded (if available).*

Patient-Reported Outcome Measures (PROMs)

PROs are important for evaluation of the lymphedema patient as well as for longitudinal assessment in response to nonsurgical or surgical intervention. Several scales have been validated for the measurement of PROs specific for lymphedema and are increasingly being used in the routine clinical setting. The lymphedema-specific scales that have been evaluated most in studies include the Lymphedema Quality of Life (LYMQOL) questionnaire, the Lymphedema Life Impact Scale (LLIS), and the Upper Limb Lymphedema 27 (ULL-27); other questionnaires include the Lymphedema Quality of Life Inventory (LyQLI), the Freiburg Life Quality Assessment for Lymphedema (FLQA-L), and the Lymphoedema Functioning, Disability and Health Questionnaire for Lower Limb Lymphedema (Lymph-ICF-LL), and recently the LYMPH-Q [29, 30]. The LLIS (version 2), which includes 18 questions about the past week distributed across physical, functional, and psychological domains [31], was found to correlate highly with the ULL-27 and was more sensitive in measuring physical and functional disability [1]. The LLIS (v2) is therefore recommended for assessment of PROs, for which the MCID is 7.31 points [31–33]. Although commonly used, one study found no correlation between the LYMQOL score and the International Society of Lymphology (ISL) stage or L-Dex score for both upper and lower extremity lymphedema [34].

Recommendation: *At each interval, a validated lymphedema-specific questionnaire should be administered.*

Physiological Restaging Imaging

Physiological lymphedema staging can be performed using ICG fluorescent lymphography to evaluate the lymphatic transport, the presence of functional lymphatic vessels, and the pattern and distribution of dermal backflow. Validated staging systems include the Dermal Backflow staging scale and the MD Anderson Cancer Center (MDACC) ICG lymphedema staging scale [6, 7]. ICG lymphography is currently regarded as the most sensitive test for lymphedema, with one study finding that all affected upper limbs with a limb volume of >10% had abnormal ICG patterns; when compared with lymphoscintigraphy, ICG lymphography has greater sensitivity in both the upper and lower extremities [35]. Physiological restaging may be performed at standardized intervals, or as indicated depending on the clinical progression postoperatively.

Radionuclide lymphoscintigraphy can also be used for restaging [36, 37]. Validated staging scales such as the Taiwan Lymphoscintigraphy Staging system evaluate the lymph nodes, lymphatic ducts, and the presence and distribution of dermal backflow [8]. Studies though are inconsistent regarding the reliability of lymphoscintigraphy [1, 36, 38], with one study finding that the sensitivity and specificity with a minimum limb volume excess of 10% were 88% and 41.4%, respectively, and the positive and negative predictive values were 72.1% and 66.7%, respectively [1]; these results are likely affected by the experience of the radiologist and interpreter, as well as definitions of normal and abnormal lymphoscintograms. MRL enables visualization of the anatomical and functional status of lymphatic vessels, lymph nodes, and dermal backflow in patients with lymphedema, and in one study MRL was found to have greater sensitivity and specificity than lymphoscintigraphy across a range of measures [39]. The main disadvantages of MRL, however, are the operator dependence and necessity for a radiologist with expertise in postprocessing and in evaluation of patients with lymphedema. There is also a paucity of validated staging scales. Lymphoscintigraphy or MRL may also be used to evaluate the physiological functioning of the transplanted lymph nodes postoperatively; however, these may be limited in contrast enhancement of proximal orthotopic VLNT [9, 10].

Recommendation: *Physiological restaging postoperatively may be performed at annual intervals or as clinically indicated depending on disease response.*

Limb Functional Assessment Instruments

Limb functional assessment instruments validated in other domains can provide complementary information regarding the physical disability resulting from lymphedema. These tools include the Disabilities of the Arm, Shoulder, and Hand Questionnaire (DASH/Quick-DASH), Lower Extremity Functional Scale (LEFS), Upper Extremity Functional Index (UEFI), and Upper Limb Disability Questionnaire (ULDQ). One study, however, found no correlation between the DASH and LEFS scores and ISL stage or L-Dex score in upper and lower extremities, respectively [34]. Further research is needed to validate their use in lymphedema due to their non-disease specificity.

A summary of these recommendations is presented in Table 24.1.

References

1. Wiser I, Mehrara BJ, Coriddi M, Kenworthy E, Cavalli M, Encarnacion E, Dayan JH. Preoperative assessment of upper extremity secondary lymphedema. Cancers (Basel). 2020;12:135.
2. Sun F, Hall A, Tighe MP, Brunelle CL, Sayegh HE, Gillespie TC, Daniell KM, Taghian AG. Perometry versus simulated circumferential tape measurement for the detection of breast cancer-related lymphedema. Breast Cancer Res Treat. 2018;172:83–91.
3. Pappalardo M, Patel K, Cheng MH. Vascularized lymph node transfer for treatment of extremity lymphedema: an overview of current controversies regarding donor sites, recipient sites and outcomes. J Surg Oncol. 2018;117:1420–31.
4. Patel KM, Lin CY, Cheng MH. A prospective evaluation of lymphedema-specific quality-of-life outcomes following vascularized lymph node transfer. Ann Surg Oncol. 2015;22:2424–30.
5. Fu MR, Axelrod D, Cleland CM, Qiu Z, Guth AA, Kleinman R, Scagliola J, Haber J. Symptom report in detecting breast cancer-related lymphedema. Breast Cancer (Dove Med Press). 2015;7:345–52.
6. Chang DW, Suami H, Skoracki R. A prospective analysis of 100 consecutive lymphovenous bypass cases for treatment of extremity lymphedema. Plast Reconstr Surg. 2013;132:1305–14.
7. Yamamoto T, Yamamoto N, Doi K, et al. Indocyanine green-enhanced lymphography for upper extremity lymphedema: a novel severity staging system using dermal backflow patterns. Plast Reconstr Surg. 2011;128:941–7.
8. Cheng MH, Pappalardo M, Lin C, Kuo CF, Lin CY, Chung KC. Validity of the novel Taiwan lymphoscintigraphy staging and correlation of Cheng lymphedema grading for unilateral extremity lymphedema. Ann Surg. 2018;268:513–25.
9. Cheng MH, Chen SC, Henry SL, et al. Vascularized groin lymph node flap transfer for postmastectomy upper limb lymphedema: flap anatomy, recipient sites, and outcomes. Plast Reconstr Surg. 2013;131:1286–98.
10. Becker C, Assouad J, Riquet M, Hidden G. Postmastectomy lymphedema: long-term results following microsurgical lymph node transplantation. Ann Surg. 2006;243:313–5.
11. Seward C, Skolny M, Brunelle C, Asdourian M, Salama L, Taghian AG. A comprehensive review of bioimpedance spectroscopy as a diagnostic tool for the detection and measurement of breast cancer-related lymphedema. J Surg Oncol. 2016;114:537–42.
12. Coroneos CJ, Wong FC, DeSnyder SM, Shaitelman SF, Schaverien MV. Correlation of L-Dex bioimpedance spectroscopy with limb volume and lymphatic function in lymphedema. Lymphat Res Biol. 2019;17:301–7.
13. Armer JM, Ballman KV, McCall L, Armer NC, Sun Y, Udmuangpia T, Hunt KK, Mittendorf EA, Byrd DR, Julian TB, Boughey JC. Lymphedema symptoms and limb measurement changes in breast cancer survivors treated with neoadjuvant chemotherapy and axillary dissection: results of American College of Surgeons

Oncology Group (ACOSOG) Z1071 (Alliance) substudy. Support Care Cancer. 2019 Feb;27(2):495–503.
14. Armer JM, Hulett JM, Bernas M, Ostby P, Stewart BR, Cormier JN. Best-practice guidelines in assessment, risk reduction, management, and surveillance for post-breast cancer lymphedema. Curr Breast Cancer Rep. 2013;5:134–44.
15. Armer JM, Stewart BR. Post-breast cancer lymphedema: incidence increases from 12 to 30 to 60 months. Lymphology. 2010;43(3):118–27.
16. Sharkey AR, King SW, Ramsden AJ, Furniss D. Do surgical interventions for limb lymphoedema reduce cellulitis attack frequency? Microsurgery. 2017;37(4):348–53.
17. Lee D, Piller N, Hoffner M, et al. Liposuction of postmastectomy arm lymphedema decreases the incidence of erysipelas. Lymphology. 2016;49:85–92.
18. Brodovicz KG, McNaughton K, Uemura N, Meininger G, Girman CJ, Yale SH. Reliability and feasibility of methods to quantitatively assess peripheral edema. Clin Med Res. 2009;7(1–2):21–31.
19. Thomis S, Dams L, Fourneau I, De Vrieze T, Nevelsteen I, Neven P, Gebruers N, Devoogdt N. Correlation between clinical assessment and lymphofluoroscopy in patients with breast cancer-related lymphedema: a study of concurrent validity. Lymphat Res Biol. 2020;25
20. Adriaenssens N, Buyl R, Lievens P, Fontaine C, Lamote J. Comparative study between mobile infrared optoelectronic volumetry with a Perometer and two commonly used methods for the evaluation of arm volume in patients with breast cancer related lymphedema of the arm. Lymphology. 2013;46:132–43.
21. Jain MS, Danoff JV, Paul SM. Correlation between bioelectrical spectroscopy and perometry in assessment of upper extremity swelling. Lymphology. 2010;43:85–94.
22. Cormier JN, Xing Y, Zaniletti I, Askew RL, Stewart BR, Armer JM. Minimal limb volume change has a significant impact on breast cancer survivors. Lymphology. 2009;42(4):161–75.
23. Fu MR, Cleland CM, Guth AA, Kayal M, Haber J, Cartwright F, Kleinman R, Kang Y, Scagliola J, Axelrod D. L-dex ratio in detecting breast cancer-related lymphedema: reliability, sensitivity, and specificity. Lymphology. 2013;46:85–96.
24. Ridner SH, Dietrich MS, Spotanski K, Doersam JK, Cowher MS, Taback B, McLaughlin S, Ajkay N, Boyages J, Koelmeyer L, DeSnyder S, Shah C, Vicini F. A prospective study of L-Dex values in breast cancer patients pretreatment and through 12 months postoperatively. Lymphat Res Biol. 2018;16:435–41.
25. Levenhagen K, Davies C, Perdomo M, Ryans K, Gilchrist L. Diagnosis of upper quadrant lymphedema secondary to cancer: clinical practice guideline from the Oncology Section of the American Physical Therapy Association. Phys Ther. 2017;97:729–45.
26. Szuba A, Strauss W, Sirsikar SP, Rockson SG. Quantitative radionuclide lymphoscintigraphy predicts outcome of manual lymphatic therapy in breast cancer-related lymphedema of the upper extremity. Nucl Med Commun. 2002;23:1171–5.
27. Czerniec SA, Ward LC, Refshauge KM, Beith J, Lee MJ, York S, Kilbreath SL. Assessment of breast cancer-related arm lymphedema-comparison of physical measurement methods and self-report. Cancer Investig. 2010;28:54–62.
28. Norman GR, Sloan JA, Wyrwich KW. Interpretation of changes in health-related quality of life. Med Care. 2003;41:582–92.
29. Coriddi M, Dayan J, Sobti N, Nash D, Goldberg J, Klassen A, Pusic A, Mehrara B. Systematic review of patient-reported outcomes following surgical treatment of lymphedema. Cancers (Basel). 2020 Feb 29;12(3):565.
30. Beelen LM, van Dishoeck AM, Tsangaris E, Coriddi M, Dayan JH, Pusic AL, Klassen A, Vasilic D. Patient-reported outcome measures in lymphedema: a systematic review and COSMIN analysis. Ann Surg Oncol. 2020;
31. Weiss J, Daniel T. Validation of the lymphedema life impact scale (LLIS): a condition-specific measurement tool for persons with lymphedema. Lymphology. 2017;48:128–38.
32. Weiss J, Daniel T. Validation of the lymphedema life impact scale version 2: a condition specific measurement tool for persons with lymphedema. Lymphology. 2015;48:128–38.
33. Beederman M, Garza RM, Agarwal S, Chang DW. Outcomes for physiologic microsurgical treatment of secondary lymphedema involving the extremity. Ann Surg. 2020;
34. Lee TS, Morris CM, Czerniec SA, Mangion AJ. Does lymphedema severity affect quality of life? Simple question. Challenging answers. Lymphat Res Biol. 2018;16:85–91.
35. Mihara M, Hara H, Araki J, Kikuchi K, Narushima M, Yamamoto T, Iida T, Yoshimatsu H, Murai N, Mitsui K, Okitsu T, Koshima I. Indocyanine green (ICG) lymphography is superior to lymphoscintigraphy for diagnostic imaging of early lymphedema of the upper limbs. PLoS One. 2012;7:e38182.
36. Maclellan RA, Zurakowski D, Voss S, Greene AK. Correlation between lymphedema disease severity and lymphoscintigraphic findings: a clinical-radiologic study. J Am Coll Surg. 2017;225:366–70.
37. Kleinhans E, Baumeister RG, Hahn D, et al. Evaluation of transport kinetics in lymphoscintigraphy: follow-up study in patients with transplanted lymphatic vessels. Eur J Nucl Med. 1985;10:349–52.
38. Hassanein AH, Maclellan RA, Grant FD, Greene AK. Diagnostic accuracy of lymphoscintigraphy for lymphedema and analysis of false-negative tests. Plast Reconstr Surg Glob Open. 2017;5:e1396.
39. Bae JS, Yoo RE, Choi SH, Park SO, Chang H, Suh M, Cheon GJ. Evaluation of lymphedema in upper extremities by MR lymphangiography: comparison with lymphoscintigraphy. Magn Reson Imaging. 2018;49:63–70.

New and Emerging Therapies for Lymphedema: Part I

26

Alex K. Wong and Anjali C. Raghuram

Introduction

The pathophysiology of lymphedema involves cellular responses to initial lymphatic injury and the accumulation of interstitial fluid, which ultimately result in impaired lymphatic function and fibroadipose tissue changes [1]. Chronic interstitial fluid stasis activates inflammatory pathways and causes tissue remodeling, lymphatic hyperplasia, and adipocyte deposition [1, 2]. CD4+ cells are the hallmark inflammatory effectors involved in progressing the disease course. Through CD4+ facilitation of a Th2-biased mixed Th1/Th2 response, surrounding fibroblasts are triggered to compensatorily initiate matrix repair via autocrine upregulation of transforming growth factor-β1 (TGF-β1), myofibroblast differentiation, and increased collagen production [2]. Additionally, the Th2 response inhibits lymphangiogenic collateral vessel formation and impairs lymphatic pumping function. The positive feedback loop of chronic inflammation in lymphedema ultimately results in disease sequelae of altered soft tissue compliance, lymphatic vessel obliteration, and patient symptomatology of limb heaviness, tightness, and/or pitting edema [1, 3].

Consequently, patients with lymphedema experience advanced stages of disease through pro-inflammatory, pro-fibrotic, and anti-lymphangiogenic mechanisms. Therapeutically targeting these mechanisms to prevent Th2-propagated inflammation provides an important clinical focus for disease management. The variability in patient incidence, degree of lymphedematous swelling, time course, and symptoms further add to the challenges associated with caring for patients facing this debilitating and distressing disease [4]. Over the past decade, there has been a concerted effort to identify specific gene, protein, lipid, and cellular targets for pharmacologic intervention. Given the frequently subtle symptoms and physiologic limb size changes in early lymphedema [4], there is a growing interest in these novel therapies with prophylactic and symptom-alleviating properties to better treat patients and minimize morbidity with lymphedema.

A. K. Wong (✉) · A. C. Raghuram
Division of Plastic Surgery, City of Hope National Medical Center, Duarte, CA, USA
e-mail: alexwong@coh.org

Lymphangiogenic Therapeutic Approaches

Lymphangiogenesis is the primary mode of lymphatic growth and involves vessel formation from preexisting vessels. There have been several identified lymphangiogenic signaling pathways, and an illustration of these target-receptor interactions is presented in Fig. 26.1. Given the lymphatic vessel obliteration and compromise seen in patients with lymphedema, lymphangiogenic mechanisms provide a key therapeutic opportunity to restore lymphatic function and provide for better interstitial fluid drainage, lipid absorption, and immune response [5]. An overview of the following lymphangiogenic therapies is presented in Table 26.1.

Vascular Endothelial Growth Factor (VEGF)

Among the central lymphangiogenic pathways, signaling via the interactions of vascular endothelial growth factor-C (VEGF-C) with vascular endothelial growth factor receptor 3 (VEGFR3) is recognized as essential for endothelial cell sprouting from embryonic veins committed to the lymphatic lineage [5]. VEGFs are also known to interact with VEGFR2, although producing less significant lymphangiogenic results of vessel enlargement and limited sprouting [6]. Via VEGF-C-mediated phosphorylation of serine kinases AKT and ERK, lymphatic endothelial cells (LECs) are able to proliferate, migrate, and survive [7]. Moreover, inhibition of VEGFR3 signaling during lymphatic vessel formation results in lymphatic regression and consequent lymphedema in mouse embryos and neonates [8]. In 70% of patients with Milroy disease, an autosomal dominant primary congenital

M. V. Schaverien, J. H. Dayan (eds.), *Multimodal Management of Upper and Lower Extremity Lymphedema*,
https://doi.org/10.1007/978-3-030-93039-4_26

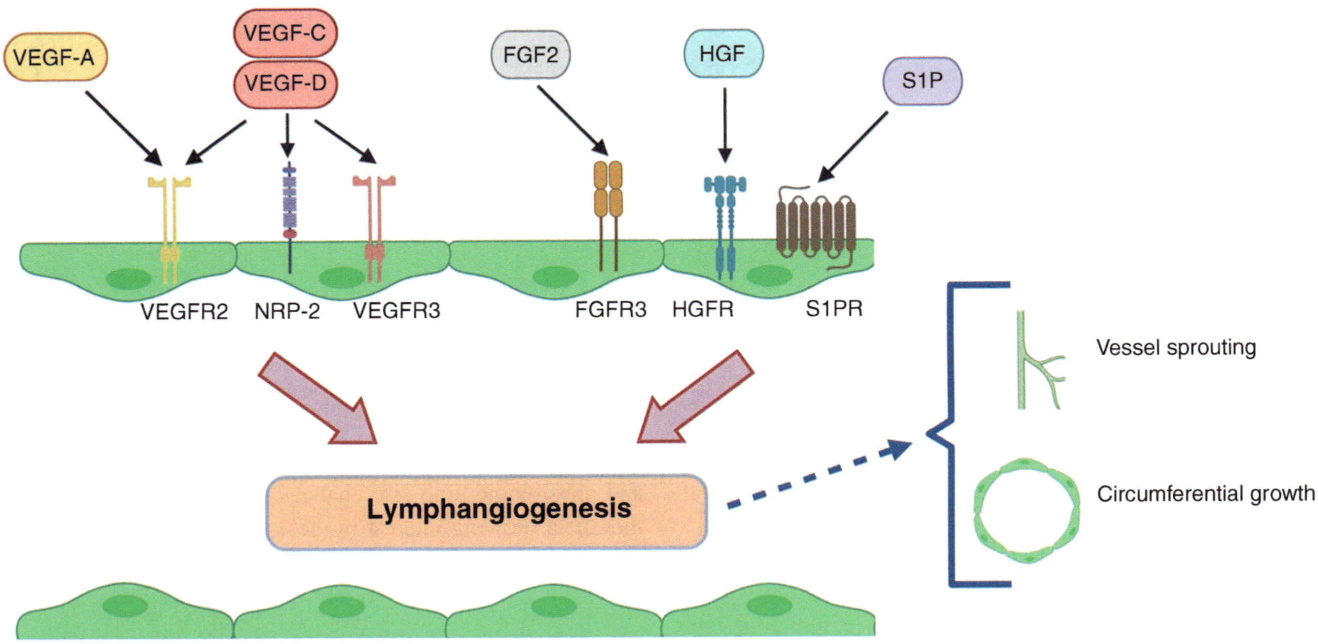

Fig. 26.1 An overview of lymphangiogenic signaling pathways

lymphedema, missense mutations are identified in the tyrosine kinase domain of VEGFR3 [9].

Given the critical and specific role of VEGF-C in lymphangiogenesis, it stands to reason that exogenous delivery of this growth factor can result in symptomatic improvement in patients with lymphedema. Experimental murine and porcine models of lymphedema have demonstrated that VEGF-C treatment, in combination with lymph node transfer, produces a superior lymphangiogenic response than treatment with other VEGF family members, such as VEGF-A and VEGF-D [10, 11]. Further, in pigs treated with VEGF-C, the structure of the transferred lymph nodes is optimally preserved, and unlike pigs treated with VEGF-D, the operated inguinal donor region does not encounter postoperative seroma [11]. Although these results are promising, clinical translation of VEGFs is limited by their concern for tumor metastatic behavior along with recruitment and migration of tumor-associated macrophages [12]. Additionally, expression of VEGF-C is found to be markedly increased in lymphedematous tissues, indicating that T-cell-derived cytokines in this inflammatory environment decrease the responsiveness of LECs to lymphangiogenic growth factors [13]. Consequently, a pilot study of VEGF-C inhibition was performed in patients with breast cancer-related lymphedema (BCRL). While patients experienced decreased interstitial fluid pressures and extracellular fluid volumes, the inhibitor pazopanib displayed an unfavorable toxicity profile [14]. It is clear that the role of VEGFs in promoting or hindering lymphangiogenesis is multifaceted and necessitates further investigation to characterize their safe and effective therapeutic use.

Fibroblast Growth Factor-2 (FGF-2) and Hepatocyte Growth Factor (HGF)

Two additional growth factor therapies for lymphedema include fibroblast growth factor-2 (FGF-2) and hepatocyte growth factor (HGF). Either in combination with VEGF-C or alone, FGF-2 induces LEC proliferation, migration, and survival, along with lymphangiogenesis in the mouse cornea [5]. FGF-2 has also demonstrated the ability to bind lymphatic vessel endothelial receptor-1 (LYVE-1) and promote signaling activation with lymphangiogenesis [5]. In a rat tail model of lymphedema, topical application of basic FGF results in decreased tail volume, upregulation of VEGF-C mRNA and protein levels, and higher lymphatic vessel density than is seen in control rat tails treated with saline [15]. Along a similar vein of effort, hepatocyte growth factor (HGF) treatment of mouse upper limbs simulated to achieve BCRL results in significantly decreased limb volume and increased lymphatic flow [16]. While this is a relatively novel application of HGF, previously encouraging work with HGF gene therapy in patients with critical limb ischemia has demonstrated no adverse systemic or local inflammatory reactions, tumor development, or progression of diabetic retinopathy [16]. However, increased use of FGF-2 and HGF is limited by the nonspecific activity of these growth factors. Both activate angiogenesis, in addition to lymphangiogenesis, and therefore are not ideal candidates for further therapeutic development focused on specifically inducing lymphangiogenic activity.

Table 26.1 Overview of lymphangiogenic therapies

Target	Mechanisms of action	Therapeutic approaches
Vascular endothelial growth factor (VEGF)	VEGF-C interacts with VEGFR2/3 to promote endothelial cell sprouting and lymphatic vessel enlargement VEGF-C phosphorylates serine kinases AKT and ERK to promote LEC proliferation, migration, and survival VEGF-C levels are elevated when LECs are nonresponsive in lymphedema	Supplementation produces a lymphangiogenic response in murine and porcine models When administered alongside lymph node transfer in pigs, there is preserved lymph node structure VEGF-C inhibition in BCRL patients decreases interstitial fluid pressures and extracellular fluid volumes
Fibroblast growth factor-2 (FGF-2) and hepatocyte growth factor (HGF)	FGF-2 induces LEC proliferation, migration, and survival FGF-2 and HGF bind to LYVE-1 and activate lymphangiogenic signaling	Topical FGF-2 in a rat tail model decreases tail volume, upregulates VEGF-C mRNA/protein levels, and increases lymphatic vessel density HGF treatment of mouse upper limbs with lymphedema decreases limb volume and increases lymphatic flow
Neuropilin-2 (NRP-2)	NRP-2 complexes with VEGFR3 and facilitates lymphangiogenic signaling NRP-2 is expressed in embryonic veins prior to and during lymphatic vessel formation	Mice deficient in NRP-2 have reduced numbers of lymphatic vessels and capillaries, so supplementation may promote lymphangiogenesis
Notch-1 and ephrin B2 (EPB2)	Conditional deletion of Notch-1 from LECs during embryonic development results in increased LEC number and size EPB2 mutations result in hypoplastic lymphatic vessels without intraluminal valves EPB2 promotes VEGFR3 internalization and signaling	Regulation of Notch-1 and EPB2 activity may serve to modulate lymphangiogenesis and quality of lymphatic vessel formation
Sphingosine-1-phosphate (S1P)	In vitro, S1P induces LEC migration and tube formation via the S1P1/G_i/PLC/Ca^{2+} pathway In vivo, S1P stimulates LEC secretion of ANG2 and contributes to normal lymphatic patterning	In a mouse tail model, S1P receptor modulation blocks CD4+ release and prevents secondary lymphedema
Hyaluronic acid (HA)	Elevated levels of HA are found in lymphedematous limbs	Treatment of mouse lymphedematous limbs with hyaluronidase reduces edema and promotes formation of denser, more elongated, LYVE+ and VEGFR3+ lymphatic vessels
Transforming growth factor-beta (TGF-β)	Threefold levels of TGF-β1are found in lymphedematous tissue with resultant fibrosis	Blocking TGF-*β* with a monoclonal antibody or soluble, defective receptor decreases tissue fibrosis and increases lymphangiogenesis and lymphatic function TGF-β inhibition decreases inflammation and recruitment of Th2 cells
Bone morphogenetic protein-9 (BMP-9) and activin receptor-like kinase 1 (ALK-1)	BMP-9 and ALK-1 upregulate the function of LEC genes involved in lymphatic valve formation	Deletion of BMP-9 results in decreased number and maturation of lymphatic valves Blocking ALK-1 in neonatal mice leads to reduction in lymphatic capillary density Augmenting function of both BMP-9 and ALK-1 can improve lymphangiogenesis
Interleukin-8 (IL-8)	IL-8 stimulates LEC proliferation, tube formation, and migration IL-8 downregulates $p57^{Kip2}$ to promote lymphangiogenesis	IL-8 supplementation can enhance lymphangiogenic activity
9-cis retinoic acid (9-cis RA)	9-cis RA upregulates expression of IL-8 mRNA to promote lymphangiogenesis 9-cis RA stimulates LEC proliferation, migration, and tube formation via signaling through FGFR	Intraperitoneal, single-use depot drug delivery or oral administration of 9-cis RA results in decreased postsurgical lymphedema after lymphatic vessel injury in murine models
Stem cells	Stem cells secrete growth factors, regulate inflammatory processes, and have the capacity for differentiation into multiple cell types to combat lymphedema Bone-marrow-derived MAPCs promote restoration of the lymphatic system at the capillary, pre-collector, and collector levels, along with functional reintegration of transplanted lymph nodes	BMMSCs and ADSCs decrease limb volume and pain in patients with lymphedema

Neuropilin-2 (NRP-2)

Neuropilin-2 (NRP-2) is found to be expressed in embryonic veins prior to lymphatic vessel formation as well as in later stages of lymphatic vessel development [5]. VEGF-C and VEGF-D can both bind to NRP-2 and induce its co-internalization with VEGFR3, but NRP-2 is also able to complex with the receptor in the absence of these growth factors. Mechanistically, NRP-2 is thought to facilitate VEGFR3 signaling [5]. Consequently, mice deficient in NRP-2 are found to have absent or reduced numbers of lymphatic vessels and capillaries. NRP-2 deficiency results in both increased fluid retention and worsened lymphedema from decreased lymphatic vessel drainage [17]. The NRP-2 pathway therefore has the potential to be a useful target for attenuating post-inflammatory edematous tissue changes.

Notch-1 and Ephrin B2 (EPB2)

LECs receive paracrine regulation via growth factors but additionally communicate among themselves through the Notch-1 and ephrin (Eph) pathways [5]. LECs in the dermis, as well as in tumors, have been found to express Notch-1 and Notch-4. The conditional deletion of Notch-1 from LECs during embryonic development has been found to result in increased numbers of LECs and increased lymph sac size [5]. Among the Eph pathways, mutations in the ephrin B2 (EPB2) pathway result in mice lymphatic vessels that are hypoplastic and deficient in intraluminal valves; these mice are susceptible to developing chylothorax. EPB2 enables more efficient VEGFR3 signaling by promoting receptor internalization [5]. While there is less known about the post-embryonic targeting of the Notch-1 and EPB2 pathways, these signaling targets may very well be important to comprehensively consider aberrant signaling in lymphedema pathophysiology.

Sphingosine-1-Phosphate (S1P)

A bioactive lysophospholipid, sphingosine-1-phosphate (S1P) has demonstrated the ability to induce LEC migration and tube formation in vitro via the S1P1/Gi/PLC/Ca2+ pathway [18]. S1P additionally stimulates LEC secretion of angiopoietin 2 (ANG2), an essential growth factor for lymphangiogenesis [5]. In vivo, S1P appears to additionally function in an autocrine manner and contribute to normal lymphatic patterning [5]. Following tail skin and lymphatic excision in mice, blocking lymph node release of CD4+ cells via an S1P receptor modulator, FTY720, prevents the development of secondary lymphedema [19]. With improved understanding of the spatiotemporal behavior of CD4+ cells in causing lymphedema, S1P shows promise as a prophylactic target following patient lymph node dissection.

Hyaluronic Acid

The role of hyaluronic acid (HA), a key component of extracellular matrix, in lymphedematous pathology has been recently reported [20]. In contrast with normal tissues that have not been subjected to lymphatic injury, lymphedematous regions are found to accumulate higher levels of HA. Moreover, HA has demonstrated varied functions depending on the molecular mass size of its fragments as it is degraded by hyaluronidase. In lymphedematous mice hind limbs treated with hyaluronidase, there is a significant reduction in edema, compared to that seen with control treatment of phosphate-buffered saline (PBS). Additionally, hyaluronidase degradation of HA supports the formation of denser and newly elongated LYVE-1+ and VEGFR3+ lymphatic vessels that differ from the large, dilated, and dysfunctional lymphatic vessels seen in untreated limbs [20]. In order to clinically translate the role of hyaluronidase in treating lymphedema in patients, further studies are needed to assess the signaling mechanisms of various-sized HA fragments produced by enzymatic digestion.

Transforming Growth Factor-Beta (TGF-β)

In response to the chronic inflammation associated with lymphedema, TGF-β1 is upregulated and results in tissue fibrosis. In comparison with normal, uninjured tissue, lymphedematous tissue demonstrates nearly threefold expression levels of TGF-β1 [21]. Consequently, blocking TGF-β function either systemically with a monoclonal antibody or locally via a soluble, defective TGF-β receptor leads to markedly decreased tissue fibrosis, increased lymphangiogenesis, and improved lymphatic function [21]. TGF-β inhibition has an additional advantage of decreasing inflammation and the associated recruitment of Th2 cells with their pro-fibrotic cytokines. Consistent with in vivo findings, TGF-β levels are elevated in patient lymphedematous regions as well [21]. Blocking this growth factor's pro-fibrotic and pro-inflammatory sequelae may therefore transform the regional environment to favor improved lymphatic vessel development after lymph node injury.

Bone Morphogenetic Protein-9 (BMP-9) and Activin Receptor-Like Kinase 1 (ALK-1)

Among members of the TGF-β family, bone morphogenetic protein-9 (BMP-9) and activin receptor-like kinase 1 (ALK-1) have also demonstrated roles in lymphangiogenesis [5]. BMP-9 upregulates the function of LEC genes involved in lymphatic valve formation. Accordingly, deletion of BMP-9 results in decreased number and overall maturation of lymphatic valves, with consequently impaired lymphatic drainage [5]. In neonatal mice, blocking ALK-1 with either a specific antibody or via the soluble extracellular receptor domain also leads to a reduction in lymphatic capillary density and lymphangiogenesis. While TGF-β blockade provides an opportunity to mitigate the fibrotic pathology of lymphedema, alleviating BMP-9 and ALK-1 inhibition can improve the formation of new lymphatic vessels.

Interleukin-8 (IL-8)

Although interleukin-8 (IL-8) is a cytokine with pro-inflammatory activity, it uniquely has a role in stimulating LEC proliferation, tube formation, and migration [22]. In vivo, IL-8 promotes embryonic lymphangiogenesis in mice and can further mitigate surgically induced lymphedema via increased lymphatic regeneration [22]. To promote lymphatic vessel formation, IL-8 downregulates p57Kip2, a major cell cycle inhibitor, through the activity of PROX1, a known master regulator of lymphatic development. As IL-8 downregulates p57Kip2's positive regulator, PROX1, there is resultant suppression of this cell cycle inhibitor to allow for enhanced lymphangiogenesis. Given that the mechanistic role of IL-8 in mediating LEC proliferation has been elucidated, future clinical studies are needed to characterize the role of this cytokine in activating lymphangiogenesis in patients with regional lymphedema.

9-cis Retinoic Acid (9-cis RA)

Over the last decade, retinoic acids (RAs) have been studied for their promotion of LEC proliferation, migration, and tube formation via signaling through the FGF receptor [23]. Comprised of biologically active vitamin A metabolites, RAs facilitate PROX1-mediated cell cycle control of the checkpoint regulators, p27Kip1, p57Kip2, and the aurora kinases. In in vivo mouse trachea, Matrigel plug, cornea pocket, and mouse tail lymphedema assays, 9-cis retinoic acid (9-cis RA) demonstrates enhanced lymphangiogenesis [23]. 9-cis RA particularly upregulates the expression of IL-8 mRNA in primary LECs to further augment lymphangiogenic activity [22]. Of note, 9-cis RA is also referred to as alitretinoin (Panretin) and has received clinical approval by the US Food and Drug Administration (FDA) for the treatment of Kaposi's sarcoma and chronic hand eczematous lesions. The compound can therefore be repurposed for the safe and effective treatment of lymphedema.

The role of 9-cis RA in the treatment of postsurgical lymphedema in the mouse hind limb model has been thoroughly explored. After lymphedema induction via irradiation injury followed by popliteal lymphadenectomy and lymphatic vessel ablation, mice hind limbs treated with intraperitoneal 9-cis RA demonstrated decreased postsurgical edema, significantly less paw lymphedema, faster lymphatic drainage, and increased lymphatic vessel density [24]. Moreover, the application of a single-use depot 9-cis RA drug delivery system (DDS) implanted at the site of lymphatic injury for sustained release of the metabolite resulted in faster lymphatic clearance, increased lymphatic density, reduced lymphatic vessel size, reduced epidermal hyperplasia, and reduced collagen staining [25]. Most recently, the authors have found that oral 9-cis RA treatment can prevent the development of postsurgical lymphedema after mouse tail lymphatic excision (Fig. 26.2). 9-cis RA thus offers versatility in treatment administration and promising therapeutic efficacy for the prevention of secondary lymphedema in patients.

Stem Cells

Recently, the application of mesenchymal stem cells (MSCs), adipose tissue-derived stem cells (ADSCs), pluripotent stem cells, and bone marrow-derived endothelial cell precursors has been investigated for therapeutic potential in the treatment of lymphedema. Considering cell availability and ethical constraints, MSCs and ADSCs have been regarded as the most promising candidates [26, 27]. In a non-randomized control study of patients with BCRL treated with either bone marrow-derived MSCs or complete decongestive therapy (CDT), patients who received stem cell therapy demonstrated decreased arm volume and pain at 3 and 12 months post-treatment [28]. Similarly, a prospective randomized study of patients with chronic lower limb lymphedema treated with bone marrow-derived mononuclear cells demonstrated significant reduction in ankle circumference, improved lymphatic capillary density, and improved symptomatology of pain and walking ability [29].

The role of ADSCs in lymphatic regeneration has been primarily explored in patients with BCRL. A prospective pilot control study of ADSC injection in breast cancer patients with secondary lymphedema from axillary lymph node dissection revealed decreased limb circumference at 4, 8, and 12 weeks after treatment, as well as significant reduction in pain and improved mobility and sensitivity [30]. When ADSC injection was combined with scar-releasing fat grafting procedures for patients with BCRL, patients reported decreased need for conservative treatment and improved symptomatology as well [31]. Although favorable results have been demonstrated with various stem cell therapy applications, there is a paucity of studies demonstrating this therapy's ability to restore lymphatic vasculature from the capillary to the collector level, a regenerative capacity that is essential for effective lymphedema treatment [32]. In contrast, bone marrow-derived multipotent adult progenitor cells (MAPCs) have the ability to promote

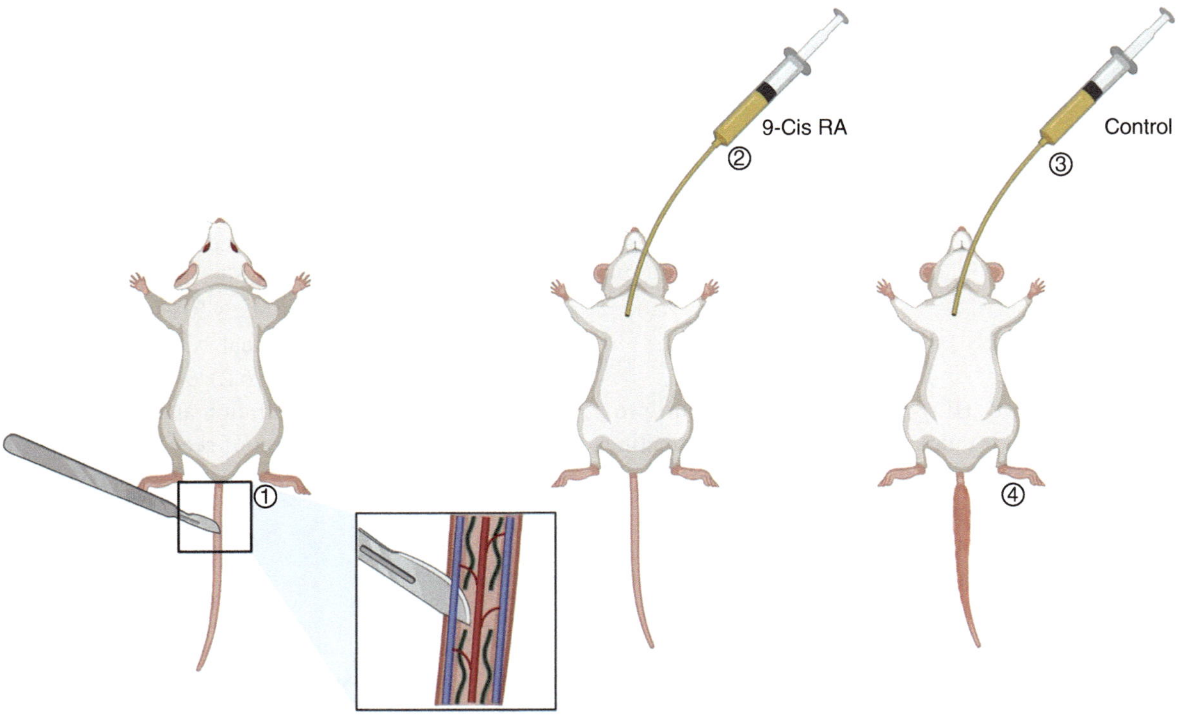

Fig. 26.2 The administration of oral 9-cis retinoic acid (9-cis RA) prevents the development of postsurgical lymphedema. (**a**) Mouse tail lymphatic excision was performed 20 mm from the tail base. (**b**) Oral gavage was performed with either 9-cis RA dissolved in sunflower oil (treatment) or sunflower oil alone (control). (**c**) Compared to those receiving control treatment, mice treated with 9-cis RA demonstrated decreased postsurgical lymphedema at postoperative days 14 and 42

restoration of a functional lymphatic system at the capillary, pre-collector, and collector levels, along with functional reintegration of transplanted lymph nodes [32]. While stem cell therapies have perhaps the most clearly characterized benefits for testing in randomized clinical trials, MAPCs may emerge as a superior treatment option in terms of their lymphvasculogenic and lymphangiogenic properties.

Anti-inflammatory and Anti-fibrotic Therapeutic Approaches

In addition to promoting lymphangiogenic recovery in the treatment of lymphedema, there is a growing interest in attenuating the chronic inflammation and fibrotic ramifications associated with this disease course. Experimental and clinical studies have recognized inflammation as a key driver in lymphedema, and upregulation of inflammatory genes has been implicated in more severe patient symptomatology as well [3]. In recognition of the feed-forward effects of inflammation and fibrosis on one another in lymphedema, targeting these pathways provides an alternative therapeutic consideration in caring for these patients. An overview of the following anti-inflammatory and anti-fibrotic therapies is presented in Table 26.2.

Ketoprofen

Ketoprofen is a nonsteroidal anti-inflammatory drug (NSAID) that reduces inflammation via cyclooxygenase inhibition and upregulates TNF-α levels to promote pro-lymphangiogenic activity (Fig. 26.3). In the mouse tail lymphedema model, subcutaneous ketoprofen treatment results in normalization of histologic changes, including restored dermal-epidermal architecture, disappearance of dilated microlymphatic vessels, and resolution of inflammatory tissue changes [33]. Consistent with these favorable in vivo findings, an exploratory open-label trial found that ketoprofen treatment resulted in improved histopathology and skin thickness in patients with both primary and secondary lymphedema at 4 months compared to baseline [34]. A follow-up, double-blind, placebo-controlled trial further substantiated these encouraging results by showing that treated patients had reduced skin thickness, improved composite histopathology measures, and decreased plasma granulocyte CSF (G-CSF) expression [34]. Barring the black box warning of cardiovascular toxicity with chronic ketoprofen use, this pharmacotherapy has significant potential for restoring compromised lymphatic circulation.

Through its anti-inflammatory properties, ketoprofen also inhibits the 5-lipoxygenase metabolite, leukotriene B4

Table 26.2 Overview of anti-inflammatory and anti-fibrotic therapies

Target	Mechanisms of Action	Therapeutic Approaches
Ketoprofen	Ketoprofen is a NSAID that inhibits cyclooxygenase to reduce inflammation. Ketoprofen inhibits LTB4, a metabolite of 5-lipoxygenase and inflammatory mediator elevated in patients with lymphedema.	In a mouse tail lymphedema model, ketoprofen normalizes histology, dermal-epidermal architecture, and resolves inflammatory tissue changes In patients with lymphedema, ketoprofen leads to reduced skin thickness and improved histopathology
Tacrolimus	Tacrolimus is an anti-T cell macrolide that decreases CD4+ infiltration in lymphedematous regions.	In murine models, tacrolimus prevents the development of postsurgical lymphedema and alleviates ongoing pathologic changes Tacrolimus also leads to improved lymphatic vessel formation and lymphatic vessel pumping
Sodium selenite	Sodium selenite is an inorganic, anti-inflammatory salt.	Patients with BCRL who received sodium selenite experienced reduction in lymphedematous volume, erysipelas index, and improved skinfold index and mobility
Pirfenidone	Pirfenidone inhibits TGF-β1 to decrease fibrotic sequelae in lymphedema.	In murine lymphedema models, pirfenidone treatment leads to decreased limb/tail volume, inflammation, and collagen deposition Pirfenidone also leads to improved lymphatic pumping frequency, collateral vessel formation, interstitial fluid transport, and decreased dermal backflow

NSAID non-steroidal anti-inflammatory drug, *LT* leukotriene, *TGF* transforming growth factor, *BCRL* breast cancer-related lymphedema

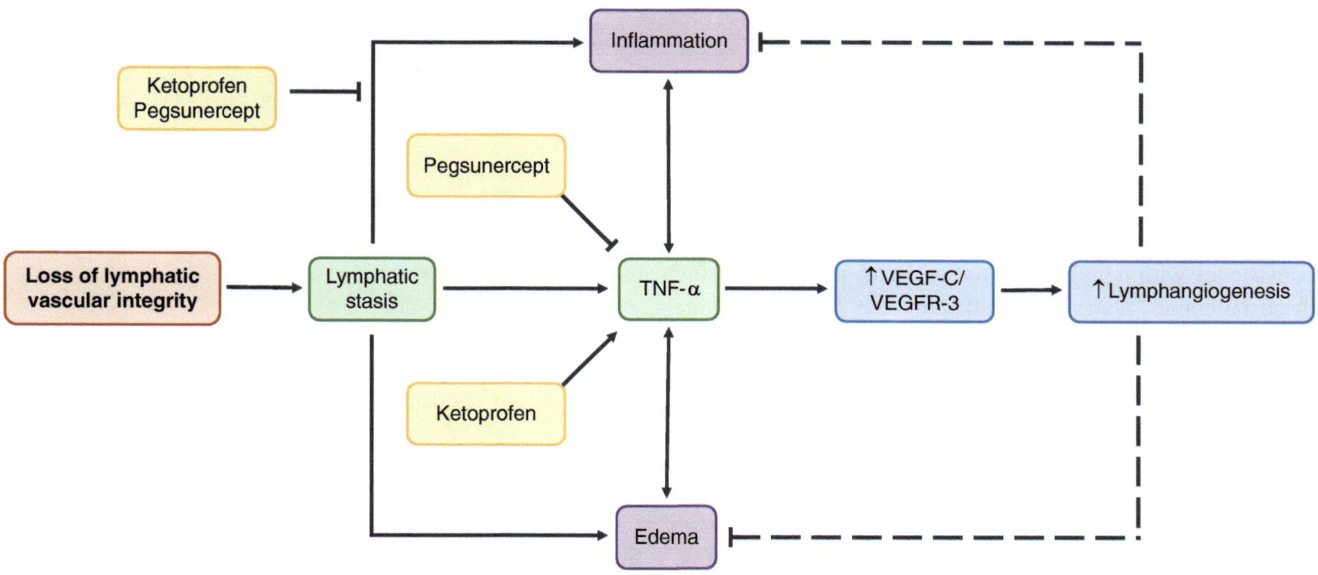

Fig. 26.3 Ketoprofen is a non-steroidal anti-inflammatory drug (NSAID) that reduces inflammation associated with lymphatic stasis by inhibiting cyclooxygenase activity. Additionally, ketoprofen increases TNF-α levels, resulting in increased VEGF-C and VEGFR3. The upregulation of this pro-lymphangiogenic signaling pathway results in lymphangiogenesis, mitigating the edema associated with lymphatic stasis. Pegsunercept is a modified soluble form of the TNF-α receptor 1 (R1) and inhibits inflammation like ketoprofen. However, pegsunercept also directly inhibits TNF-α activity and disrupts pro-lymphangiogenic activity. (Adapted from Nakamura et al. [33]. Copyright (2009) by Nakamura et al.)

(LTB4), an inflammatory mediator found to be significantly elevated in patients with postsurgical lymphedema [27]. Produced by macrophages, LTB4 further recruits macrophages and other inflammatory cells, such as neutrophils and CD4+ cells, to lymphedematous tissue. In in vitro work looking at the functional bimodality of LTB4, low levels are found to promote human LEC sprouting and growth, while high concentrations inhibit lymphangiogenesis and induce apoptosis [35]. As LTB4 has been identified as a specific anti-lymphangiogenic target with its pro-inflammatory effects, future clinical studies can aim to more precisely antagonize this leukotriene, such as with the administration of leukotriene A4 hydrolase (LTA4H), a biosynthetic enzyme with anti-LTB4 activity [27].

Tacrolimus

Tacrolimus is an anti-T cell macrolide that has been FDA-approved in a topical formulation to treat cutaneous inflam-

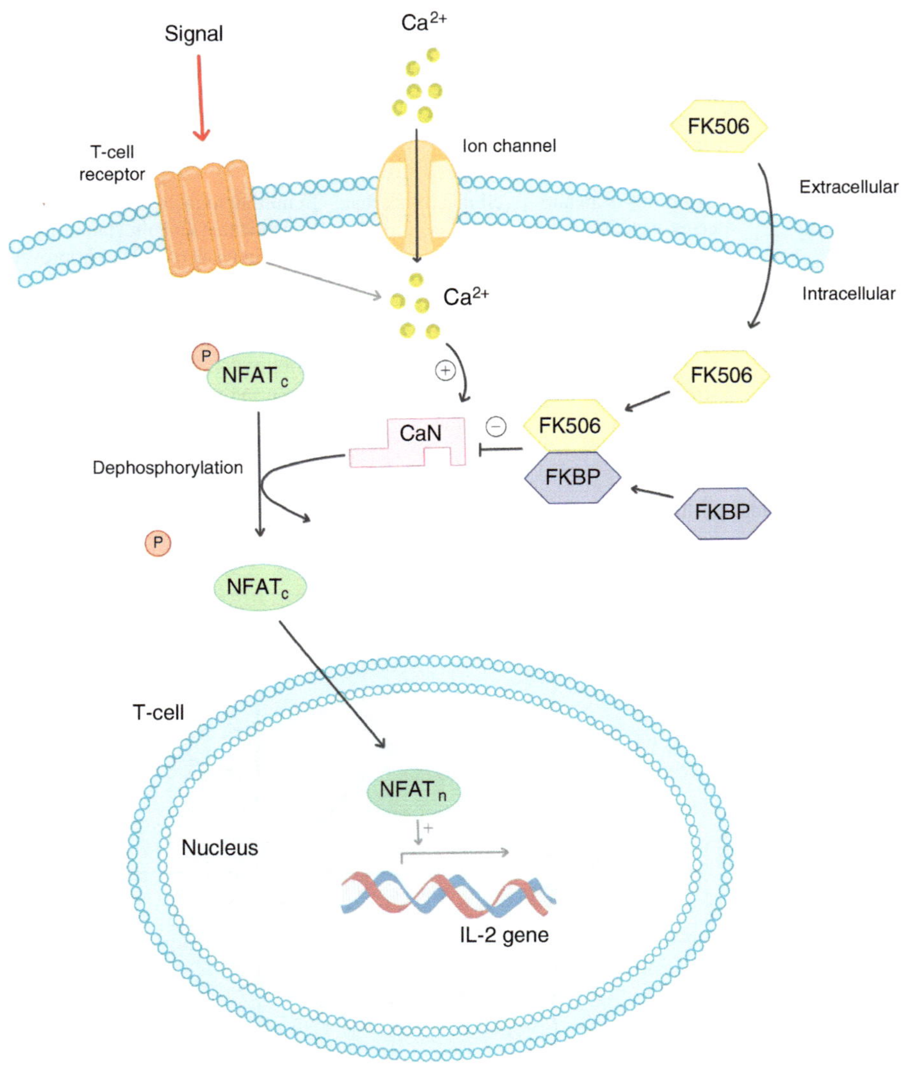

Fig. 26.4 Tacrolimus (FK506) binds to FK506-binding protein (FKBP) in the cytoplasm. This resultant complex binds to the enzyme calcineurin (CaN), preventing the dephosphorylation of the cytoplasmic nuclear factor of activated T cells ($NFAT_c$). $NFAT_c$ is thus unable to enter the nucleus, preventing the binding of the nuclear NFAT ($NFAT_n$) to the IL-2 gene promoter. Without the production of IL-2, full T-cell activation does not take place. (Adapted from Bennett et al. [40]. Copyright (2016) by Bennett et al.)

matory and fibrotic diseases, such as atopic dermatitis, psoriasis, and localized scleroderma [36]. Tacrolimus works to inhibit a calcineurin-mediated pathway that thereby prevents IL-2 expression and full T cell activation (Fig. 26.4). Given the critical role of CD4+ T cells in lymphedema, the use of tacrolimus for both the prevention and treatment of lymphedema has been investigated. In both the mouse tail and popliteal lymph node dissection lymphedema models, topical application of tacrolimus prevents the development of secondary lymphedema and alleviates pathologic changes inherently taking place with established lymphedema [36]. In addition to its anti-inflammatory and anti-fibrotic effects via decreased CD4+ cell infiltration, tacrolimus increases the formation of lymphatic collaterals and improves lymphatic collecting vessel pumping. Future clinical trials are needed to further validate the enhanced lymphatic function in response to tacrolimus therapy, but this compound is nevertheless unique in its low systemic absorption but potent decrease of dermal and subcutaneous T cell infiltration and tissue fibrosis following lymphatic injury [36].

Sodium Selenite

Sodium selenite (Na2SeO3) is an inorganic salt with anti-inflammatory properties. In a placebo-controlled, double-blind clinical study of patients with BCRL, patients treated with sodium selenite had reduction in lymphedematous arm volume and erysipelas incidence, along with improved skin-fold index and mobility [37]. Additionally, clinical studies of patients with either arm or head and neck lymphedema have demonstrated volume reduction with sodium selenite treatment [37]. The ease of sodium selenite's clinical translation is due in part to its low cost and nontoxic profile, making this compound a particularly favorable candidate for further testing as a lymphedema treatment.

Pirfenidone

More recently, the use of pirfenidone, an anti-fibrotic medication previously approved for the treatment of idiopathic pulmonary fibrosis, has been explored in the treatment of postsurgical lymphedema. Via inhibition of TGF-β1, pirfenidone treatment results in significantly decreased mouse tail and hind limb volume, inflammation, and collagen deposition [38]. Following popliteal lymph node dissection to induce hind limb lymphedema, mice treated with pirfenidone exhibited significantly improved collecting lymphatic pumping frequency, decreased dermal backflow, increased collateral lymphatic formation, and increased interstitial fluid transport [38]. While anti-inflammatory pharmacotherapy for lymphedema often confers anti-fibrotic benefits as well, pirfenidone emerges as a novel, anti-fibrotic agent that has the potential to mitigate the disfiguring sequelae of advanced disease.

Discussion

As lymphedema notoriously burdens patients with chronic illness in the absence of a definitive cure, it is necessary to offer patients effective treatment strategies with the goal of primary prevention or symptomatic attenuation. Among the nonsurgical treatment approaches that are often used as standalone or in conjunction with surgically reductive techniques or physiologic methods, pro-lymphangiogenic, anti-inflammatory, and anti-fibrotic therapies are emerging due to enhanced understanding of the cellular and tissue-specific behaviors in lymphedema. There is thought that the more fine-tuned, molecular regulation of this disease process will even diminish the need for future surgical intervention and reduce patient morbidity as a result of advanced and frequently irreversible symptomatology.

Lymphangiogenic agents such as growth factors, receptors, lipids, enzymes, cytokines, and more broadly cell-based therapies and overall signaling pathways confer favorable therapeutic benefits in restoring interstitial fluid drainage and lymphatic function after lymph node dissection or lymphatic injury. Anti-inflammatory and consequently anti-fibrotic therapies, many of which have been approved for the treatment of other diseases with a similarly chronic course, act to prime the environment for lymphangiogenesis. As a result, optimal yet tailored use of these multimodal agents is likely to result in the greatest patient improvement. More widespread use of these various compounds is contingent on robust clinical testing, as well as patient and provider education regarding their realistic capacity to alter the disease course and/or address existing symptoms.

On the horizon of new lymphedema treatments is the use of nanofibrillar collagen scaffolds to promote lymphangiogenesis and reduce inflammation. Human microvascular endothelial cells demonstrate the ability to morphologically organize along nanopatterned scaffolds, with improved cell survival and decreased inflammation [39]. In a porcine lymphedema model, the use of nanofibrillar collagen scaffolds, either alone or when supplemented with lymph node transfer, resulted in a significant increase in lymphatic collectors near the scaffolds and reduction in extracellular fluid volume [27]. The scaffolds augment microlymphatic vascular engraftment, and the favorable fibril alignment decreases excessive fibroblast proliferation, resulting in less scar formation [39]. In vivo demonstration of scaffold-facilitated lymphangiogenesis has encouraged investigators in pilot clinical studies to examine the role of BioBridge (Fibralign Corporation, Union City, CA) collagen scaffolds, along with non-vascularized lymph node transfer, vascularized lymph node transfer, and lymphaticovenous anastomosis (LVA) for the treatment of secondary lymphedema [39]. These scaffolds can additionally be seeded with ADSCs to further support LEC survival, maintenance, and function. Compared to patients who underwent lymph node transfer or LVA alone, the use of the collagen scaffolds resulted in significantly decreased edema and enhanced lymphatic regeneration.

Conclusions

Promising developments in knowledge of lymphedema pathophysiology have provided for a wide array of potential therapeutics, with varying yet interrelated mechanisms of action. Further understanding of specific molecular and cellular targets for intervention will improve the ability to treat patients facing this prevalent yet incurable disease. The combined and judicious use of medical and nonsurgical therapies offers the opportunity to improve lymphangiogenesis, decrease inflammation and fibrosis, and ultimately bolster patient lymphatic function.

References

1. Dayan JH, Ly CL, Kataru RP, Mehrara BJ. Lymphedema: pathogenesis and novel therapies. Annu Rev Med. 2018;69:263–76. https://doi.org/10.1146/annurev-med-060116-022900.
2. Rutkowski JM, Swartz MA. A driving force for change: interstitial flow as a morphoregulator. Trends Cell Biol. 2007;17(1):44–50. https://doi.org/10.1016/j.tcb.2006.11.007.
3. Ly CL, Kataru RP, Mehrara BJ. Inflammatory manifestations of lymphedema. Int J Mol Sci. 2017;18(1):171. https://doi.org/10.3390/ijms18010171.
4. Norman SA, Localio AR, Potashnik SL, Simoes Torpey HA, Kallan MJ, Weber AL, et al. Lymphedema in breast cancer survivors: incidence, degree, time course, treatment, and symptoms. J Clin Oncol. 2009;27(3):390–7. https://doi.org/10.1200/JCO.2008.17.9291.
5. Zheng W, Aspelund A, Alitalo K. Lymphangiogenic factors, mechanisms, and applications. J Clin Invest. 2014;124(3):878–87. https://doi.org/10.1172/JCI71603.
6. Wirzenius M, Tammela T, Uutela M, He Y, Odorisio T, Zambruno G, et al. Distinct vascular endothelial growth factor signals for lymphatic vessel enlargement and sprouting. J Exp Med. 2007;204(6):1431–40. https://doi.org/10.1084/jem.20062642.
7. Makinen T, Veikkola T, Mustjoki S, Karpanen T, Catimel B, Nice EC, et al. Isolated lymphatic endothelial cells transduce growth, survival and migratory signals via the VEGF-C/D receptor VEGFR-3. EMBO J. 2001;20(17):4762–73. https://doi.org/10.1093/emboj/20.17.4762.
8. Makinen T, Jussila L, Veikkola T, Karpanen T, Kettunen MI, Pulkkanen KJ, et al. Inhibition of lymphangiogenesis with resulting

lymphedema in transgenic mice expressing soluble VEGF receptor-3. Nat Med. 2001;7(2):199–205. https://doi.org/10.1038/84651.
9. Gordon K, Spiden SL, Connell FC, Brice G, Cottrell S, Short J, et al. FLT4/VEGFR3 and Milroy disease: novel mutations, a review of published variants and database update. Hum Mutat. 2013;34(1):23–31. https://doi.org/10.1002/humu.22223.
10. Tervala TV, Hartiala P, Tammela T, Visuri MT, Yla-Herttuala S, Alitalo K, et al. Growth factor therapy and lymph node graft for lymphedema. J Surg Res. 2015;196(1):200–7. https://doi.org/10.1016/j.jss.2015.02.031.
11. Lahteenvuo M, Honkonen K, Tervala T, Tammela T, Suominen E, Lahteenvuo J, et al. Growth factor therapy and autologous lymph node transfer in lymphedema. Circulation. 2011;123(6):613–20. https://doi.org/10.1161/circulationaha.110.965384.
12. Shiao SL, Ganesan AP, Rugo HS, Coussens LM. Immune microenvironments in solid tumors: new targets for therapy. Genes Dev. 2011;25(24):2559–72. https://doi.org/10.1101/gad.169029.111.
13. Rutkowski JM, Moya M, Johannes J, Goldman J, Swartz MA. Secondary lymphedema in the mouse tail: lymphatic hyperplasia, VEGF-C upregulation, and the protective role of MMP-9. Microvasc Res. 2006;72(3):161–71. https://doi.org/10.1016/j.mvr.2006.05.009.
14. Miller K, Brown C, Perkins S, Schneider B, Storniolo A, Sledge G. A pilot study of vascular endothelial growth factor inhibition with pazopanib in patients (pts) with lymphedema following breast cancer treatment. Cancer Res. 2010;70(24):P2-14-02.
15. Onishi T, Nishizuka T, Kurahashi T, Arai T, Iwatsuki K, Yamamoto M, et al. Topical bFGF improves secondary lymphedema through lymphangiogenesis in a rat tail model. Plast Reconstr Surg Glob Open. 2014;2(8):e196-e. https://doi.org/10.1097/GOX.0000000000000154.
16. Saito Y, Nakagami H, Kaneda Y, Morishita R. Lymphedema and therapeutic lymphangiogenesis. Biomed Res Int. 2013;2013:804675. https://doi.org/10.1155/2013/804675.
17. Mucka P, Levonyak N, Geretti E, Zwaans BMM, Li X, Adini I, et al. Inflammation and lymphedema are exacerbated and prolonged by neuropilin 2 deficiency. Am J Pathol. 2016;186(11):2803–12. https://doi.org/10.1016/j.ajpath.2016.07.022.
18. Yoon CM, Hong BS, Moon HG, Lim S, Suh P-G, Kim Y-K, et al. Sphingosine-1-phosphate promotes lymphangiogenesis by stimulating S1P1/Gi/PLC/Ca2+ signaling pathways. Blood. 2008;112(4):1129–38. https://doi.org/10.1182/blood-2007-11-125203.
19. Garcia Nores GD, Ly CL, Cuzzone DA, Kataru RP, Hespe GE, Torrisi JS, et al. CD4(+) T cells are activated in regional lymph nodes and migrate to skin to initiate lymphedema. Nat Commun. 2018;9(1):1970. https://doi.org/10.1038/s41467-018-04418-y.
20. Roh K, Cho S, Park J-H, Yoo BC, Kim W-K, Kim S-K, et al. Therapeutic effects of hyaluronidase on acquired lymphedema using a newly developed mouse limb model. Exp Biol Med (Maywood). 2017;242(6):584–92. https://doi.org/10.1177/1535370216688570.
21. Avraham T, Daluvoy S, Zampell J, Yan A, Haviv YS, Rockson SG, et al. Blockade of transforming growth factor-beta1 accelerates lymphatic regeneration during wound repair. Am J Pathol. 2010;177(6):3202–14. https://doi.org/10.2353/ajpath.2010.100594.
22. Choi I, Lee YS, Chung HK, Choi D, Ecoiffier T, Lee HN, et al. Interleukin-8 reduces post-surgical lymphedema formation by promoting lymphatic vessel regeneration. Angiogenesis. 2013;16(1):29–44. https://doi.org/10.1007/s10456-012-9297-6.
23. Choi I, Lee S, Kyoung Chung H, Suk Lee Y, Eui Kim K, Choi D, et al. 9-cis retinoic acid promotes lymphangiogenesis and enhances lymphatic vessel regeneration: therapeutic implications of 9-cis retinoic acid for secondary lymphedema. Circulation. 2012;125(7):872–82. https://doi.org/10.1161/circulationaha.111.030296.
24. Bramos A, Perrault D, Yang S, Jung E, Hong YK, Wong AK. Prevention of postsurgical lymphedema by 9-cis retinoic acid. Ann Surg. 2016;264(2):353–61. https://doi.org/10.1097/sla.0000000000001525.
25. Daneshgaran G, Paik CB, Cooper MN, Sung C, Lo A, Jiao W, et al. Prevention of postsurgical lymphedema via immediate delivery of sustained-release 9-cis retinoic acid to the lymphedenectomy site. J Surg Oncol. 2020;121(1):100–8. https://doi.org/10.1002/jso.25587.
26. Chen CE, Chiang NJ, Perng CK, Ma H, Lin CH. Review of preclinical and clinical studies of using cell-based therapy for secondary lymphedema. J Surg Oncol. 2020;121(1):109–20. https://doi.org/10.1002/jso.25661.
27. Schaverien MV, Aldrich MB. New and emerging treatments for lymphedema. Semin Plast Surg. 2018;32(1):48–52. https://doi.org/10.1055/s-0038-1632403.
28. Hou C, Wu X, Jin X. Autologous bone marrow stromal cells transplantation for the treatment of secondary arm lymphedema: a prospective controlled study in patients with breast cancer related lymphedema. Jpn J Clin Oncol. 2008;38(10):670–4. https://doi.org/10.1093/jjco/hyn090.
29. Ismail AM, Abdou SM, Abdelnaby AY, Hamdy MA, El Saka AA, Gawaly A. Stem cell therapy using bone marrow-derived mononuclear cells in treatment of lower limb lymphedema: a randomized controlled clinical trial. Lymphat Res Biol. 2018;16(3):270–7. https://doi.org/10.1089/lrb.2017.0027.
30. Maldonado GE, Perez CA, Covarrubias EE, Cabriales SA, Leyva LA, Perez JC, et al. Autologous stem cells for the treatment of post-mastectomy lymphedema: a pilot study. Cytotherapy. 2011;13(10):1249–55. https://doi.org/10.3109/14653249.2011.594791.
31. Toyserkani NM, Jensen CH, Andersen DC, Sheikh SP, Sorensen JA. Treatment of breast cancer-related lymphedema with adipose-derived regenerative cells and fat grafts: a feasibility and safety study. Stem Cells Transl Med. 2017;6(8):1666–72. https://doi.org/10.1002/sctm.17-0037.
32. Beerens M, Aranguren XL, Hendrickx B, Dheedene W, Dresselaers T, Himmelreich U, et al. Multipotent adult progenitor cells support lymphatic regeneration at multiple anatomical levels during wound healing and lymphedema. Sci Rep. 2018;8(1):3852. https://doi.org/10.1038/s41598-018-21610-8.
33. Nakamura K, Radhakrishnan K, Wong YM, Rockson SG. Anti-inflammatory pharmacotherapy with ketoprofen ameliorates experimental lymphatic vascular insufficiency in mice. PLoS One. 2009;4(12):e8380-e. https://doi.org/10.1371/journal.pone.0008380.
34. Rockson SG, Tian W, Jiang X, Kuznetsova T, Haddad F, Zampell J, et al. Pilot studies demonstrate the potential benefits of antiinflammatory therapy in human lymphedema. JCI Insight. 2018;3(20):e123775. https://doi.org/10.1172/jci.insight.123775.
35. Tian W, Rockson SG, Jiang X, Kim J, Begaye A, Shuffle EM, et al. Sci Transl Med. 2017;9(389) https://doi.org/10.1126/scitranslmed.aal3920.
36. Gardenier JC, Kataru RP, Hespe GE, Savetsky IL, Torrisi JS, Nores GDG, et al. Topical tacrolimus for the treatment of secondary lymphedema. Nat Commun. 2017;8:14345. https://doi.org/10.1038/ncomms14345.
37. Forte AJ, Boczar D, Huayllani MT, Lu X, McLaughlin SA. Pharmacotherapy agents in lymphedema treatment: a systematic review. Cureus. 2019;11(12):e6300. https://doi.org/10.7759/cureus.6300.
38. Savetsky IL, Hespe GE, Gardenier JC, Torrisi JS, García Nores GD, Nitti MD, et al. Pirfenidone decreases fibrosis and improves lymphatic function in mouse models of lymphedema. J Am Coll Surg. 2015;221(4):e121–e2. https://doi.org/10.1016/j.jamcollsurg.2015.08.224.
39. Rochlin DH, Inchauste S, Zelones J, Nguyen DH. The role of adjunct nanofibrillar collagen scaffold implantation in the surgical management of secondary lymphedema: review of the literature and summary of initial pilot studies. J Surg Oncol. 2020;121(1):121–8. https://doi.org/10.1002/jso.25576.
40. Bennett J, Cassidy H, Slattery C, Ryan MP, McMorrow T. Tacrolimus modulates TGF-β signaling to induce epithelialmesenchymal transition in human renal proximal tubule epithelial cells. J Clin Med. 5(50):3.

New and Emerging Therapies for Lymphedema: Part II

27

Robert C. Sibley and Stanley G. Rockson

Introduction

Understanding the intricate roles of inflammation, fibrosis, and adipose deposition in response to lymph stasis is critical to providing excellent medical care for patients with lymphedema. The overarching hypothesis has been that lymph stasis leads to inflammation. This inflammation then leads to progressive tissue fibrosis and adipose deposition, which in turn decreases lymphatic function, creating a pathologic feedback loop [1]. The complex role of inflammation in lymphedema likely explains the phenomenon of late symptom onset in breast cancer-related lymphedema (BCRL), often occurring 1–5 years after initial therapy. Lymph stasis results in the induced expression of danger signals, with upregulated functional gene expression within pathways related to acute inflammation, immunity, complement cascade, wound healing, and fibrosis [2]. Six biomarkers characteristic of lymphatic vascular insufficiency have been identified; these participate in lymphangiogenesis, inflammation, fibrosis, and adipocytokine signaling [3]. In many ways, progressive fibrosis of the superficial tissues can be conceptualized as end-organ failure of the lymphatic system, in analogy with progressive inflammatory disease processes in other organ systems, where parenchymal replacement with scar tissue occurs. Before we discuss new therapies that target inflammation and fibrosis, we must first briefly review our current understanding of the key targets in the inflammatory and fibrotic mechanisms associated with lymphedema. Many of the pathways have been characterized in mouse models of acquired lymphedema; these simulate the histopathology, altered immune trafficking, abnormal lymphoscintigraphic patterns, and volume responses seen in human lymphedema [2, 4].

R. C. Sibley · S. G. Rockson (✉)
Stanford Center for Lymphatic and Venous Disorders, Division of Cardiovascular Medicine, Stanford University School of Medicine, Stanford, CA, USA
e-mail: rockson@stanford.edu

The Key Targets of Inflammation and Fibrosis in Lymphedema

Vascular Endothelial Growth Factor (VEGF)-C, Cytokines, and Leukotriene B4 (LTB4)

Vascular endothelial growth factor (VEGF)-C regulates differentiation, survival, and migration of lymphatic endothelial cells (LECs) through VEGF receptor-3 (VEGFR3). Milroy's disease is an autosomal dominant primary lymphedema that occurs when a heterozygous missense mutation of the VEGFR3 gene causes partial inactivation. When VEGF-C is delivered locally or through gene therapy in animal models of primary or secondary lymphedema, the defect is overcome, lymphangiogenesis is increased, and edema diminishes [5]. However, VEGF-C has been demonstrated to play a role in tumor lymphangiogenesis, so there is understandable concern that administration of this growth factor might have the capacity to initiate tumor recurrence or metastasis.

Interleukin (IL)-4 and IL-13 are T helper (T_h) 2 cytokines that participate significantly in allergic diseases such as asthma. IL-4 and IL-13 have been demonstrated to inhibit lymphangiogenesis and diminish LEC survival, proliferation, migration, and tube formation [6, 7]. Tumor necrosis factor (TNF)-α is an inflammatory cytokine and acute phase protein. In a mouse lymphedema model, TNF- α inhibition increases tissue edema, decreases VEGF-C expression, and increases with disease severity [8]. Ketoprofen is a non-steroidal anti-inflammatory drug (NSAID) that increases TNF-α expression and is discussed later. Leukotriene B4 (LTB4) is an eicosanoid inflammatory mediator. LTB4 production is elevated in preclinical and clinical lymphedema. LTB4 regulates lymphangiogenesis by altering human lymphatic endothelial cell function and survival. Ubenimex inhibits LTB4 production and is discussed below.

M. V. Schaverien, J. H. Dayan (eds.), *Multimodal Management of Upper and Lower Extremity Lymphedema*,
https://doi.org/10.1007/978-3-030-93039-4_27

T Cells

CD4+ cells, also known as T helper (T_h) cells, participate actively in the lymphedema inflammatory response. Nearly 70% of all inflammatory cells in lymphedematous tissues are CD4+ positive, and CD4+ cell number correlates positively with increasing disease severity [9]. IL-2 expression is necessary for T cell activation and for the differentiation of CD4+ cells. IL-2 expression is decreased by calcineurin inhibitors such as tacrolimus, discussed below. T_h2 cells predominate in lymphedema-associated inflammation. Blocking T_h2 differentiation has been demonstrated to prevent and reverse lymphedema in animal models [10]. In addition, inhibiting T_h2 differentiation (not generalized inflammation) markedly decreases initiation and progression of fibrosis and improves lymphatic function [10].

In addition to T_h2 cells, regulatory T (Treg) cells are also increased in human lymphedema. Treg cells are immunosuppressive cells that inhibit T cell responses and suppress regional proinflammatory neutrophils. In the mouse model of lymphedema, Treg cells decrease T_h1/T_h2 immune response, fibrosis, and expression of interferon (IFN)-γ, IL-13, IL-4, and transforming growth factor (TGF)-ß1 [11]. T_h1 and T_h17 cells may play a complex role: chronic lymphedema develops through the ability of these cells to promote the excessive generation of leaky neo-lymphatic vessels, mediated by increased macrophage generation of VEGF-C. This has been demonstrated in an axillary lymph node dissection model of lymphedema. Atorvastatin modulates the function of T_h1 and T_h17 as discussed below [12].

Macrophages

Lymphedematous tissues contain increased numbers of macrophages [9, 13]. This increase is mediated, at least in part, by CD4+ cells [10]. Macrophages exercise a complex role in lymphangiogenesis and fibrosis. Microphages can be categorized into two groups. M1 macrophages promote inflammation, whereas M2 macrophages decrease inflammation and promote wound healing. Macrophages contribute significantly to inflammatory lymphangiogenesis. These cells have been demonstrated to promote lymphedema in the acute setting [12]. M2 macrophages predominate in the mouse tail model of acquired lymphedema [13]. M2 macrophages regulate lymphangiogenesis through VEGF-C production and by promotion of tissue remodeling through the regulation of collagen and matrix metalloproteinases [14]. It has been proposed that coumarin, a benzopyrone, increases the proteolytic activity of macrophages; this is discussed below as a therapeutic option [15]. In a lymphedema model, when macrophages are depleted, VEGF-C expression is decreased, fibrosis is increased, and lymphatic function is impaired [13]. Toll-like receptor deficiency results in hindered lymphangiogenesis and lymphatic vascular repair in the mouse tail model of lymphedema; this likely results from decreased recruitment of macrophages [16].

Fibrosis and the Extracellular Matrix

The fibrosis in lymphedema appears to result from T cell inflammation and, more specifically, from T_h2 differentiation, rather than from inflammation in general [10]. Fibrosis proceeds in two stages: fibroblast proliferation and activation. Fibroblasts are regulated by T_h1 and T_h2 cells. T_h2 cells promote fibrosis, whereas T_h1 cells stimulate healing and counteract fibrosis.

The profibrotic factor, TGF-ß1, also plays an interactive and independent role in fibrosis. TGF-ß1 regulates extracellular matrix synthesis and accumulates excessively in the lymphedematous limb in patients with postsurgical lymphedema. Radiation induces fibrosis through TGF-ß1 expression, and this diminishes lymphatic function. Blocking TGF-ß1 results in improved lymphatic function, decreased T cell inflammation, and decreased expression of IL-4 and IL-13 [17]. TGF-ß1 impairs lymphatic endothelial proliferation, migration, and tubule formation.

Hyaluronic acid (HA) is a major component of the extracellular matrix. HA accumulates in lymphedematous tissues. Concentrations have been reported to be approximately eight times greater than in the contralateral limb. HA exists in varying molecular sizes; the function of HA depends on the size of the fragment. Hyaluronidase is the enzyme that breaks down high-molecular-weight (HMW) HA into low-molecular-weight (LMW) HA and is discussed below. HA has a high water-binding capacity and has been used in soft tissue augmentation. The primary HA receptor is CD44; binding of HA to this receptor promotes T_h1 cell differentiation. LMWHA is required for lymphatic growth as it binds lymphatic vessel endothelial HA receptor (LYVE)-1 [18]. LYVE-1 plays a vital role in lymphatic endothelial cell (LEC) biogenesis and in lymphangiogenesis. 4-mer HA upregulates IL-12, which promotes differentiation of T_h1 and TNF-α.

Adipose Deposition

In the later stages of lymphedema, adipose hypertrophy accompanies fibrous tissue deposition. These tissue changes are less likely to respond to conventional therapies. The relationship between lymphatic dysfunction and adipose biology is complex. In the mouse tail model, depletion of T_h2 cell inflammation inhibits adipose tissue deposition [10]. IL-6 has been demonstrated to correlate with the presence of adipose tissue depots in obese patients. Both primary and secondary models of lymphedema demonstrate increased expression of IL-6. Il-6 is increased in lymphedematous tissues and peripheral serum of human lymphedema patients [19]. However, when IL-6 is lost or inhibited, adipose deposition is increased and inflammation is decreased. This suggests that IL-6 decreases adipose deposition and contributes to chronic inflammation in order to maintain adipose homeostasis [19].

Summary of Key Targets

T_h1, T_h2, M1 macrophages, LTB4, IL-4, and IL-13 demonstrate an injurious immune response resulting in decreased lymphatic function. Treg cells, M2 macrophages, and VEGF-C function as a reparative immune response to promote lymphatic function [20].

Anti-inflammatory and Anti-fibrotic Therapies

Ketoprofen

Ketoprofen is an NSAID with a unique dual anti-inflammatory mechanism of action that inhibits both cyclooxygenase and 5-lipoxygenase (5-LO). Systemic administration of ketoprofen in an acquired lymphedema mouse model led to reversal of disease burden and normalization of histopathology [8]. In the murine model, ketoprofen reduced inflammation and tissue edema through induction of TNF-α and an increase in VEGF-C expression [8]. In a prospective, randomized, double-blind, placebo-controlled study, 4 months of ketoprofen treatment markedly improved skin histopathology and reduced skin thickness. However, limb volume and bioimpedance were not significantly altered. One patient withdrew from the study secondary to rectal bleeding from hemorrhoids. Another patient experienced dyspepsia but was able to complete the trial [21]. After patient enrollment was completed, a black box warning for NSAIDs (unrelated to this specific trial) was issued regarding the risk of heart attack and stroke.

Ubenimex

Ubenimex, also known as bestatin, is a competitive, reversible inhibitor of leukotriene A4 hydrolase that converts LTA4 to LTB4. In leukotriene biosynthesis, activation of this enzyme results from the upstream activation of 5-LO expression that is inhibited by ketoprofen. Thus, the therapeutic benefit of ketoprofen is thought to be primarily a result of reduced LTB4 synthesis [22]. High concentrations of LTB4 inhibit lymphangiogenesis and induce human lymphatic endothelial cell (HLEC) death. In the mouse model, ubenimex results in improved lymphatic clearance, diminished tissue inflammation, improved blood vessel integrity, and improved anatomic integrity. Additionally, concentrations of IL-6, IL-4, and IL-13 were significantly decreased after ubenimex treatment. Of note, ibuprofen exacerbated edema in this model [22].

Tacrolimus

Tacrolimus inhibits calcineurin and decreases the IL-2 expression that is necessary for T cell activation and differentiation. A topical formulation of tacrolimus is FDA-approved and used to treat cutaneous inflammatory/fibrotic diseases. In a mouse tail model, topical tacrolimus had a reversing effect on lymphedema without depletion of systemic T cell counts. T cell, CD4+, and macrophage counts in the lymphedematous tissues were decreased. When fibrosis was assessed, type I collagen was decreased in the dermal, subcutaneous, and peri-lymphatic tissues. Lymphangiogenesis was also increased with increased VEGF-C and decreased TGF-β1, IFN-γ, IL-4, and IL-13. Lymphatic function improved with tacrolimus therapy when assessed by near infrared fluorescence and lymphoscintigraphy [23]. However, additional studies will be required to determine the optimal concentration and delivery method for topical tacrolimus for the treatment of lymphedema.

Atorvastatin

HMG-CoA reductase inhibitors (statins) can modulate the function of T cells, including T_h1 and T_h17 cells [24]. In an axillary lymph node dissection mouse model, atorvastatin was demonstrated to suppress early, leaky neo-lymphangiogenesis by inhibiting the interaction between T_h1 cells, T_h17 cells, and macrophages in lymphedema. Additionally, thickened dermis, fibrosis, and adipogenesis were decreased in later stages in this model [12]. There has been no human, clinical assessment of the lymphedema response to statins.

Hyaluronidase

Subcutaneous injection of hyaluronidase into lymphedematous tissues of a mouse model resulted in a decrease in the total concentration of HA and an increased proportion of LMWHA when compared to control subjects. The group treated with hyaluronidase demonstrated decreased swelling and improved histologic features. Additionally, the treated group demonstrated increased lymphatic vessel density and increased VEGFR3 expression. Lymphoscintigraphy demonstrated enhanced lymphatic drainage [25]. Pro-fibrotic cytokines, TGF-β and IL-4, are significantly downregulated, whereas anti-fibrotic cytokines, IL-12 and IFN-γ, are upregulated, resulting in suppressed fibrogenesis in mice treated with hyaluronidase [26]. Hyaluronidase has also been demonstrated to decrease lymphedema volume and reduce neutrophils in the mouse tail model [27].

Benzopyrones

The therapeutic mechanism of benzopyrones is poorly understood. However, it has been proposed that α-benzopyrones (e.g., coumarin) activate proteolytic activity of macrophages, and γ-benzopyrones (e.g., diosmin) increase oncotic pressure and the frequency and intensity of lymphatic vessel contraction. Benzopyrones are a group of drugs that have been reported to successfully treat lymphedema, especially when combined with complete decongestive therapy (CDT). However, a Cochrane review found insufficient evidence to support treatment of patients with lymphedema with benzopyrones [28]. A recent prospective randomized controlled trial in BCRL demonstrated that a product containing coumarin, diosmin, and arbutin (a diuretic) combined with CDT was more effective than CDT alone in producing limb volume reduction. While hepatoxicity has been reported with coumarins in the past, this complication is likely dose dependent; no hepatotoxicity was identified in this study [29].

A Few Notes on Non-pharmacologic Therapies

The risk factors for lymphedema, including surgery, radiation, infection, and obesity, are all associated with inflammation and should be minimized whenever possible. Lymphedema therapists should be encouraged to use exercise and other physical techniques to reduce fibrosis. Low-level laser therapy (LLLT) demonstrates anti-inflammatory and anti-fibrotic effects in the mouse model, and a systemic review and meta-analysis of patient with breast cancer-related lymphedema found that patients treated with LLLT, alone or in combination with other treatments, had significantly decreased pain and swelling [30]. Finally, the inflammation associated with lymphedema is decreased by CDT, and this standard of care should be optimized for all patients with lymphedema.

References

1. Avraham T, Daluvoy S, Zampell J, Yan A, Haviv YS, Rockson SG, Mehrara BJ. Blockade of transforming growth factor-beta1 accelerates lymphatic regeneration during wound repair. Am J Pathol. 2010;177:3202–14.
2. Tabibiazar R, Cheung L, Han J, Swanson J, Beilhack A, An A, Dadras SS, Rockson N, Joshi S, Wagner R, Rockson SG. Inflammatory manifestations of experimental lymphatic insufficiency. PLoS Med. 2006;3:e254.
3. Lin S, Kim J, Lee MJ, Roche L, Yang NL, Tsao PS, Rockson SG. Prospective transcriptomic pathway analysis of human lymphatic vascular insufficiency: identification and validation of a circulating biomarker panel. PLoS One. 2012;7:e52021.
4. Schneider M, Ny A, Ruiz de Almodovar C, Carmeliet P. A new mouse model to study acquired lymphedema. PLoS Med. 2006;3:e264.
5. Hartiala P, Saarikko AM. Lymphangiogenesis and lymphangiogenic growth factors. J Reconstr Microsurg. 2016;32:10–5.
6. Savetsky IL, Ghanta S, Gardenier JC, Torrisi JS, García Nores GD, Hespe GE, Nitti MD, Kataru RP, Mehrara BJ. Th2 cytokines inhibit lymphangiogenesis. PLoS One. 2015;10:e0126908.
7. Shin K, Kataru RP, Park HJ, Kwon BI, Kim TW, Hong YK, Lee SH. TH2 cells and their cytokines regulate formation and function of lymphatic vessels. Nat Commun. 2015;6:6196.
8. Nakamura K, Radhakrishnan K, Wong YM, Rockson SG. Anti-inflammatory pharmacotherapy with ketoprofen ameliorates experimental lymphatic vascular insufficiency in mice. PLoS One. 2009;4:e8380.
9. Zampell JC, Yan A, Elhadad S, Avraham T, Weitman E, Mehrara BJ. CD4(+) cells regulate fibrosis and lymphangiogenesis in response to lymphatic fluid stasis. PLoS One. 2012;7:e49940.
10. Avraham T, Zampell JC, Yan A, Elhadad S, Weitman ES, Rockson SG, Bromberg J, Mehrara BJ. Th2 differentiation is necessary for soft tissue fibrosis and lymphatic dysfunction resulting from lymphedema. FASEB J. 2013;27:1114–26.
11. Gousopoulos E, Proulx ST, Bachmann SB, Scholl J, Dionyssiou D, Demiri E, Halin C, Dieterich LC, Detmar M. Regulatory T cell transfer ameliorates lymphedema and promotes lymphatic vessel function. JCI Insight. 2016;1:e89081.
12. Ogata F, Fujiu K, Matsumoto S, Nakayama Y, Shibata M, Oike Y, Koshima I, Watabe T, Nagai R, Manabe I. Excess lymphangiogenesis cooperatively induced by macrophages and CD4(+) T cells drives the pathogenesis of lymphedema. J Invest Dermatol. 2016;136:706–14.
13. Ghanta S, Cuzzone DA, Torrisi JS, Albano NJ, Joseph WJ, Savetsky IL, Gardenier JC, Chang D, Zampell JC, Mehrara BJ. Regulation of inflammation and fibrosis by macrophages in lymphedema. Am J Physiol Heart Circ Physiol. 2015;308:H1065–77.
14. Zampell JC, Yan A, Avraham T, Daluvoy S, Weitman ES, Mehrara BJ. HIF-1α coordinates lymphangiogenesis during wound healing and in response to inflammation. FASEB J. 2012;26:1027–39.
15. Casley-Smith JR, Morgan RG, Piller NB. Treatment of lymphedema of the arms and legs with 5,6-benzo-[alpha]-pyrone. N Engl J Med. 1993;329:1158–63.
16. Zampell JC, Elhadad S, Avraham T, Weitman E, Aschen S, Yan A, Mehrara BJ. Toll-like receptor deficiency worsens inflammation and lymphedema after lymphatic injury. Am J Physiol Cell Physiol. 2012;302:C709–19.
17. Avraham T, Yan A, Zampell JC, Daluvoy SV, Haimovitz-Friedman A, Cordeiro AP, Mehrara BJ. Radiation therapy causes loss of dermal lymphatic vessels and interferes with lymphatic function by TGF-beta1-mediated tissue fibrosis. Am J Physiol Cell Physiol. 2010;299:C589–605.

18. Wu M, Du Y, Liu Y, He Y, Yang C, Wang W, Gao F. Low molecular weight hyaluronan induces lymphangiogenesis through LYVE-1-mediated signaling pathways. PLoS One. 2014;9:e92857.
19. Cuzzone DA, Weitman ES, Albano NJ, Ghanta S, Savetsky IL, Gardenier JC, Joseph WJ, Torrisi JS, Bromberg JF, Olszewski WL, Rockson SG, Mehrara BJ. IL-6 regulates adipose deposition and homeostasis in lymphedema. Am J Physiol Heart Circ Physiol. 2014;306:H1426–34.
20. Jiang X, Nicolls MR, Tian W, Rockson SG. Lymphatic dysfunction, leukotrienes, and lymphedema. Annu Rev Physiol. 2018;80:49–70.
21. Rockson SG, Tian W, Jiang X, Kuznetsova T, Haddad F, Zampell J, Mehrara B, Sampson JP, Roche L, Kim J, Nicolls MR. Pilot studies demonstrate the potential benefits of antiinflammatory therapy in human lymphedema. JCI Insight. 2018;3:e123775.
22. Tian W, Rockson SG, Jiang X, Kim J, Begaye A, Shuffle EM, Tu AB, Cribb M, Nepiyushchikh Z, Feroze AH, Zamanian RT, Dhillon GS, Voelkel NF, Peters-Golden M, Kitajewski J, Dixon JB, Nicolls MR. Leukotriene B4 antagonism ameliorates experimental lymphedema. Sci Transl Med. 2017;9:eaal3920.
23. Gardenier JC, Kataru RP, Hespe GE, Savetsky IL, Torrisi JS, Nores GD, Jowhar DK, Nitti MD, Schofield RC, Carlow DC, Mehrara BJ. Topical tacrolimus for the treatment of secondary lymphedema. Nat Commun. 2017;8:14345.
24. Ulivieri C, Baldari CT. Statins: from cholesterol-lowering drugs to novel immunomodulators for the treatment of Th17-mediated autoimmune diseases. Pharmacol Res. 2014;88:41–52.
25. Roh K, Cho S, Park JH, Yoo BC, Kim WK, Kim SK, Park K, Kang H, Ku JM, Yeom CH, Lee K, Lee S. Therapeutic effects of hyaluronidase on acquired lymphedema using a newly developed mouse limb model. Exp Biol Med (Maywood). 2017;242:584–92.
26. Cho S, Roh K, Park J, Park YS, Lee M, Cho S, Kil EJ, Cho MJ, Oh JS, Byun HS, Cho SH, Park K, Kang H, Koo J, Yeom CH, Lee S. Hydrolysis of hyaluronic acid in lymphedematous tissue alleviates fibrogenesis via TH1 cell-mediated cytokine expression. Sci Rep. 2017;7:35.
27. Jeong HJ, Roh KH, Kim GC, Kim YO, Lee JH, Lee MJ, Sim YJ. Hyaluronidase treatment of acute lymphedema in a mouse tail model. Lymphology. 2013;46:160–72.
28. Badger C, Preston N, Seers K, Mortimer P. Benzo-pyrones for reducing and controlling lymphoedema of the limbs. Cochrane Database Syst Rev. 2004:CD003140.
29. Cacchio A, Prencipe R, Bertone M, De Benedictis L, Taglieri L, D'Elia E, Centoletti C, Di Carlo G. Effectiveness and safety of a product containing diosmin, coumarin, and arbutin (Linfadren®) in addition to complex decongestive therapy on management of breast cancer-related lymphedema. Support Care Cancer. 2019;27:1471–80.
30. Smoot B, Chiavola-Larson L, Lee J, Manibusan H, Allen DD. Effect of low-level laser therapy on pain and swelling in women with breast cancer-related lymphedema: a systematic review and meta-analysis. J Cancer Surviv. 2015;9:287–304.

Lymphatic Education and Research Network Centers of Excellence: A Multidisciplinary Approach to Lymphatic Care

28

Melisa D. Granoff, Rosie Friedman, Arin K. Greene, and Dhruv Singhal

The Lymphatic Education & Research Network (LE&RN) is an international nonprofit organization with a mission to "fight lymphatic diseases and lymphedema through education, research and advocacy" [1]. The number of lymphatic patients is rising as the amount of cancer survivors grows, with some estimates projecting a disease burden of 7% or more of the entire US population [2]. This increase in prevalence brings with it a surge in unmet needs of patients and increasingly overwhelmed lymphatic caretakers, as general healthcare professionals are often unfamiliar with the diagnosis and treatment of lymphatic diseases (LD) [3]. To keep up with this demand, LE&RN established the Centers of Excellence (COE) in the Diagnosis and Treatment of Lymphatic Disease [4]. Previously, individual chapters of LE&RN were meeting patient demand by curating individual ad hoc lists of lymphatic providers, collected by word of mouth [2]. However, patients struggled to determine which LD specialists could best meet their specific needs. The COE designation helps patients navigate healthcare systems by identifying pre-vetted institutions with qualified providers that are not only prepared to treat LD but also are able to connect patients with resources for addressing various comorbidities. By establishing COE criteria, LE&RN crafted the blueprints for standards that institutions must meet. By making these criteria transparent, the COE designation encourages prospective institutions to evolve and strive for excellence in lymphatic treatment, leading to optimization in care of patients [2].

A COE is a designation awarded by LE&RN to institutions that offer comprehensive care for lymphedema [5]. For centers that do not offer comprehensive care but do have services for patients with lymphedema, other designations can be given, including Networks of Excellence, Referral Networks of Excellence, LD Surgery COE, and LD Conservative Care COE (Fig. 28.1) [4]. These address the overall shortfall of qualified institutions for lymphedema care because some institutions offer high-quality services for the care of patients with LD, but not comprehensive care. There are 13 major categories by which LE&RN uses to evaluate applicants, each with multiple criteria, most of which must be met to achieve the COE designation. The categories used to evaluate potential centers include diagnosis, imaging, nonoperative management, assessment tools, interventional therapies, surgical treatments, genetics evaluation, interdisciplinary consulting ability, research, accountability, collegiality, administration, and community [4]. Once a center has applied for and been awarded a designation, their information appears on the LE&RN website, which acts as a centralized, pre-vetted, and reputable source for patients.

The Boston Lymphatic Center is an example of a LE&RN COE. We were proud to be named a COE in 2020, and we hope that by sharing our experience, other institutions might have insight into the process of applying for and attaining this designation. The foundation of our center's approach to lymphedema care is a multidisciplinary effort. This begins with a shared vision that guides the goals of every department involved, best summarized by our mission statement: "The Boston Lymphatic Center provides compassionate care and advocacy for individuals with lymphatic disorders while uniting health care providers and researchers from all disciplines to advance our knowledge of lymphatic disease and therapy." Our weekly multidisciplinary conferences, which bring together nursing, diagnostic radiology, interventional radiology, nuclear medicine, vascular medicine, lymphatic

M. D. Granoff · R. Friedman · D. Singhal (✉)
Boston Lymphatic Center, Division of Plastic and Reconstructive Surgery, Beth Israel Deaconess Medical Center, Harvard Medical School, Boston, MA, USA
e-mail: dsinghal@bidmc.harvard.edu

A. K. Greene
Boston Lymphatic Center, Department of Plastic and Oral Surgery, Boston Children's Hospital, Harvard Medical School, Boston, MA, USA

M. V. Schaverien, J. H. Dayan (eds.), *Multimodal Management of Upper and Lower Extremity Lymphedema*,
https://doi.org/10.1007/978-3-030-93039-4_28

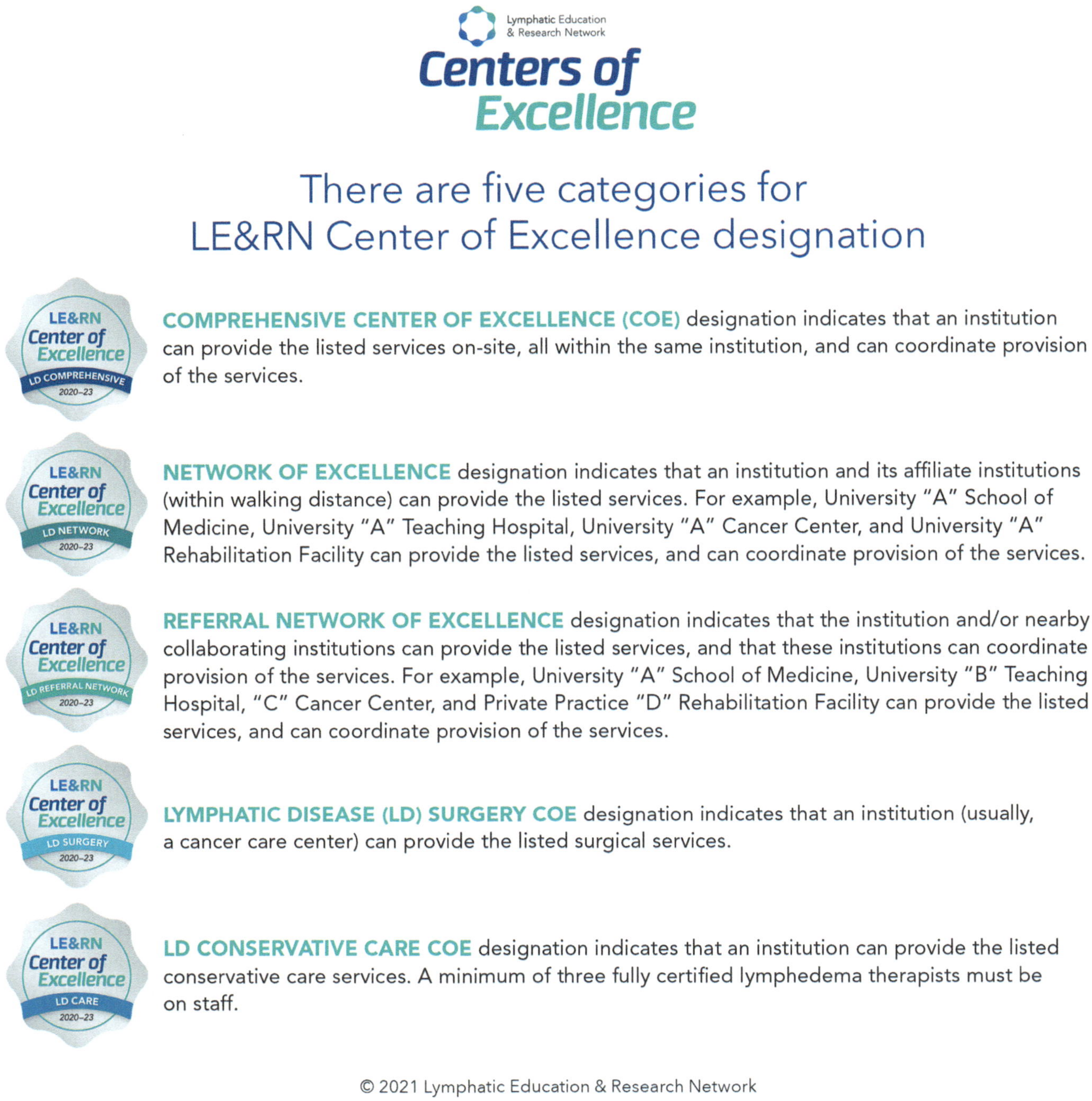

Fig. 28.1 Designations awarded to Lymphatic Education & Research Network (LE&RN) Centers of Excellence corresponding to the level of care provided

surgery, physical therapy, data analytics, and research, are central to patient care. Furthermore, our principles as a center are best illustrated by our nonclinical activity. We believe sharing knowledge is critical to furthering the field of lymphatics and therefore began hosting the Boston Lymphatic Symposium in 2017, which runs both a patient and clinical program simultaneously. In addition, to contribute what we have learned to the medical literature, the Singhal Laboratory is a clinical and translational research group focused on elucidating the role that lymphatic anatomy variations play in the development of secondary lymphedema. The Greene Laboratory is focused on identifying novel mutations for primary lymphedema as well as understanding the pathophysiology of capillary and arteriovenous malformations that can be associated with primary lymphedema. We also believe that engagement with the community is central to furthering our goal of bringing awareness to lymphatic disease. Through collaboration with the Massachusetts chapter of LE&RN and their work with Governor Charlie Baker, we officially began celebrating World Lymphedema Day on March 6, 2018, by annually lighting the Zakim Bridge in Boston teal.

In order to simplify the experience for pediatric and adult patients, the Boston Lymphatic Center has a single toll-free call line. However, patients ultimately have slightly different courses based on whether they are an adult or pediatric patient. For adult patient care, the Boston Lymphatic Center is composed of a clinical triad that includes lymphatic surgery, lymphatic medicine, and lymphatic treatment clinics (physical therapy). Upon initial evaluation by these clinics, patients are pipelined into personalized care plans based on our institutional algorithm, which has been previously described [6].

Patients presenting with chronic lymphedema are evaluated by lymphatic medicine to confirm the diagnosis and optimize medical management, by lymphatic therapy to optimize conservative therapies, and by imaging specialists (nuclear medicine, diagnostic radiology, interventional radiology) to further characterize their individual disease. The patient is then presented at the weekly multidisciplinary meeting, where the determination of whether or not they are a good surgical candidate is made. Patients with fat-dominant lymphedema are offered debulking surgery, and patients with fluid-dominant lymphedema are offered a physiologic procedure, which includes vascularized lymph node transfer or lymphovenous bypass [7, 8].

Patients presenting for a risk-reducing procedure are evaluated by the lymphatic surgery and lymphatic treatment clinics prior to nodal dissection to establish a baseline measure of their at-risk extremities. After undergoing oncologic surgery with immediate lymphatic reconstruction (ILR), they are surveilled regularly by the lymphatic treatment clinic for a minimum of 4 years. Any patients who develop lymphedema are transferred into the chronic lymphedema arm of our center, as previously described.

In the first year of the adult program at the Boston Lymphatic Center, nearly half of our patients were referred from outside institutions within New England, and many had bypassed other tertiary care centers in closer proximity to their home residences to seek care through our program [6]. The population consisted primarily of breast cancer patients who were seeking ILR at the time of axillary lymph node dissection for the prevention of secondary lymphedema. Fourteen percent of all patients who were referred to our program for the treatment of chronic lymphedema did not actually have lymphedema and were found to have an alternative diagnosis by our lymphatic medicine team [6]. Adherence to follow-up was optimized through targeted patient outreach and coordination with other oncologic appointments. However, social determinants, financial factors, and variable insurance coverage affected patients' ability to present for a return visit.

Patients referred to the pediatrics arm of the Boston Lymphatic Center tend to have different presentations and medical needs than the adult program. Between 2009 and 2019, most patients referred to the center were females with congenital lymphedema [9]. Under a quarter of referred patients had secondary lymphedema, and 16% had obesity-induced lymphedema (OIL) [9]. The remainder were found to have diagnoses other than lymphedema upon evaluation, underscoring the need for greater understanding of lymphedema by the general medical community. Upon referral, lymphedema diagnosis is similarly confirmed by lymphatic medicine as in the adult program, and individuals receive counseling and education about their condition, including ways to prevent progression and complications. All patients are initially managed by the lymphatic treatment clinic with nonoperative medical therapies such as compression garments, placing focus on volume maintenance and infection prevention. In contrast to the adult pipeline, only 6% of patients in the pediatric program were treated with surgical intervention [9]. Those that were treated surgically underwent debulking surgery with suction-assisted lipectomy. Patients with OIL were referred to bariatric surgical centers, as OIL does not respond to typical lymphedema treatments, and lymphatic function cannot be improved without significant weight loss. Regardless of lymphedema etiology, every patient that was referred had a tailored approach to treatment that was made possible by a collaborative effort of the multidisciplinary team.

Summary

At the Boston Lymphatic Center, we are proud to offer comprehensive care to patients both with and without lymphedema and to have earned the LE&RN COE designation. We hope by sharing our experience, including the specifics of our multidisciplinary approach for both children and adults, other centers may have insight into how to offer comprehensive care for patients with lymphatic disorders and how to secure a COE designation.

References

1. Mission | Lymphatic Education & Research Network. https://lymphaticnetwork.org/about/mission. Accessed 20 Feb 2021.
2. Chang D, Dayan J, Fried P, et al. Establishing standards for centers of excellence for the diagnosis and treatment of lymphatic disease. Lymphat Res Biol. 2021;19:4–10.
3. Rockson SG, Granger DN, Skeff KM, Chaite W. Lymphatic biology and disease: is it being taught? Who is listening? Lymphat Res Biol. 2004;2(2):86–95.
4. Lymphatic Education & Research Network. https://lymphaticnetwork.org/centers-of-excellence-standards. Accessed 20 Feb 2021.

5. Lymphatic Education & Research Network. https://lymphaticnetwork.org/centers-of-excellence. Accessed 20 Feb 2021.
6. Johnson A, Fleishman A, Tran BN, et al. Developing a lymphatic surgery program: a first-year review. Plast Reconstr Surg. 2019;144(6):975e–85e.
7. Granoff M, Johnson A, Shillue K, et al. A single institution multidisciplinary approach to power-assisted liposuction for the management of lymphedema. Ann Surg. 2020.
8. Johnson AR, Bravo MG, Granoff MD, et al. Flow-through omental flap for vascularized lymph node transfer: a novel surgical approach for delayed lymphatic reconstruction. Plast Reconstr Surg Glob Open. 2019;7(9):e2436.
9. Sudduth CL, Maclellan RA, Greene AK. Study of 700 referrals to a lymphedema program. Lymphat Res Biol. 2020;18(6):534–8.

Index

M. V. Schaverien, J. H. Dayan (eds.), *Multimodal Management of Upper and Lower Extremity Lymphedema*,
https://doi.org/10.1007/978-3-030-93039-4

GPSR Compliance

The European Union's (EU) General Product Safety Regulation (GPSR) is a set of rules that requires consumer products to be safe and our obligations to ensure this.

If you have any concerns about our products, you can contact us on ProductSafety@springernature.com

In case Publisher is established outside the EU, the EU authorized representative is:

Springer Nature Customer Service Center GmbH
Europaplatz 3
69115 Heidelberg, Germany

Batch number: 10731524

Printed by Printforce, the Netherlands